This is the first in a new series in child and adolescent psychiatry, bringing together aspects of normal development and psychopathology. Each volume will concentrate on those topics where the growth of knowledge has had the greatest impact on the understanding and treatment of mental illness. This establishing volume provides an account of the nature and characteristics of depression in children and adolescents. Experts in the field provide a unique approach through discussion of the historical development of the concept and provide a synthesis of existing knowledge on the normal development of emotion in young children and the onset of depression in the older child.

With equal attention being given to both theory and practice, this volume is certain to appeal widely to child psychiatrists and psychologists, developmental psychologists and related professions in developmental science and mental health, including neuroscientists.

The Depressed Child and Adolescent:
Developmental and Clinical Perspectives

MONOGRAPHS IN CHILD AND ADOLESCENT PSYCHIATRY

Child and adolescent psychiatry is an important and growing area of clinical psychiatry. The last decade has seen a rapid expansion of scientific knowledge in this field and has provided a new understanding of the underlying pathology of mental disorders in these age groups. This series is aimed at practitioners and researchers both in child and adolescent mental health services and developmental and clinical neuroscience. Focusing on psychopathology, it highlights those topics where the growth of knowledge has had the greatest impact on clinical practice and on the treatment and understanding of mental illness. Individual volumes benefit both from the international expertise of their contributors and a coherency generated through a uniform style and structure for the series. Each volume provides firstly an historical overview and a clear descriptive account of the psychopathology of a specific disorder or group of related disorders. These features then form the basis for a thorough critical review of the aetiology, natural history, management, prevention and impact on later adult adjustment. Whilst each volume is therefore complete in its own right, volumes also relate to each other to create a flexible and collectable series that should appeal to students as well as experienced scientists and practitioners.

CAMBRIDGE MONOGRAPHS IN CHILD AND ADOLESCENT PSYCHIATRY

The Depressed Child and Adolescent: Developmental and Clinical Perspectives

Edited by
IAN M. GOODYER

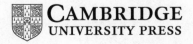

CAMBRIDGE
UNIVERSITY PRESS

Published by the Press Syndicate of the University of Cambridge
The Pitt Building, Trumpington Street, Cambridge CB2 1RP
40 West 20th Street, New York, NY 10011-4211, USA
10 Stamford Road, Oakleigh, Melbourne 3166, Australia

First published 1995

Printed in Great Britain at the University Press, Cambridge

A catalogue record for this book is available from the British Library

Library of Congress cataloguing in publication data

The Depressed child and adolescent : developmental and clinical
perspectives / edited by Ian M. Goodyer.
   p.   cm. – (Cambridge monographs in child and adolescent psychiatry)
Includes bibliographical references (p.   ).
ISBN 0 521 43326 6
1. Depression in children.   2. Depression in adolescence.
I. Goodyer, Ian M.   II. Series.
RJ506.D4D44 1995
618.92′8527 – dc20   94–31399 CIP

ISBN 0 521 43326 6 hardback

TAG

Contents

Contents

Contents

Contributors

Adrian Angold
> Department of Psychiatry
> Duke University Medical Center
> Box 3454
> Durham
> North Carolina 27710–3454, USA

Leo J. Bastiaens
> Allegheny Neuropsychiatric Institute
> 7777 Steubenville Pike
> Oakdale, PA 15071, USA

Jeanne Brooks-Gunn
> Director Center for Children and Families
> Teachers College
> New York
> NY 10027, USA

Bruce E. Compas
> Department of Psychology
> John Dewey Hall
> University of Vermont
> Burlington
> VT 05405-0134, USA

Contributors

Elizabeth J. Costello
    Department of Psychiatry
    Duke University Medical Center
    Box 3454
    Durham
    NC 27710-3454, USA

R. F. W. Diekstra
    Psychosocial Department
    Department of Paediatrics
    University of Utrecht
    Wilhelmina Children's Hospital
    PO Box 18009
    3501 CA Utrecht
    The Netherlands

Ian M. Goodyer
    Developmental Psychiatry
    University of Cambridge
    Douglas House
    18b Trumpington Road
    Cambridge CB2 2AH, UK

Richard Harrington
    University Department of Child Psychiatry
    Royal Manchester Children's Hospital
    Pendlebury
    Manchester M27 1HA, UK

Kim Kendall
    Adolescent Health Training Program
    Department of Pediatrics, WJ-10
    University of Washington Medical School
    Seattle,
    WA 98195, USA

C. W. Kienhorst
    Psychosocial Department
    Department of Paediatrics
    University of Utrecht
    Wilhelmina Children's Hospital
    PO Box 18009
    3501 CA Utrecht
    The Netherlands

Israel Kolvin
    Department of Child/Adolescent Psychiatry
    University of London
    Tavistock Clinic
    120 Belsize Lane
    London NW3 5BA, UK

Maria Kovacs
    University of Pittsburgh Medical Center
    Western Psychiatric Institute and Clinic
    3811 O'Hara Street
    Pittsburgh
    PA 15213-2593, USA

Stan Kutcher
    Head, Division of Adolescent Psychiatry
    Sunnybrook Hospital University of Toronto Clinic
    2075 Bayview Avenue
    North York
    Ontario
    Canada M4N 3M5

Elizabeth McCauley
    Department of Psychiatric and Behavioural Sciences
    University of Washington School of Medicine
    Division of Child & Adolescent Psychiatry, CH-13
    Seattle
    Washington 98195, USA

Contributors

Mark Meerum Terwogt
Department of Developmental Psychology
Free University
Van der Boechorststraat 1
1081 BT, Amsterdam
The Netherlands

William Ll. Parry-Jones
Department of Child and Adolescent Psychiatry
University of Glasgow
Royal Hospital for Sick Children
Yorkhill
Glasgow G3 8SJ, UK

Karen Pavlidis
Department of Psychology, NI-25
University of Washington
Seattle
WA 98195, USA

Anne C. Petersen
The Graduate School
University of Minnesota
101 Pleasant Street S.E.
Minneapolis MN 55455, USA

Professor Helmut Remschmidt
Klinik für Kinder und Jugendpsychiatrie
Philipps-Universität
Hans-Sachs-Str 6
D-3550 Marburg
Germany

Eberhard Schulz
Klinik für Kinder und Jugendpsychiatrie
Philipps-Universität
Hans-Sachs-Strasse 6
D-3550 Marburg
Germany

Hedy Stegge
    Department of Developmental Psychology
    Free University
    Van der Boechorststraat 1
    1081 BT, Amsterdam
    The Netherlands

Stephen Sokolov
    Mood Disorders Unit
    Clarke Institute of Psychiatry
    University of Toronto
    Ontario
    Canada, M4N 3M5

Michael Strober
    Neuropsychiatric Institute
    UCLA
    760 Westwood Plaza
    Room 48-240
    Los Angeles
    California 90024, USA

Panos Vostanis
    Department of Psychiatry
    University of Birmingham
    Queen Elizabeth Psychiatric Hospital
    Birmingham B15 2QZ, UK

E. J. de Wilde
    Department of Paediatrics
    University of Utrecht
    Wilhelmina Children's Hospital
    PO Box 18009
    3501 CA Utrecht
    The Netherlands

Monographs in child and adolescent psychiatry

The 20th century has witnessed substantial progress in the understanding of child and adolescent development. Psychologists have established that cognitive, emotional, and social development are active processes, arising in the context of diverse social experiences in the home, school and peer group. In addition, the unique individuality and rights of children and adolescents have been recognised increasingly, and despite growing dependence on the state and the intrusion of specialist agencies, parents have attained fuller acknowledgement that they have responsibilities towards, as well as expectations of, their offspring. These scientific and social advances have been associated with the emergence of more sophisticated services for children and adolescents with emotional and behavioural difficulties. During the last 30 years, academic and clinical child and adolescent psychiatry and psychology have become established specialities, with the recognition that treating and managing mental disorder in young people requires expertise which is not available readily in general psychiatry or psychology, or in paediatrics. Similar professional advances have characterised other child-related health care professions. In particular, the expansion of academic centres to foster research and teaching in child development and in the psychiatric disorders of childhood and adolescence has had considerable impact on the training and education of scientists, social scientists and practitioners in the field of child and adolescent mental health. The predominant feature of theory and clinical practice has been to emphasise the role of the family and social factors in the causation and management of child and adolescent psychiatric disorder. Towards the close of the 20th century, however, there is a growing awareness that the nature of child and adolescent mental disorders is highly complex, involving brain function as well as social and psychological processes. Three new major areas of endeavour have emerged, complementing existing research strategies investigating the aetiology, nature and outcome of mental disorders in young people, namely the role of genetic factors, the importance of neurobiology and the effectiveness of existing services. Associations between brain, mind and the environment will become fully understood only through interdisciplinary collaboration, bridging the gap between basic and clinical science and clinical practice. Fundamental advances in the understanding of neural structure and function are being accompanied rapidly by fuller interplay between neurochemistry and human behaviour. Combining behavioural measurement with non-invasive neuro-imaging procedures will provide more detailed information about the integrity of brain function in health and disease. Innovative neuroscientific approaches, combined with new techniques of behavioural genetic research, will result in a clearer definition of the important psychosocial mechanisms in the onset and outcome of psychiatric disorders, as well as providing new insights into pathogenesis. In addition, the need to determine what service provisions are in the best interests of children and their families and which treatments are the most effective under different service delivery conditions, becomes an increasingly important topic in clinical and public health research. The search for new methods to evaluate treatment outcome and the need to equate costs with the benefits of child mental health care are emerging as basic elements in health service planning and provision. Such ideas, in combination with research, educational and clinical advances, are fostered through closer collaboration between basic and clinical neuroscience and clinical practice in only a few centres around the world and, therefore, require dissemination to reach a wider scientific and clinical audience. Textbooks are an essential medium for the diffusion of research and clinical information. In child and adolescent psychiatry, a few comprehensive, multi-author textbooks, designed for library reference and for experienced postgraduate use, have become well-established as standard texts. These have been augmented by in-depth volumes devoted to a single topic. Some of the latter incorporate valuable introductory overviews of major disorders, usually intended for undergraduate or postgraduate readership. Others have reviewed specific areas, relevant to both student and specialist. As the scientific basis of child and adolescent psychiatry and the methods of treatment has widened, in-depth coverage by single authors has become correspondingly difficult.

Over recent years, a number of key advances in developmental science and child and adolescent psychiatry research have provided the stimulus for the evolution of a new developmental approach to the study of psychopathology. Continuities and discontinuities between normative developmental processes and the onset of emotional and behavioural disorders have been a growing focus of research. The identification of social risk factors for mental disorder is being supplanted by the need to determine the mechanisms and processes that arise from such factors and which are responsible for the onset and maintenance of disorder. There has been a recognition that such mechanisms will not be fully elucidated without new interdisciplinary research collaboration. Thus, the close relationship fostered between social, psychological and psychiatric researchers in the behavioural sciences will be promoted by collaboration with neuroscientists in the laboratory, in the clinical settings and the neuro-imaging centres. Determining mechanisms, involving brain and mind as well as psychosocial processes, will then assume an increasing reality.

This book is the first volume in a new series entitled Monographs in Child and Adolescent Psychiatry. The series is aimed at practitioners in child and adolescent mental health services and researchers in development and clinical neuroscience. Each volume will be dedicated to a specific topic within the field of child and adolescent psychopathology. While the general aim is to provide comprehensive coverage of the major syndromes, it is intended that there should be detailed consideration of topics less commonly dealt with in standard texts. In order to provide coherence within the series, a uniform style and structure will be utilised throughout, with due recognition of specialised aspects of such topics as are essential for inclusion, but which do not readily fit the standard structure. Each volume will open with a historical account of the topic, providing a perspective on the evolution of concepts and practices in present day usage. Since child and adolescent psychiatry has experienced rapid growth during the latter part of the 20th century, there is a tendency for the pace of change to obscure the contributions from previous generations. The historical chapters focus mainly on 18th to 20th century developments. Following this, there is a thorough exposition of the normal and the developmental biology pertinent to each topic. This will provide the necessary framework for comparing normal and abnormal mechanisms and processes, as well as continuities and discontinuities of thoughts, feelings and behaviours over time. These chapters will discuss, where appropriate, physio-chemical and neural, as well as social and psychological, aspects of normal behaviour.

The clinical components will include detailed expositions on the prevalence, nature, characteristics, evolution and outcome of the disorder. A life-span approach will be adopted to trace the course of childhood disorders into adult life. Recent advances in the classification of disorders, including comorbidity and the influence of development on presenting signs and symptoms, together with syndrome definition and recognition, will receive close attention. The application of behavioural genetics and the importance of gene–environment interaction will be covered, as well as environmental contribution to psychiatric syndromes. Family and peer group influences on onset, recovery and relapse will be discussed. Pathophysiological and pathopsychological accounts of the topic will be highlighted and, wherever possible, allocated separate chapters. Clinical chapters will include accounts of treatment and current public health policies. The differential impact of single and recurrent episodes on subsequent child and adult adjustment will form an important component of these clinical sections. Although the chapters will be written by international experts from widely different backgrounds and areas of expertise, each volume will conform to the overall structure of the series, providing a coherent approach to each topic. While complete in its own right, each volume will relate to the others in style and structure, creating a flexible and collectable series, which should appeal to students, as well as experienced scientists and practitioners.

Preface

It is increasingly apparent that depressive disorders in young people are more common than previously considered. The depressed child or adolescent is not however easily recognised, either by the youngsters themselves, their parents or their teachers. Even when recognition does occur many adolescents are reluctant to seek help and many children are dependent on the motivation and insight of others to seek help on their behalf. In many respects depression in children and adolescents represents a 'private illness', but one which carries a substantial risk of recurring during the formative years of youth and young adulthood. In addition to further episodes of depression, high rates of marital and friendship difficulties and employment problems are being documented in many adults depressed in their childhood years. One implication of these recent findings is that for some individuals childhood depression may alter the trajectory of development for the worse perhaps through decreasing the resilience required for dealing with the subsequent tasks in adult life.

Much of the recent advances over the past three decades concerning the nature, characteristics and outcome of depression have come about through the application of standard diagnostic criteria such as the Diagnostic and Statistical Manual of the American Psychiatric Association and the International Classification of Diseases of the World Health Authority. These criteria have provided a common language and framework for scientific investigation. As a result advances in our understanding of the causes and consequences of depression in childhood and adolescence have been substantial. In recent years, however, child psychologists and psychiatrists have come to question the overarching reliance on these nosological frameworks, which are derived, in the main, from a consideration of the clinical signs and symptoms of depression in adults. It is becoming apparent, for example, that adult criteria for eliciting an episode of major depressive disorder are neither sensitive nor specific enough to detect clinical depression in the pre-school years. The pattern of depressive symptoms varies with age and future research must take this into account when investigating the evolution, nature and outcome of depressive disorders in young people.

Indeed advances in human developmental biology have illustrated how normal components of development exert marked influences on children's emotional and behavioural repertoire. Research on children's cognitive development and interpersonal relationships in the pre-school and early school years, continues to inform us about the complexities of emotional development. Similarly a greater understanding of the physiological parameters of human emotions and the genetics of human behaviour has resulted in a more succinct understanding of person–environment interactions. Children influence their environments as well as being influenced by them because of their personal characteristics. These advances provide the opportunity for a more detailed investigation of the complex interplay between social, psychological, physiological and genetic aspects of normal development, and their relative contributions to the onset of depressive disorders, than has hitherto been achieved. The internationally distinguished group of researchers who have contributed to this volume do so from different but related perspectives within child and adolescent psychology and psychiatry. Each author has focused, wherever possible, on the continuities and discontinuities between normal emotional states and clinical depression. As well as the emphasis on the interplay between normal and abnormal aspects of development there is a reaffirmation of the importance of studying the systems biology of depression which, by definition, requires an investigation of the role of environmental, psychological, physiological and genetic perspectives in the onset and outcome of disorder. Such an approach makes it clear that depression is a heterogeneous condition in which the pattern and relative contribution of different extrinsic, intrinsic and interpersonal elements exert a variety of effects on the nature, characteristics and outcome of disorder. It is only through such an approach that a greater understanding of both the general components and the specific individual differences of depressive disorders in children and adolescents can be achieved. In so doing our knowledge about

depression will be advanced and more effective and efficient programmes of prevention and treatment will be devised. This volume, by
providing a coherent account of current knowledge, indicates that whilst
much has been learnt, many questions about the nature of depressive
disorders in children and adolescents remain unanswered. It is the hope
of all the contributors that this account acts as a stimulus for further
scientific research and clinical effort into a complex mental disorder on
behalf of those who often suffer in private.

Ian M. Goodyer   Cambridge

1

Historical aspects of mood and its disorders in young people

William Ll. Parry-Jones

INTRODUCTION

The last 20 years have witnessed rapid expansion of clinical and theoretical interest in affective disorders in children and adolescents. While reference is often made to the controversy surrounding the concept, even to the existence of depression and mania in children before this time, extensive historical examination of the subject has been minimal. The primary aims of the chapter, therefore, are to assemble evidence about the wider historical background and to set some current clinical and research issues in perspective. The methodology and interpretation of historical research on affective disorder in young people needs to take into consideration a number of factors.

Growth of interest in juvenile mental disorder

Prior to the mid-nineteenth century, little systematic attention was given to juvenile lunatics and the existence of insanity in early life was disputed or denied. A picture of their disorders and care has to be assembled, therefore, from diverse sources, mainly reports of unusual cases (Parry-Jones, 1993). Subsequently, insanity in children and adolescents featured increasingly in asylum practice and in textbooks and journals, although it was not until the 1920s and 1930s that a recognisably separate discipline of child psychiatry emerged. The multidisciplinary specialty that took shape was the product of the confluence of expertise

1

from paediatrics, asylum medicine, the training and custodial care of the mentally retarded, psychoanalysis, psychology, psychiatric social work, remedial education and criminology. Later, influenced by the new medical psychology and by psychoanalytic thinking, the developing specialty moved away from asylum-based psychiatry, with its concepts of organ pathology, heredity, phenomenological syndromal description and physical treatments, towards psychosocial and psychodynamic models. In the process, it distanced itself from the most severely disturbed juveniles, particularly adolescents.

Following the Second World War, there was rapid growth of hospital-based out-patient clinics, first inaugurated in the 1920s and 1930s, and the development of in-patient wards. From the mid-1960s, increasing acceptance of the need for separate services for adolescents arose out of concern about their care with adults in mental hospitals. The last 30 years have seen the emergence of British child and adolescent psychiatry as a well-established scientific specialty, accompanied by the slow expansion, from the 1970s, of academic departments.

Changing theories of child mental development

The theories of Locke and Rousseau continued to influence concepts of child development in the first half of the nineteenth century. Darwin's theory of evolution, however, raised new problems concerning development and variation that were alien to the older psychology. By the last quarter of the century, major new interest in child study was developing rapidly in Europe and America, associated with biographical accounts of infant development. Such interest had clinical implications, for example Clouston (1891) catalogued disorders associated with development up to the end of adolescence (interpreted as occurring between the ages of 18 and 25) when reproductive functions were developed and full growth attained. A recurrent theme at this time was ancestral recapitulation, whereby, during an individual's development, stages were passed through which characterised those of the race. Early twentieth century theories of child development were influenced principally by Sigmund and Anna Freud and subsequent child psychoanalytical theorists, and by Claparède, Piaget, Kohlberg, Vygotsky and Erikson.

Theories concerning the nature, development and expression of emotion

Accounts of the history of the psychology of emotion are fraught with difficulties, since 'the field is replete with theory and scantily covered with relevant experimental evidence' (Mandler, 1979). Consideration needs to be given to the influence of concepts arising from a number of different theoretical viewpoints (Gardiner *et al.*, 1937), including theological and philosophical perspectives, psychoanalytical and experiential theories, ethological concepts, physiological and neurobiological explanations and behavioural and cognitive interpretations. Darwin's observation (1872) that there was universal similarity of facial expression of emotions and that expressions of sadness and stress had an adaptive function was highly influential, until the advent of the James–Lange theory of emotion in the late 1880s and its subsequent critique by Cannon in the 1920s. In order to elucidate the psychology and physiology of normal emotional life, Thalbitzer (1926) drew upon the study of 'mood-psychoses', suggesting that, in children and 'very naive, primitive and uncivilised people', these states tended to be 'simple and uncomplicated'. For many years, theories of emotional development (Bridges, 1932) indicated that emotional expressions change and become more complex and differentiated until about 2 years of age. Relatively recently, there has been an upsurge of human- and animal-based research into emotional development (Strongman, 1987) (see Chapter 2).

Changing conceptions of childhood

Historical studies illustrate the changing role and status of children in the family and society (Parry-Jones, 1993). The principal issues bearing on the recognition and classification of childhood mental disorders concern the extent to which children were regarded as miniature adults, the awareness of the psychological component in children's lives and interest in the deterministic significance of early life experiences.

Terminological and conceptual confusion

A wide variety of words have been used, over the centuries, to describe and define emotional experience, expression and disturbance, generating a confusing array of theoretical concepts. 'Mania', for example, has been used for diverse excited states. In addition to the core term 'melancholia', a range of alternatives has been used to refer to depressive states, such as 'the vapours', hypochondriasis, spleen, 'hip', 'lypemania' and 'tristimania'. During the last century, the situation has been complicated by inconsistent use and definition of the terms 'affect', 'mood', 'emotion' and 'feeling'. In particular, application of 'affect' and 'mood' has suffered from sustained confusion because of variation in the reliance placed, in definition, on the duration of an emotional state or the distinction between subjective and objective components.

History of affective disturbance in adults

In view of the limited consideration given to childhood disorders until the mid-nineteenth century, the field is dominated by issues concerned with affective disorders in adults. Although the extensive history of this subject is receiving increasing notice (Jackson, 1986; Berrios, 1992), aspects relating to children and young people, before the mid-twentieth century, have attracted minimal attention.

Diversity and variability of source material

There is only sporadic survival of heterogeneous manuscript material before 1800 and little in the way of consecutive patient-related records. With the growth of theoretical interest in childhood insanity, the availability of printed source material expanded progressively during the nineteenth century. Primary sources, including patient records, are increasingly available from the second half of the century.

Limited historiography of child and adolescent mental disorders

Historical accounts of child and adolescent psychiatry have been concerned mainly with its development as a medical speciality and with innovative therapeutic techniques. Very limited attention has been given to the history of clinical syndromes or to the wider implications of childhood insanity (Parry-Jones, 1992).

PRE-NINETEENTH CENTURY

Despite copious discussion of the phenomenon of melancholia from the time of Hippocrates, the condition was very rarely alluded to among juveniles. An exception was the Greek physician, Rufus of Ephesus in the opening years of the second century AD, who stated that melancholia 'did not occur in adolescents, but it occasionally occurred in infants and in young boys' (Jackson, 1986). Before the nineteenth century, the term 'melancholia' was used to refer to 'a rag-bag of insanity states', not necessarily including sadness and low affect, and was a sub-type of mania (Berrios, 1992). Depressive states without delusions were designated by terms such as 'hypochondria', 'vapours' and 'spleen'. Although there were occasional references in the seventeenth century to 'depression' or 'defection' of spirits and 'depressed', it was only in the latter part of the eighteenth century that such terms began to feature more specifically in discussions of melancholia.

Specific references to childhood insanity and its treatment are elusive and outwardly relevant early texts covering the topics of 'melancholy', 'frensie' and 'madness', such as those by Bright in 1586 and Willis in 1683, contribute little of relevance. Burton's comprehensive work on melancholy (Burton, 1827, p. 215), first published in 1621, was not concerned primarily with depressive disorders in the modern sense, but he made some observations that were pertinent to childhood. He referred to education, for example, as a source of melancholy, especially when conducted by parents. In this context, he criticised parents who were both 'too stern, alway threatning, chiding, brawling, whipping or striking; by means of which, their poor children are so disheartned and cowed, that they never after have any courage, a merry hour in their lives, or take pleasure in any thing'. At the other extreme, he criticised parents who were too indulgent. Among the other causes of melancholy in relation to children, Burton referred to melancholic parents producing offspring who inherited their characteristics. In the case of the mother, this could occur even during pregnancy and, similarly, a wet nurse could transmit melancholic tendencies to the infant. Finally, Burton emphasised that severe terror and fright could cause melancholy in the young, describing two little girls near Basle, frightened, respec-

5

tively, by a body on a gibbet and a corpse in an open grave, who 'could not be pacified, but melancholy died' (Burton, 1827, p. 219).

In the eighteenth century, neither Sauvage's seminal nosology nor Arnold's detailed account of classification and causation afforded examples of childhood melancholy, apart from a passing reference by the latter to vulnerability of young people to 'nostalgic insanity', when away from their homes (Arnold, 1782). This condition was first described clinically in the late seventeenth century by Hofer, whose cases included a young peasant girl, pining in hospital from parental separation. Whytt (1767) described a 14-year-old boy, who become low-spirited before the onset of an eating disorder. Perfect (1791), a private madhouse owner in Kent, England, provided a comprehensive account of an 11-year-old boy treated without admission to the madhouse. He displayed 'depression and lowness', alternating with confusion and acutely disturbed 'obstreporous' states, in which he was irrational and furious, behaving like a 'raving maniac'. The disorder, which Perfect thought had no clear causation, lasted for 4 to 5 months and was treated with the customary polypharmacy of the period.

NINETEENTH CENTURY

Melancholia and depression

Changes began to take place in the classical usage of the term melancholia, with its connotations of humoral physiology (black bile), leading to its emergence more specifically as a primary disorder of the emotions, which, in turn, became referred to as mental depression or simply depression (Berrios, 1988). Early nineteenth century classificatory developments in France were particularly influential in defining new disorders. Esquirol (1845, pp. 29, 33–4)), for example, coined the term 'lypemania' for a condition characterised by 'delirium with respect to one or a small number of objects, with predominance of a sorrowful and depressing passion', although this term did not gain widespread European popularity. Esquirol considered lypemania to be 'rather the lot of adult age' whereas 'In youth, mania and monomania burst forth in all their varieties and forms'. In Germany, classifications by Griesinger, Kahlbaum and Krafft-Ebing remained influential until the publication of Kraepelin's seminal work (1921). In Britain, by the end of the nineteenth century, melancholia was defined clearly as a disorder characterised by 'a feeling of misery which is in excess of what is justified by the circumstances in which the individual is placed' (Mercier, 1892). Numerous forms were recognised, broadly grouped into those with and without delusions, including a hysterical form 'occurring principally in young girls' and a pubertal variant in which 'the patient often evinces a listless and moody apathy and perverseness of conduct' (Tuke, 1892). By the close of the century, the term depression had gained greater currency, becoming a synonym for melancholia.

The growing number of case reports of juvenile lunatics in the first half of the century rarely included melancholia and it was not until the second part of the century that there was consistent evidence of the identification, description and discussion of abnormal mood states in children and young people. Crichton-Browne (1860) made the significant observation that although melancholia 'appears incompatible with early life ... it is so only in appearance, for the buoyancy and gladness of childhood may give place to despondency and despair and faith and confidence may be superseded by doubt and misery'. He recognised a range of disorders, principally 'pure, abstract indefinite depression' and also religious melancholy. Other forms, including hypochondriasis, were less common before puberty, 'as their existence implies subjectivity of thought'. Finally, 'simple melancholia a mere exaggeration of that feeling of depression to which we are all at times liable, may, in youth, as in mature life, exist without at all involving the intellectual faculties'.

Maudsley (1867, pp. 259–93) included melancholia among the 7 forms of childhood insanity. In his view, depression occurred in children 'with and without definite delusion or morbid impulse'. In some cases, depressive symptoms marked 'a constitutional defect of nervous element whereby an emotional or sensational reaction of a painful kind follows all impressions; the nervous or cyclical tone is radically infected with some vice of constitution so that every impression is painful'. Maudsley went on to suggest that this was often due to inherited syphilis. Deep melancholic depression was associated in older children with delusions and could lead to suicide. The concept of moral insanity, first described by Prichard (1835), was quite widely applied to young people and Maudsley referred to it as 'affective insanity' to convey 'the fundamental condition of nerve element which shows itself in affections of the mode of feeling generally, not of the special mode of moral feeling only' (Maudsley, 1879, p. 280). In fact, he used the term 'affective derangement' to comprise both moral insanity and mental depression.

Maudsley's principal contribution lay in the elucidation of the early onset and forms taken by childhood melancholic states and in his attempt to relate the type of melancholia to the level of development reached by the child at the time of onset. In infants, 'Feeling going before thought in the order of mental development', melancholic expression was by a 'primitive language of cries, grunts, exclamations, tones of sounds, gestures and features'. Older children aged 4 or 5 might have 'fits of moaning melancholy and apprehensive fears' and later, features of typical melancholy could occur, sometimes with suicidal ideas (Maudsley, 1895, pp. 163–233). This developmental sequence differed from that of many other writers, which generally only included melancholia from the age of 10 or 12 years (e.g. Hurd, 1895). The form taken by melancholia after puberty was generally thought to resemble that in adults, including, for example, the commonly occurring presentation with hypochondriacal delusions relating to bodily conditions. According to Mills (1893), delusions commonly occurring in adults, 'as of self condemnation, of the unpardonable sin, of coming to want, or of fatal organic disease' were often absent, although children brought up 'in a morbidly religious, or in distressing surroundings, sometimes exhibit a delusional state of a religious and painful character'.

In Europe, similar references to affective disorders in children began to be made. Griesinger (1867) stated that all forms of insanity occurred before puberty, albeit infrequently, including 'melancholic forms in all their varieties'. He drew specific attention to the occurrence of hypochondria, 'especially where the parents manifest excessive care of the health of the child', and to 'simple melancholic states . . . whose foundation is a general feeling of anxiety'. Later, in his influential work on 'psychic disturbance of childhood', Emminghaus (1887) demonstrated a clear understanding of the difference between child and adult disorders and identified four forms of childhood melancholia, including juvenile suicide.

Growing interest in childhood insanity in the mid-nineteenth century was slow to be reflected in paediatric literature. Although West (1854, pp. 185–206), for example, referred to hypochrondriasis, malingering and moral insanity in children, no specific mention was made to mood disorder. In the early twentieth century, however, notable paediatric authors began to devote attention to functional nervous diseases of childhood, reflecting increasing awareness of the effects of emotional health, the problems of neurotic children and possible consequences in adulthood. Guthrie (1909), for example, drew attention to manifestations of fretting and home-sickness and to the effects of 'hospitalism', later studied by Spitz (1946) and Cameron (1929) recognised recurrent depression in children including *folie circulaire*.

Mania and manic-depressive insanity

During the second half of the nineteenth century, there was increasing clarification of the concept of mania as an emotional disorder, characterised by elated affect, and its separation from general madness. By the end of the century, Maudsley (1895, pp. 234–96) divided mania, or 'insanity with excitement', into a simple form (without delusions), acute and chronic mania and 'alternating recurrent insanity'. The association between melancholic and manic states had a long history and an intimate connection between these conditions had been made as early as the second century AD by both Aretaeus and Soranus. In the medieval period, melancholia and mania were usually listed together under diseases of the head (Jackson, 1986). The position was clarified, in the mid-nineteenth century, by two French alienists, Falret and Baillarger, who, respectively, described and named the alternating sequence as *la folie circulaire* and *la folie à double forme*. When Kraepelin (1921, pp. 167–74) correlated the various forms, he confirmed that adolescence carried a predisposition for manic-depressive insanity, as well as dementia praecox, and observed that 0.4% of manic-depressive patients experienced their first episode at 10 years of age or younger.

Throughout the nineteenth century, a steady stream of published case reports recorded the occurrence of mania in children and young people, usually portrayed as early onset examples of the 'adult-type' disorder (Morison, 1848; Mills, 1893; Fletcher, 1895). Down (1887) gave examples of infantile mania and cases 'where the various phases of insanity in the adult have been well represented'. In many of the reported cases it is difficult to distinguish primary affective disorders from states of excitement and confusion forming part of other psychotic disorders. For example, Greves (1884) gave a detailed account of 'acute mania' in a 5-year-old child, with a history of 2 to 3 weeks of acute disturbance but, in fact, this condition was more likely to have been a symptomatic psychotic state rather than an affective disorder. During the last quarter of the century, many cases of *folie circulaire* in children were described. Ireland (1875), for example, reported a 13-year-old German boy, who 'had been so often punished at school ... that he became deeply melancholy and tried

9

to kill himself. The melancholy alternated with mania, in which he whistled and sang day and night, tore his clothes and was filthy in his habits'. Such a case was regarded as 'very rare at such an early age'. Hurd (1895, p. 14) was in no doubt, however, that most cases of *folie circulaire* began at puberty, 'due to an original unstable state of the nervous system, as is shown by the mental failure which follows an attempt to take on the second stage of physical and mental development'.

Pubescent and adolescent insanity

Puberty became accepted as an important physiological cause of mental disturbance and pubescent or adolescent insanity was referred to frequently during the second half of the nineteenth century. Generally, the disorders of children over the age of 12 years were thought to differ little from adult manifestations. The diverse 'insanities' of this period included abnormalities of feeling and conduct, with impaired self-control, waywardness, irritability and irresponsibility. In his entry on the 'developmental insanities' in Tuke's *Dictionary of psychological medicine*, Clouston (1892) detailed the special characteristics of pubescent or adolescent mania and melancholia. In summary, 'the mania of adolescence is acute, but seldom delirious; the melancholia is stuperous, and not very suicidal. Each maniacal attack is short in duration, while the melancholic attacks are longer, the mania recurs from two to twenty times while the depression also recurs, but not so often. The chief complications are masturbation in the males and hysterical symptoms in the females.'

Theories of causation

Melancholia and mania in juveniles have always attracted a wide range of causative explanations, generally reflecting contemporary clinical and scientific interests. Prevailing ideas of causation in the nineteenth century fall into four groups.

Physical causes

Causes thought to act primarily on the brain and nervous system included disorders such as epilepsy, febrile episodes, infections including meningitis, scarlet fever, typhoid fever and measles, intestinal parasites and trauma, particularly head injury and over-exposure to the sun.

Psychological (or moral) causes

Severe shocks and frights, anxiety and distress, disappointments, bereavements, jealousy, faulty education, excessive study, religious excitement and parental brutality were the most commonly cited psychological causes. Actual or perceived loss was a recurrent theme, the consequences being particularly related to depressive states, with frequent reference to the effects of bereavement, separation and other adverse life events, such as failure in relationships and in school. Such adverse influences could be mediated by the parents. For example, Spitzka was reported to have seen 'constitutionally melancholic children in whom no other predisposing cause could be discovered than that the mother was struggling with direct or indirect results of financial crisis. In several cases the death of the father was a contributory cause of maternal depression' (Talbot, 1898, p. 60). Over the last 20 years, earlier object loss and life-stress explanations have been complemented by more specific models based on behavioural theories, the concepts of learned helplessness, and cognitive distortion and, most recently, limbic-diencephalic dysfunction.

Early experience and education

The consequences of adverse early experiences, especially during child-rearing, and faulty educational practices, generated increasing comment during the nineteenth century and the role of parents and families was of special concern to many writers. Parkinson (1807), for example, drew attention to the potentially harmful effects of both 'excessive indulgence' and parental inconsistency on children. He argued that the over-indulged, manipulative child could later discover his shortcomings and become depressed, 'suffering under an accumulation of real and fancied ills, his misery becomes so great and insupportable, that sullen or furious insanity, or dreadful suicide may soon be expected to succeed'. Harsh educational methods, over-emphasis on scholastic attainment and the dangers of excessive 'mental exertion' in school, also attracted increasing attention, especially in relation to suicide.

11

Hereditary transmission

The established belief in the connection between heredity and mental disease in children and adolescents was reiterated in the eighteenth century and was an enduring feature of nineteenth century lay and medical writings and case material, with considerable preoccupation with concepts of degeneration. Distinction was made between connate disorders and hereditary susceptibilities, which could generate either disposition to disorder, for which hopes for prevention were poor, or predisposition, where the disorder was triggered by external causes and, therefore, carried the best prognosis. The role of hereditary predisposition in melancholia was recognised widely by notable alienists, including Esquirol, Heinroth, Bucknill, D.H. Tuke and Mercier.

Juveniles in asylums

Throughout the nineteenth century, severely disturbed children and adolescents were treated routinely in adult asylum wards. Mania and melancholia were common diagnoses. For example, among 592 young people admitted to Bethlem Royal Hospital, from 1815 to 1899, who were given definite diagnoses, 345 were suffering from mania and 109 from melancholia (Wilkins, 1987). In a study of Oxfordshire asylums, Parry-Jones (1990) found evidence of a small number of young people presenting with clear evidence of depression and manic-depressive disorders.

TWENTIETH CENTURY

'Adultomorphic' descriptions of childhood affective disorders

A small number of essentially anecdotal case reports were published of manic and depressive states in children and adolescents (Brill, 1926; Kasanin & Kaufman, 1929), but the rarity of these early-onset adult-type disorders was acknowledged. Kasanin (1931), for example, described ten cases under the age of 16, the youngest being 11 years, and emphasised their extreme rarity, citing the fact that only two to three children with affective psychoses presented among the 1900 new patients seen annually at the Boston Psychopathic Hospital. In the late 1930s, there was some interest in tracing aspects of the pre-morbid personality back to childhood (Bowman, 1934). The 1940s and 1950s, however, reflected the search for specific juvenile forms and it is noteworthy that, in 1952, a special issue of the journal, *The Nervous Child*, was devoted to manic-depressive illness in childhood. Despite such reports, however, it is significant that these disorders were not included routinely in the general text-books of psychiatry or child psychiatry. Creak & Shorting (1944) made no reference to childhood affective disorders in their review of child psychiatry over the period of the Second World War.

Isolated descriptions of mania and hypomania, phenomenologically similar to the adult disorder, continued to appear, more frequently among adolescents than among pre-pubertal children. Bleuler (1934), for example, reported on mania in children and Rice (1944) described manic features in a 14-year-old boy. However, the number of cases recorded was small. In 1951, Creak could recall seeing only two typically manic children, one recovering from acute encephalitis and the other, a boy of borderline intelligence, in whom 'the manic flight appeared to be a defence built around his very inadequate capacity'. In a review of world literature on juvenile manic states, Anthony & Scott (1960) found only three cases satisfying their strict inclusion criteria. More recently, however, the argument has swung in the other direction and, using a retrospective study of published cases during the period 1809 to 1982, Weller *et al.* (1986) sought to demonstrate that mania had been under-diagnosed in pre-pubertal children. Although the possibility of depression in adolescents was always in less doubt than in younger children, it was often argued that it posed diagnostic and treatment problems not present in adult patients, because of the alleged admixture of atypical, age-related features.

Deprivation reactions: effects of separation and loss

A separate theme is discernible concerned with the effects of separation and loss in infants and small children. Studies from the 1920s onwards began to draw attention to the behavioural consequences of sensory and social deprivation in institutionalised infants and the production of a syndrome, with depressive elements, resembling adult retarded depression (Levy, 1937; Freud & Burlingham, 1944; Scott, 1948; Winnicott, 1945). Spitz (1946) developed the concept of 'anaclitic depression' as a reaction, in children aged 6 to 12 months, to separation from their mothers, the 'love object', with features of misery, lack of expression

13

and withdrawal. Analogies were drawn between such states and classical descriptions of mourning, pathological mourning and melancholia by Abraham (1911) and Sigmund Freud (1917), which had generated a new explanatory model of depression following the loss of a loved person. Spitz made a clear distinction between anaclitic depression and Klein's concept of the 'depressive position', which formed an integral element of the infantile psyche, arising when the infant perceives and introjects the mother as a whole person (Klein, 1991).

The description of deprivation-related depression drew comparison with the effects of separation experiences in non-human primates (Hinde & Spencer-Booth, 1971). It also raised questions about the role of maternal–infant bonding and led to a rapid expansion of interest in the effects of maternal deprivation, a topic pursued by many authors. Emde et al. (1965) provided a detailed account of a depressed infant in a residential nursery and, from the 1950s, influential studies were reported by the Robertsons, describing the affective response in young children detached from their mothers (Robertson & Robertson, 1971). Bowlby (1960) drew heavily on James Robertson's institutional data in his own descriptions of hospitalism and child reactions to maternal loss. In addition to these issues, the concept of anaclitic or deprivation-related depression in infants raised many other questions, especially whether or not it represented a prototype of depression in older children. Further, it was at this time that studies also commenced on the impact of early parental loss on the development of adult depression.

Doubts, challenge and denial concerning childhood depression

The developmental factors that altered a child's susceptibilities to depression, as well as the different patterns of childhood emotional responses compared with those of adults, such as increased lability of mood, received acknowledgement during the first half of the twentieth century. Although perceptive by modern standards, such views could also generate a very cautious approach to the significance of mood lowering. For example, Gillespie (1939) was in no doubt that 'the fact that, following some disappointment, a child is found to be depressed and to have suicidal preoccupations, does not justify us in thinking of that child in the same terms as we would think of a similar condition in an adult. Such depressive reactions are more akin to those of psychopathic adolescents and young adults, i.e. emotionally immature people, than they are to depressions (melancholia) of constitutional type'. From the late 1940s to the 1960s, doubts about affective disorder in pre-pubescent children increased and its existence as a clinical entity was challenged, even denied, by many writers (Bradley, 1945; Anthony & Scott, 1960).

In the first edition of his influential textbook, Kanner (1935, p. 506) emphasised only the extreme rarity of 'Full-fledged thymergastic reactions' before 15 or 16 years, although he did draw attention to mood variation occurring in normal healthy children. Even in the second edition, depression received only passing reference in the chapter on suicide. Harms (1952), however, challenged forcefully 'the present autocratic opinion of academic psychiatry that there does not exist manic-depressive disease pattern among children', in the course of which he claimed that Meyer's influence in discarding Kraepelinian concepts of manic-depression had created nosological and terminological confusion. Circumspect authors, such as Schachter (1952), sought to explain diametrically opposed views in terms of the consequences of 'reducing' adult disorders to the infantile scale, confusing 'periodic psychoses' in children with personality disturbances and, above all, the absence of any long-term observation.

The strongest views that the dynamics of adult depression, 'a superego phenomenon', could not be applied to children, came from a number of prominent psychoanalytic theorists. They argued that this was the case because, before the end of the latency period, children lacked well-developed superegos (Rochlin, 1959); they were unable to tolerate the affect of hopelessness for any length of time (Rie, 1966) and lacked experience of separation till the end of adolescence (Wolfenstein, 1966). Negative views were expressed authoritatively. For example, Mahler (1961), contended, with great conviction, that, 'the systematized affective disorders are unknown in childhood ... the immature personality structure of the infant or older child is not capable of producing a state of depression such as that seen in the adult. It cannot survive in an objectless state for any length of time'. An exception to this trend was provided by the work of Sandler & Joffe (1965), who examined the psychoanalytic records of 100 children and collated features associated commonly with depressed affect. This constituted an important step forward, confirming that depression was seen in children and characterised by sad affect, withdrawal, discontent, a feeling of being rejected or unloved, passivity and insomnia.

Concept of masked depression

In order to explain the apparent difficulty in recognising depression in children, the concept of 'masked depression' was propounded. This proposed that an underlying dysphoric mood could be masked by other symptoms not usually associated with depression, e.g. somatic complaints, behavioural problems and delinquent behaviour, school phobia and learning difficulties. In fact, such complaints covered a large part of child and adolescent psychopathological nosology (Toolan, 1962; Glaser, 1967; Bakwin, 1972). Depression in the mentally retarded could also be concealed in this way and Glaser emphasised that feelings of inadequacy, helplessness, hopelessness and rejection might be expressed in acting-out behaviour rather than depression in the mentally retarded. This view was in keeping with the longstanding recognition of the possibility of intercurrent mania and melancholia in this group. It had been reported by Ireland (1898) and Barr (1904) suggested that insanity in the mentally deficient could take the specific form of melancholia or 'nervous excitability developing into acute mania'.

By recognising that depressive affect occurred, albeit rarely observable, the concept of masked depression advanced understanding of affective disturbance in children, but it remained controversial and unsatisfactory. The diagnosis lacked operational criteria and it was impossible to tell whether or not a common symptom was pathognomonic of depression as a 'depressive equivalent'.

Trend towards diagnostic uniformity across age groups

Depression in childhood, in both acute and chronic forms, was included for the first time in a major classification system by the Group for the Advancement of Psychiatry (1966). It emphasised that it presented 'in ways somewhat different from those manifested by adults', but childhood depression was not mentioned in DSM-II in 1968. The early 1970s, however, saw a dramatic shift in thinking, with increasing interest in phenomenology and diagnosis. There was acceptance of the existence of childhood affective disorders, especially in the pre-pubertal period, as distinct clinical entities, albeit rare before adolescence, and possessing some unique features distinguishing them from adult states (Frommer, 1967; Poznanski & Zrull, 1970; Malmquist, 1971; Anthony, 1975). This development involved growing recognition of age-related changes in language and behaviour influencing clinical expression in children, responsible for the divergence from common adult presentations (Cytryn & McKnew, 1979). Increasing reliance was now placed on the child as the best single source of information, as opposed to the conventional use of parental reports.

The recognition of the heterogeneous group of juvenile affective disorders encouraged new approaches to the specification of operational criteria for their diagnosis and classification (Cytryn & McKnew, 1972). In this context, it is interesting to note that there was a trend among American investigators to continue to claim that psychotic affective disorder was virtually non-existent till mid-adolescence, although this was not the prevailing European view. The development of new assessment methods, using structured and semi-structured interviews and rating scales, and reliable diagnostic criteria, such as Research Diagnostic Criteria, was critical in resolving confusion, particularly the differentiation between depressive affects and depressive syndromes. Epidemiological studies also began to be undertaken and the first attempts were made to clarify the pathophysiology of affective disorder. For a period, the view was sustained that child and adult depression were isomorphic, with no distinction in the diagnostic criteria for pre-pubertal, adolescent and adult depression, allowing the use of the same classification systems (Puig-Antich et al., 1978). The most recent studies, however, have focused again on developmental differences and age-specific features, emphasising the necessity for their consideration during assessment and classification.

CHILDHOOD SUICIDE AND ITS RELATION TO DEPRESSION

Archival evidence indicates that there was a high incidence of 'self-killing' by children and adolescents in early modern England, despite the fact that by the mid-seventeenth century, legal authorities held that children under 14 years were not mentally capable of committing felo de se. From 1485 to 1714, for example, over 16% of recorded suicides were in juveniles under 15 years and 27% were aged 15 to 24 years, proportionally higher than their number in the general population (MacDonald & Murphy, 1990). According to Murphy (1986), youthful suicide at this time was an impulsive, retaliatory response to an alienating and rejecting social structure.

In the nineteenth century, the rarity of suicide in early childhood, but its increasing frequency thereafter, was well recognised. Winslow (1840), for example, referred to a small number of suicides in children of 12 or under, mentioning 'correction for a trifling fault' as a common precipitant. In 1845, Esquirol noted that although suicide usually occurred after puberty, he had seen 'school-children terminating their existence, the victims of a vicious education, which teaches that a state of nothingness lies beyond the limits of this life, and it is lawful for a man to deprive himself of his existence, whenever it becomes disagreeable to him'. Later, a study of suicide in children, by a French physician, Durand-Fardel (1855), attracted widespread interest. The adverse effects that parents and teachers could have on a child's feelings were emphasised and attention drawn to the importance of the child's emotional life, as well as to its education. Maudsley incorporated considerable discussion of childhood suicide in his principal textbooks (1867, 1879, 1895). Although regarded as a definite manifestation of melancholia, Maudsley (1895) noted that suicide 'is often done without any previous depression, on a sudden impulse springing out of the sad mood of the moment and the most trifling motive; not presumably with actual realisation of the momentous consequences, but rather perhaps as an outlet of temper or in unthinking imitation of a suicide which has been lately heard or read of'.

In the late nineteenth century, child suicide was thought to be increasing (Beach, 1898; Ireland, 1898) and, while acknowledging the difficulty of obtaining reliable statistics, serious attempts were made to monitor developments. From 1861 to 1888 in England and Wales, for example, suicides in juveniles under 15 numbered 148 boys and 113 girls (Strahan, 1893). In addition to such factors as fear of reprimand or maltreatment, excessive educational pressure was thought consistently to be a contributory factor and Westcott (1885) referred to, 'several English cases of children killing themselves because unable to perform school tasks; yet it must be allowed that the most modern alteration in school life – the abolition of corporal punishment – has removed one fertile cause of suicide in childhood'.

During the first half of the twentieth century, anecdotal reports of suicide in children and young adolescents continued to appear in the psychiatric literature, but association with depression, however, tended not to be made (Bender & Schilder, 1937). Despert (1952) noted the paucity of reports of children's depressive reactions and suicide and concluded that depression was rarely associated with suicidal preoccupation as was the case in adults. Instead 'suicide in children is predominantly of an impulsive character', with multiple potential motives. More recent studies have indicated much higher rates of suicidal ideation and suicide attempts in pre-pubertal children (Pfeffer *et al.*, 1980), suggesting clearly that in the past such features were under-represented (Schaffer, 1974).

TREATMENT

There is no evidence of specific treatment regimes for children with mania or melancholia until the 1920s and 1930s and the same range of restraints, physical methods and moral management techniques employed with adults would have been applied. Institutional care was resorted to for severe states of elation or depression, and especially to provide protection against destructiveness and suicide. In mental hospitals, it has to be assumed, in the absence of positive information, that children received the same range of physical treatments and opportunities for employment and recreation as adults (Kanner, 1937). Medication was always used extensively, despite its frequently non-specific therapeutic characteristics. Antidepressants began to be given to children in the 1960s, although stimulants had been used in treating behaviourally disordered children since the 1940s. Frommer (1967), for example, reported the use of monoamine oxidase inhibitor (MAOI) drugs and Annell (1969) described the successful use of lithium for children and adolescents.

CONCLUSIONS

The rapid growth of clinical and research interest in mood disorders in juveniles over the last 20 years was preceded by a long period in which these conditions were discussed only cursorily, or not at all, in textbooks of psychiatry, child psychiatry or paediatrics. Nevertheless, it is evident that these disorders did not go unrecognised and the sweeping generalisation that, until relatively recently, 'affective disorders in childhood were completely disregarded as a clinical entity' (Cytryn & McKnew, 1979) is not, in fact, supported by the historical evidence. On the contrary, case reports and references to affective disorders in children and adolescents had been occurring sporadically in previous centuries, with increasing frequency from the mid-nineteenth century onwards. In common with all forms of juvenile insanity, however, melancholia and mania were considered to be rare before puberty and the occurrence and nature of the disorder in this age group was always more controversial than that arising in pubescence or adolescence. In general, until the last quarter of the present century, free recognition of pre-pubertal affective disorder was held back by doubts, misconceptions and lack of knowledge and awareness about the extent to which the child's limited cognitive and emotional development permitted the expression of sadness, hopelessness and depression. During the 1950s and 1960s, when the domination of child and adolescent psychiatry by psychoanalytic theory reached its peak, particularly in America, notions about superego development and its role in the definition of depression took their turn as the prime factors negating the recognition of childhood depression. With the subsequent return to near-Kraepelinian concern for descriptive diagnosis and the search for organic causes, fostered by new knowledge and pharmacological treatments, clinical and scientific interest in mood disorders and their pathophysiology began to surface. Under-diagnosis of major mood disorders in adolescents has also occurred, in part related to the alleged difficulty of their distinction from schizophrenia.

Modern reviewers of the history of child psychiatry have underestimated, or neglected, the level of awareness before the present century, of child development and the aetiological implications for mental disorder of early life experiences and other factors, such as changing parent–child relationships, influencing child behaviour. Serious attempts were made, in the second half of the nineteenth century, to clarify the distinctive nature of childhood disorders and classification was not simply an exercise in superimposing adult nosology. The influence of developmental levels and age of onset on the manifestation of the disorder was recognised, in addition to hereditary factors. This broad interest in the connections between the pattern of mental disorder and the underlying processes of normal physical and mental development, however, was not pursued actively in the early twentieth century and, since major affective morbidity in juveniles was managed in adult mental hospitals, an emphasis on adult-type disorders continued to prevail. The transition from the application to children of advances in the study of adult depression to the specific study of psychopathology in children was only to take place during the last two decades.

The historical study of mood disorders in children and adolescents draws attention to many of the issues and questions that continue to call for clinical and research attention. The complex array of meanings attached to the term depression, ranging from depressive feelings and behaviours to depressive disorders, highlights the persisting need to strive for greater definitional precision. Uncertainty about continuities and discontinuities between the mood disorders of children, adolescents and adults has been an enduring theme in the literature. This raises questions about the extent to which they represent aspects of the same spectrum of disorders, whether childhood depression leads on to, or predisposes to, adult depression and whether there are juvenile antecedents to adult disorder. The necessity for a focus on the developmental variation of disorders, therefore, is overriding, without losing sight of the continuities across age groups.

REFERENCES

Abraham, K. (1911). *On character and libido development*, pp. 15–34. W.W. Norton, New York.

Annell, A.L. (1969). Lithium in the treatment of children and adolescents. *Acta Psychiatrica Scandinavica* (Supplement), **207**, 19–30.

Anthony, E.J. (1975). Childhood depression. In *Depression and human existence*, (ed. E.J. Anthony & T. Benedek), pp. 231–77. Little, Brown, Boston.

Anthony, J. & Scott, P.D. (1960). Manic-depressive psychosis in childhood. *Journal of Child Psychology and Psychiatry*, **1**, 53–70.

Arnold, T. (1782). *Observations on the nature, kinds, causes, and prevention of insanity, lunacy or madness*, Vol. 1, pp. 265–72. G. Robinson, Leicester.

Bakwin, H. (1972). Depression – a mood disorder in children and adolescents. *Maryland State Medical Journal*, **21**, 55–61.

Barr, M.W. (1904). *Mental defectives their history, treatment and training*. P. Blakiston's Son & Co., Philadelphia.

Beach, F. (1898). Insanity in children. *Journal of Mental Science*, **44**, 459–74.

Bender, L. & Schilder, P. (1937). Suicidal preoccupations and attempts in children. *American Journal of Orthopsychiatry*, **7**, 225–34.

Berrios, G. E. (1988). Melancholia and depression during the nineteenth century: a conceptual history. *British Journal of Psychiatry*, **153**, 298–304.

Berrios, G.E. (1992). History of the affective disorders. In *Handbook of affective disorders*, 2nd edn (ed. E.S. Paykel), pp. 43–56. Churchill Livingstone, Edinburgh.

Bleuler, E. (1934). *Textbook of psychiatry*. Macmillan, New York.

Bowlby, J. (1960). Grief and mourning in infancy and early childhood. *Psychoanalytic Study of the Child*, **15**, 9–52.

Bowman, K. M. (1934). A study of the pre-psychotic personality in certain psychoses. *American Journal of Orthopsychiatry*, **4**, 473–98.

Bradley, C. (1945). Psychoses in children. In *Modern trends in child psychiatry* (ed. N. Lewis & B. Pacella), pp. 135–54. International Universities Press, New York.

Bridges, K.M.B. (1932). Emotional development in early infancy. *Child Development*, **3**, 324–41.

Bright, T. (1586). *A treatise of melancholie*. T. Vautrollier, London

Brill, A.A. (1926). Psychotic children: Treatment and prophylaxis. *American Journal of Psychiatry*, **5**, 357–64.

Burton, R. (1827). *The anatomy of melancholy*, Vol. I. Longman, Rees, Orme, and Co., London

Cameron, H.C. (1929). *The nervous child*, 4th edn, pp. 77–8. Oxford University Press, London.

Clouston, T.S. (1891). *The neurosis of development, being the Morison Lectures for 1890*. Oliver & Boyd, Edinburgh.

Clouston, T.S. (1892). Developmental insanities and psychoses. In *A dictionary of psychological medicine*, Vol. 1 (ed. D. H. Tuke), pp. 357–71. Churchill, London.

Creak, M. (1951). Psychoses in childhood. *Journal of Mental Science*, **97**, 545–54.

Creak, E.M. & Shorting, B.J. (1944). Child psychiatry. *Journal of Mental Science*, **90**, 365–81.

Crichton-Browne, J. (1860). Psychical diseases of early life. *Journal of Mental Science*, **6**, 284–320.

Cytryn, L. & McKnew, D. H. (1972). Proposed classification of childhood depression. *American Journal of Psychiatry*, **129**, 149–55.

Cytryn, L. & McKnew, D. H. (1979). Affective disorders. In *Basic handbook of child psychiatry*, Vol. 2 (ed. J. D. Noshpitz) Basic Books, New York.

Darwin, C. (1872). *The expression of the emotions in man and animals*. Murray, London.

Despert, J. L. (1952). Suicide and depression in children. *Nervous Child*, **9**, 378–89.

Down, J. L. (1887). *On some of the mental affections of childhood and youth*. J. & A. Churchill, London.

Durand-Fardel, M. (1855). Étude sur le suicide chez les enfants. *Annales Médico-Psychologiques*, **1**, 61–79

Emde, R.N., Polak, P.R. & Spitz, R.A. (1965). Anaclitic depression in an infant raised in an institution. *Journal of the American Academy of Child Psychiatry*, **4**, 545–53.

Emminghaus, H. (1887). *Die Psychischen Storungen der Kindesalters*. Tubingen.

Esquirol, E. (1845). *Mental maladies. A treatise on insanity* (trans. E.K. Hunt). Lea & Blanchard, Philadelphia.

Fletcher, W.B. (1895). Mental development and insanity of children. *International Clinics*, **1**, 138–47.

Freud, A. & Burlingham, D. (1944). *Infants without families*. International Universities Press, New York.

Freud, S. (1917). *Mourning and melancholia* (trans. J. Strachey). *Standard Edition of the Complete Psychological Works of Sigmund Freud*, Vol. XIV, pp. 243–58. Hogarth Press, London (1957).

Frommer, E.A. (1967). Treatment of childhood depression with antidepressant drugs. *British Medical Journal*, **I**, 729–32.

Gardiner, H.M., Metcalf, R.C. & Beebe–Center, J.G. (1937). *Feelings and emotion: A history of theories*. American Book Company, New York.

Gillespie, R. D. (1939). Psychoses in childhood. In *A survey of child psychiatry* (ed. R.G. Gordon) p. 66. Oxford University Press, London.

Glaser, K. (1967). Masked depression in children and adolescents. *American Journal of Psychotherapy*, **21**, 565–74.

Greves E. H. (1884). Acute mania in a child of five years. *Lancet*, **ii**, 824–26.

Griesinger, W. (1867). *Mental pathology and therapeutics*, p.143. New Sydenham Society, London.

Group for the Advancement of Psychiatry (1966). *Psychopathological disorders in childhood: theoretical considerations and a proposed classification*. Report No. 62, pp. 236–7, 287. Group for the Advancement of Psychiatry, New York.

Guthrie, L. G. (1909). *Functional nervous disorders in childhood*. H. Frowde & Hodder & Stoughton, London.

Harms, E. (1952). Differential pattern of manic-depressive disease in childhood. *Nervous Child*, **9**, 326–56.

Hinde, R. A. & Spencer-Booth, Y. (1971). Effects of brief separation from mother on rhesus monkeys. *Science*, **173**, 111–18.

Hurd, H. M. (1895). *Some mental disorders of childhood and youth*. Friedenwald Co., Baltimore.

Ireland, W. W. (1875). German retrospect. *Journal of Mental Science*, **20**, 615–31.

Ireland, W. W. (1898). *The mental affections of children, idiocy, imbecility and insanity*. J. & A. Churchill, London.

Jackson, S.W. (1986). *Melancholia and depression. From hippocratic times to modern times*. Yale University Press, New Haven.

Kanner, L. (1935). *Child psychiatry*, Ballière, Tyndall & Cox, London.

Kasanin, J. (1931). The affective psychoses in children. *American Journal of Psychiatry*, **10**, 897–926.

Kasanin, J. & Kaufman, M.R. (1929). A study of the functional psychoses in childhood. *American Journal of Psychiatry*, **9**, 307–84.

Klein, M. (1991). The emotional life and ego development of the infant with special reference to the depressive position. (Paper read 1944.) In *The Freud-Klein controversies 1941–45* (ed. P. King & R. Steiner), pp. 752–97. Tavistock/Routledge, London.

Kraepelin, E. (1921). *Manic-depressive insanity and paranoia*. E. & S. Livingstone, Edinburgh.

Levy, D. M. (1937). Primary affect hunger. *American Journal of Psychiatry*, **94**, 643–52.

MacDonald, M. & Murphy, T.R. (1990). *Sleepless souls. Suicide in early modern England*, pp. 250–6. Clarendon Press, Oxford.

Mahler, M. S. (1961). On sadness and grief in infancy and childhood. *Psychoanalytic Study of the Child*, **16**, 332–54.

Malmquist, C. P. (1971). Depressions in childhood and adolescence. I. II. *New England Journal of Medicine*, **284**, 887–93, 955–61.

Mandler, G. (1979). Emotion. In *The first century of experimental psychology* (ed. E. Hearst), pp. 275–391. Lawrence Erlbaum Associates, Hillsdale, N.J.

Maudsley, H. (1867). *The physiology and pathology of the mind*. Macmillan, London.

Maudsley, H. (1879). *The pathology of mind*. Macmillan, London.

Maudsley, H. (1895). *The pathology of mind*. Macmillan, London.

Mercier, C. (1892). Melancholia. In *A dictionary of psychological medicine*, Vol. II (ed. D.H. Tuke), pp. 787–96. J. & A. Churchill, London.

Mills, C. K. (1893). Some forms of insanity and quasi-insanity in children. *Transactions of the Medical Society of Pennsylvania*, **24**, 204–13.

Morison, T. C. (1848). Case of mania occurring in a child six years old. *Journal of Psychological Medicine and Mental Pathology*, **1**, 317–18.

Murphy, T. R. (1986) 'Woful childe of parents rage': Suicide of children and adolescents in early modern England, 1507–1710. *Sixteenth Century Journal, XVII*, 259–70.

Parkinson, J. (1807). *Observations on the excessive indulgence of children, particularly intended to show its injurious effects on their health, and the difficulties it occasions in their treatment during sickness*. H. D. Symonds, London.

Parry-Jones, W. Ll. (1990). Juveniles in nineteenth-century Oxfordshire asylums. *British Journal of Clinical and Social Psychiatry*, **7**, 51–8.

Parry-Jones, W.Ll. (1992). Historical research in child and aedolescent psychiatry: scope, methods and application. *Journal of Child Psychology and Psychiatry*, **33**, 803–12.

Parry-Jones, W. Ll. (1993). History of child and adolescent psychiatry. In *Child and adolescent psychiatry, modern approaches*, 3rd edn (ed. M. Rutter, L. Hersov & E. Taylor), pp. 794–812. Blackwell Scientific, Oxford.

Perfect, W. (1791). *A remarkable case of madness, with the diet and medicines used in the cure*. For the author, Rochester.

Pfeffer, C. R., Conte, H.R., Plutchik, R. & Jerrett, I. (1980). Suicidal behavior in latency-age children: an out-patient population. *Journal of the American Academy of Child Psychiatry*, **19**, 703–10.

Poznanski, E. & Zrull, J. P. (1970). Childhood depression: clinical characteristics of overtly depressed children. *Archives of General Psychiatry*, **23**, 8–15.

Prichard, J. C. (1835). *A treatise on insanity and other disorders affecting the mind*. Sherwood, Gilbert & Piper, London.

Puig-Antich, J., Blau, S., Marx, N., Greenhill, L. & Chambers, W. (1978). Prepubertal major depressive disorder: Pilot study. *Journal of the American Academy of Child Psychiatry*, **17**, 695–707.

Rice, K. K. (1944). Regular 40 to 50 day cycle of psychotic behavior in a 14 year old boy. *Archives of Neurology and Psychiatry*, **51**, 478–80.

Rie, H. E. (1966). Depression in childhood. A survey of some pertinent contributions. *Journal of the American Academy of Child Psychiatry*, **5**, 653–85.

Robertson, J. & Robertson, J. (1971). Young children in brief separation: A fresh look. *Psychoanalytic Study of the Child*, **26**, 264–315.

Rochlin, G. (1959). The loss complex. *Journal of the American Psychoanalytic Association*, **7**, 229–316.

Sandler, J. & Joffe, W.G. (1965). Notes on childhood depression. *International Journal of Psychoanalysis*, **46**, 88–96.

Schachter, M. (1952). The cyclothymic states in the pre-pubescent child. *Nervous Child*, **9**, 357–62.

Schaffer, D. (1974). Suicide in childhood and early adolescence. *Journal of Child Psychology and Psychiatry*, **15**, 275–91.

Scott, W. C. M. (1948). The psychoanalytic concept of the origin of depression. *British Medical Journal*, **I**, 538–40.

Spitz, R. A. (1946). Anaclitic depression. *Psychoanalytic Study of the Child*, **2**, 313–42.

Strahan, S. A. K. (1893). *Suicide and insanity. A physiological and sociological study*. Swan Sonnenschein & Co., London.

Strongman, K. T. (1987). *The psychology of emotion*, 3rd edn, pp. 141–66. Wiley, Chichester.

Talbot, E .S. (1898). *Degeneracy its causes, signs and results*. W. Scott Ltd., Chichester.

Thalbitzer, S. (1926). *Emotion and insanity*, pp. 70–1. Kegan Paul, Trench, Trubner, London.

Toolan, J. H. (1962). Depression in children and adolescents. *American Journal of Orthopsychiatry*, **32**, 404–15.

Tuke, D. H. (ed.) (1892). *A dictionary of psychological medicine*, Vol. II. J. & A. Churchill, London.

Weller, R .A., Weller, E. B., Tucker, S. G. & Fristad, M. A. (1986). Mania in prepubertal children: Has it been underdiagnosed? *Journal of Affective Disorders*, **11**, 151–4.

West, C. (1854). *Lectures on the diseases of infancy and childhood*, 3rd edn. Longman, Brown, Green & Longmans, London.

Westcott, W. W. (1885). *Suicide; its history, literature, jurisprudence, causation and prevention*. H. K. Lewis, London.

Whytt, R. (1767). *Observations on the nature, causes and cures of those disorders which have been commonly called nervous, hypochondriac or hysteric.* Edinburgh.

Wilkins, R. (1987). Hallucinations in children and teenagers admitted to Bethlem Royal Hospital in the nineteenth century and their possible relevance to the incidence of schizophrenia. *Journal of Child Psychology and Psychiatry*, **28**, 569–80.

Willis, T. (1683). *Two discourses concerning the soul of brutes which is that of the vital and sensitive of man* (trans. S. Pordage). Thomas Dring, Ch. Harper & John Leigh, London.

Winslow, F. (1840). *The anatomy of suicide.* Henry Renshaw, London.

Winnicott, D.W. (1945). Primitive emotional development. *International Journal of Psychoanalysis*, **26**, 137–43.

Wolfenstein, M. (1966). How is mourning possible? *Psychoanalytic Study of the Child*, **21**, 93–123.

2

Emotional behaviour and emotional understanding: A developmental fugue

Mark Meerum Terwogt and Hedy Stegge

INTRODUCTION

Like almost any other important psychological concept, the term emotion is often used as if it is a self-evident concept that needs no further definition. In fact by scanning the psychological and psychiatric literature, Plutchik (1980) was able to quote about 30 different descriptions, stressing physiological components of emotion, motivational or cognitive aspects, emotional expression and other behavioural correlates, or a combination of two or more of these elements. The variety of definitions reflects the diversity of techniques that are applied to the study of emotion and the many different levels at which this takes place. Clearly, there is no agreement on defining emotion. As a consequence, some authors have gone as far as suggesting banning the concept from psychology altogether (e.g. Duffy, 1934). We do not share this extreme point of view, but for the moment we also do not want to add to the confusion by producing a definition of our own. We agree with Kagan (1978) that at this stage the study of emotion should focus on the different aspects of the phenomenon, rather than on its definition.

Physiological evidence indicates that some of the oldest parts of the brain play a critical role in the emotional process. In fact, emotions in their original form are archaic response syndromes that break in and take over when basic interests of the organism are at stake. For example, fear activates an acute flight reaction that may save us from danger. In this sense we share our emotions with lower animals (MacLean, 1970). However, our human emotions are also influenced by more recent evolutionary parts of the brain, such as the neo-cortex. These connections allow us some cognitive control over emotion; the possibility to adapt our primitive emotional reaction patterns to the requirements of modern society. The present chapter focuses on the question how children gradually learn to use their cognitive abilities to gain control over emotion.

THE EMOTIONAL PROCESS

Lewis & Michalson (1983) divided emotion up into five structural components: (a) the eliciting stimulus event, (b) the emotional state, (c) the receptor, i.e. the neurological system that mediates between elicitors and states, (d) the emotional expression, and (e) the emotional experience. None of these constructs is without problems. Sometimes this has to do with a lack of information. For example, we do not know whether the receptors involve specific loci and pathways or non-specific general systems, or even if they can be located at all. In other cases the problems are directly related to fundamental theoretical questions in the history of emotion research. For instance, the unresolved question of whether we have to consider emotions as states varying along a few dimensions such as pleasantness–unpleasantness and intensity (Wundt, 1903) or as a limited set of 'discrete' states (Darwin, 1872), bears great relevance to the meaning of Lewis and Michalson's state concept.

Within the context of this chapter we think it more helpful to present a short outline of the emotional *process*, rather than to elaborate any further on the structural problems of the emotion concept. Arnold (1960) describes an emotion as 'the felt tendency towards anything intuitively appraised as good (beneficial), or away from anything intuitively appraised as bad (harmful). This attraction or aversion is accompanied by a pattern of physiological changes organised towards approach or withdrawal' (Arnold, 1960, p. 182). Like a number of other leading theorists (e.g. Lazarus, 1975; Frijda, 1986), Arnold gives prominence to the appraisal process in emotion. When she uses the qualification 'intuitive' she means the appraisal to be direct, immediate and non-reflective, as in the phrase 'he knew intuitively that he had just met a friend'. Of course, not every appraisal is correct. The first intuitive impression is often supplemented or corrected by later reflection. This secondary appraisal is more cognitive by nature and resembles problem solving.

Let us try to give a chronological description of the emotional process. Whenever a stimulus has an emotional impact (that is, when it serves or threatens some personal interest) it triggers a tendency for direct action: simple stereotypical action patterns like flight or attack. This action tendency involves a mental representation of the situation, as well as physiological changes in preparation to the forthcoming action. Often, however, the direct action is blocked or frustrated by situational (often social) constraints and a reappraisal of the situation is called for. In order to cope with the situation, we may regard alternative actions, rearrange the present information or focus on new aspects of the situation. Moreover, we can search our memory after earlier experiences in similar kinds of situations or inspect our generalised knowledge about (our own) emotional performance.

A description like this suggests that coping is not different from any other problem-solving process. That is not true. In coping we have to deal with so-called 'hot cognitions' (Abelson, 1963; Zajonc, 1980). We cannot block the action impulse for ever, without doing anything about it. Secondary appraisal is pressed by the need to find a quick solution. Therefore, we often follow shaky or unrealistic appraisals that seem to serve our short-term interests. Such biased problem solving becomes even less surprising if we realise that the memories used in the process most likely have an emotional connotation themselves. The undertaking of finding a suitable response can be described as a constant interplay between cognitive appraisals, emotion, subsequent information processing, reappraisals, and so on (e.g. Lazarus, Averill & Opton, 1970; Folkman, Schaefer & Lazarus, 1979; Lazarus, Coyne & Folkman, 1982).

Figure 2.1 represents the gist of a typical appraisal theory of emotion. The black arrows in the bottom half of the process indicate that the direct action pathway is basically non-reflective. Theorists such as Izard (1977, 1991) or Plutchik (1980), who are oriented towards evolutionism, will regard this pathway as an innate automatic programme. In their view, all people are equipped with a limited number of these programmes right from the beginning: the so-called 'basic emotions'. These primitive programmes are elicited by a characteristic set of stimuli and result in universally recognisable facial expressions and stereotypical action patterns. Bonds between situations and emotional reactions are essentially fixed. Although these bonds might have been useful in the early stages of our evolutionary history, they are often inadequate in contemporary social life. For example, after having been angered by the behaviour of your superior you may get away with making a nasty remark, but acting out the stereotypical reaction, hitting one's adversary, will probably be inadvisable.

This phylogenetic claim applies also to ontogenesis. The fact that

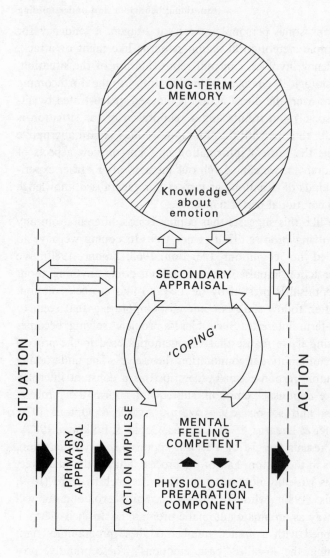

Figure 2.1. The emotional process.

young children immediately cry when experiencing distress serves a clear purpose. It attracts the attention of the caregiver, who might be able to remove the source of the trouble. Later on such a display of dependency is not permitted any more: 'big boys don't cry'.

Given such pre-existing programmes, emotional development can best be described as the development of emotional control, i.e. the enrichment of emotional experience and the growing power of secondary appraisal. Through this appraisal activity old programmes become more flexible and newly derived patterns such as 'jealousy' or 'guilt' emerge.

In order to give secondary appraisal a chance, the child has to break into a programme that is already in operation and redirect it. The appropriate tool for this – as for all automatic behaviour – is self-reflection, making the programme the object of attention. The effect of this introspective activity can be nicely demonstrated by asking someone who tries to keep his balance on a balancing beam to tell us how he manages to do so. Someone who really tries to answer this question falls off: the highly organised and automatic act of balancing is disturbed. The same phenomenon can be observed if we ask an experienced driver how he changes gears. By making the act the object of his attention he is likely to make a mistake; a mistake he otherwise never would have made. In both examples self-reflection disrupts a highly successful automatic programme. Of course, in this case such an action is counterproductive. There is no need to alter a programme like this one. In fact, if programmes, like the driving skill in the second example, become automatised during the course of development, we have given up control exactly *because* they are always successful. In the case of basic emotion programmes it is the other way round. In the course of development there are less and less situations in which the acting out of the original programmes is advisable or even permitted. If we want to cope with those social constraints we need more flexibility. We have to think before we act.

As mentioned above, the strength of the impulse provides us with limited time to find a solution. But usually we can block the impulse long enough to allow at least some secondary appraisal, given that we heed our feelings in time. A new cognitive representation of the events may elicit an impulse of different intensity (for instance, if we take into consideration that the one who hurt our feelings did not do it on purpose) or even a quite different feeling (for instance, if we realise that the remark that hurt us was made for our own good), but if the eliciting stimulus causes an extremely strong action tendency the original programme is carried out before we get the chance to break in. 'I was so angry that I couldn't help myself. I hit my boss, before I knew what I was doing'.

THE ORIGIN OF KNOWLEDGE ABOUT EMOTION

Our coping potential is partly determined by our knowledge about emotion (see Figure 2.1). The connection between knowledge and behaviour is one of the main reasons for studying the child's growing body of knowledge about emotion. Before embarking upon a discussion about knowledge and behaviour, we should specify what we mean by the phrase 'knowledge about emotion'.

The simple observation that a child gets angry in one situation and not in another does not necessarily imply that the child has knowledge of the different anger-arousing potential of both situations. Just as the ability to see depth does not imply that one is aware of the several cues that make this possible, one cannot infer children's knowledge about their own emotional functioning just from observing their behaviour. Knowledge about emotion refers to a person's cognitive *representations* concerning the origins and consequences of emotions. These representations may be relatively simple or quite complex in nature. Moreover, they may contain information that is relatively explicit and easy to verbalise as well as information that is implicit and difficult to catch in words.

How do people acquire such representations? One of the answers is by the observation of the behaviour of others in emotional circumstances. This way children may find out the causal connection between not obeying mother and her nasty behaviour, or they may come to the strategic observation that you better wait asking for a biscuit till mum is in the right mood. In this context, 'mood' refers to a complex of diverging behavioural components (characteristic facial expressions and acts). We have to keep in mind that feelings of others cannot be observed directly. Without this abstract notion that links all observable elements together it is hardly possible for the child to acquire a rich conception of emotions.

Children may learn to use emotion words correctly since others sometimes use these labels in emotional circumstances. For instance, the mother may mention her 'anger' when she acts accordingly. There are however an enormous variety of situations that can make us angry. It is a difficult task for the child to determine the exact meaning of such a word used in markedly different circumstances and with a variability of outcome. However, young children can often count on the assistance of their parents for this. For instance, parents not only tell the child that they are happy, but also that they feel that way because the child 'helped his little sister' (antecedent) and that he therefore 'deserves a biscuit' (consequence). Later on, verbal communication can also be an effective means for the direct transfer of more complex phenomena like control strategies: 'you better count to ten before you answer'.

Thus far, we have mentioned two of the three sources of information that enable the child to build a representation of emotions; in terms of Harris & Olthof (1982), they are the *behavioural model* – information transfer by the active observation of others – and the *socio-centric model* – in which the child acts as a 'passive' recipient of information provided by the (verbal) community. However, for a full grasp of emotional concepts these two sources have to be combined with the information from a third source: the *solipsistic model*, the term Harris & Olthof introduced for the observation of one's own private processes (introspection).

In the first years of life, inner signals like 'it hurts' or 'I feel good', if registered, stay relatively isolated. Young children do not relate them to the antecedents in the outside world. They do not infer that they 'feel good' because their mother just praised them. That does not necessarily mean that they do not appreciate the difference between the mental and physical environment, as Piaget (1962) once suggested. At the age of 3, at least, it is easy to demonstrate that they do. If we tell 3-year-olds a story about a child who owns a dog and a child who thinks about a dog, they know exactly which of the two dogs can be touched or stroked (Wellman & Estes, 1986; Harris *et al.*, 1991). However, at this age children usually are not yet inclined to monitor their inner signals spontaneously; the relevance of this kind of information is not acknowledged (Meerum Terwogt & Olthof, 1989). The phenomenon that other people often refer to inner processes ('How do you *feel?*', 'I feel angry *inside*') stimulates children to 'look inside' themselves. Later on, this solipsistic knowledge becomes the main factor in the identification of emotion. We *are* happy, because we *feel* happy.

It can be said that adults tend to overestimate their introspective abilities (Nisbett & Wilson, 1977). These abilities are probably limited since a lot of information processing concerning emotions seems to take place along parallel channels (Neisser, 1963) or is simply too fast to reflect upon. A more practical limitation is that we do not always heed the process as it happens. For instance, when somebody else puts forward a proposal to us in a condescending way we may not give attention to the fact that this way of presenting arouses our anger. If we detect our emotional state a few moments later it is quite possible that we try to explain our anger in terms of the content of the proposal. We are then inclined to call that proposal 'unfair'; what else could have caused our anger? Often, a *post hoc* search for plausible motives is mistaken for introspection (Nisbett & Wilson, 1977). Experientially the difference between the two phenomena is not always easy to detect. However, the subject who takes his (or her) *post hoc* reasoning for introspection will be completely convinced that he is right. He 'knows'! Moreover, he is the only one who can know for sure, since he is the only one who can look inside his own head. If he realises what has happened, he will be less sure. *Post hoc* explanations are vulnerable to mistakes. We have to link inside information (the detected anger) with the outside circumstances. In fact, this situation is quite similar to the situation in which we have to explain other people's emotions. Even if we know a person very well – as we hope we know ourselves – we feel that there is always a chance that we may make the wrong interpretation.

None the less, introspective knowledge can still be marked as an essential source for the acquisition of an adult representation of emotion. The awareness of one's own mental state fills in the missing link between emotional stimuli and emotional behaviour. Some authors claim that young children lack the introspective abilities to detect this missing link (e.g. Selman, Lavin & Brion-Meisels, 1982). Such a claim is hard to prove. But at least we may say that young children do not posses the introspective attitude that is necessary to scan the inner environment (Meerum Terwogt & Olthof, 1989). Therefore, when questioned about emotions, they seldom refer to mental states (Harris, Olthof & Meerum Terwogt, 1981). For instance, 6-year-olds typically answer the question 'How do you know that you are happy?' with statements like 'Cos it's my birthday' or 'Cos I'm laughing': observable components (antecedents as well as consequences) of the emotional state. Only one out of ten gives an answer that refers to the inner state. By the age of 10 the mental component has got a much more central position in the child's concept of emotion. Half of the 10-year-olds answered immediately with something like 'I'm happy since I *feel* happy (inside)', and including later reactions, about 90% of the 10-year-olds seem to appreciate mental state as an important identifying element. The 6-year-old 'behaviourists' have changed into 10-year-old 'mentalists' (Harris & Olthof, 1982).

KNOWLEDGE AND BEHAVIOUR

Earlier on we mentioned the relation between knowledge and behaviour. Usually we can observe a *developmental time-lag* between the two: you have to be able to do something before you know what you can (Meerum Terwogt, 1986; Meerum Terwogt & Olthof, 1989). For instance, Cole (1986) reported that even 3- to 4-year-old children are able to attenuate the overt display of disappointment if the social environment expects them to do so. Upon receiving a disappointing gift from the experimenter, they came up with a kind of half-smile; an expression which was quite different from the frank disappointment they showed when the experimenter was not around. However, when asked, the children were not aware of the display rule that governed their behaviour. Similarly, Meerum Terwogt, Schene & Harris (1986b) found that 6-year-old children used a mental strategy to control a negative emotion, without being able to report on such a strategy. In this particular experiment, children were able to manipulate the impact of a sad story which they had to 'retell' afterwards. Children who were instructed to listen carefully 'in such a way that you feel sad yourself' became more sad than children who were instructed to listen to the story 'in such a way that you don't become sad yourself'. In this case, the children were also unable to tell the experimenter what they had done to get involved or detached. There is still no sign of *reflection on the recently derived abilities.*

These examples show that children's actual behaviour precedes the understanding of the psychological determinants of that same behaviour. Of course, one may ask then what the reason is for studying children's knowledge. Why is it important? What is the function of more or less generalised knowledge? The answer to these questions is obvious: the child's 'theory of mind' (Wellman, 1990) is an important factor in the further development of the behavioural repertoire. The impact of changes in the child's naive conceptions can be compared to the consequences of a theory change in science (Wellman, 1990; Astington & Gopnik, 1991): a relatively simple reorganisation of the information causes a radical change in the way we perceive ourselves and the surrounding world. And as in science, this influences our information-seeking processes and explanatory patterns, and by that our whole development.

One of the theoretical approaches that is consistent with this view is attribution theory (e.g. Weiner, 1986). This theory claims that the causal attribution that is made (in the mind) for mentally positive or negative outcomes is critical for the emotional and behavioural reactions that follow. Attribution theory describes a two-step evaluation process. Firstly, evaluation occurs in terms of success or failure and results in 'outcome-dependent emotions' like happiness or sadness of an experience. Secondly, a more complex and cognitive causal search to explain the outcome refines or modifies this initial emotional reaction and results in 'attribution-dependent emotions' such as surprise, pride, guilt, shame or gratitude. Young children simply rely on outcome-dependent emotions. Later in development, increasingly more complex cognitions enter into the emotion process to further differentiate experience.

People may develop idiosyncratic modes of causal analysis. In that case, attribution tendencies become more or less stable personal characteristics that can have major influences. For example, if someone is inclined to ascribe failure to factors beyond personal control, he or she comes to realise that virtually nothing can be done about it. This leads to low expectancies of future success and motivational decrements. The person gives up; there is no longer anything to be done. Abramson, Seligman & Teasdale (1978) labelled this phenomenon 'learned helplessness'. Although the cognitive limitations of young children make them less susceptible to helplessness than older children (Rholes *et al.*, 1980), this reaction pattern can already settle in quite early in life.

If we ask emotionally disturbed children about their concept of emotion, we find a pattern that resembles the learned helplessness phenomenon. Earlier on we described the emotional process as an automatic programme that can be changed by cognitive appraisal processes. Emotionally disturbed children (11- to 15-year-old institutionalised children) focus mainly on the autonomous character of emotions: 'It is something that comes over you; something that just goes on by itself', whereas children of that same age group usually already appreciate the possibility of mental manipulation (Meerum Terwogt, Schene & Koops, 1990). For emotionally disturbed children, control is limited to the regulation of the emotional expression. These children were fairly confident they were able to hide their emotions from others. Although this behaviour may keep them out of immediate trouble sometimes, it does not provide them with an opportunity to let out the emotion in a socially acceptable way. Moreover, their conviction that emotions cannot be changed keeps them from looking for possible solutions and therefore inhibits their further emotional development.

To conclude this section, we will try to specify the impact of knowledge on development in more general terms. Development is often described in terms of a sequence from *simple* to more and more *complex* patterns. With respect to children's cognitive skills (and the cognitive skills involved in the emotional process) this is a sensible conclusion. In general, however, the statement is misleading. We can observe already highly organised and precisely calibrated skills in very young children. For instance, early processes like 'keeping one's balance' or 'perceiving depth' are extremely complicated. We clearly need another criterion to characterise development. Whatever the level of complexity, all early processes have one thing in common: they are tightly wired into specific types of behaviour and can be applied only to a narrow range of situations (Rozin, 1975). This is also true for the basic emotional programmes. Therefore development can better be described as a gradual change from *rigid* to *flexible* patterns. Patterns, like the emotion programmes, that prove themselves inadequate in a range of new situations during the course of development, have to be attenuated and extended.

In summary, initially the young child's emotional behaviour is determined by relatively rigid, wired-in programmes. The child has no cognitive access to these programmes and no knowledge of them. Emotional behaviour is entirely determined by environmental input. After this initial 'biological' stage, the child gradually gains insight into the determinants of emotional behaviour. Their own cognitive representation of events may now serve as an elicitor of affect (Saarni, 1978). The child's emotional behaviour is now no longer entirely 'data driven'. That is, behaviour is no longer entirely based on elements directly derived from the actual situation. Situational characteristics may trigger relevant knowledge structures; the child's emotional behaviour becomes increasingly 'knowledge driven'.

LABELLING EMOTIONS

In the remainder of this chapter we will turn to some of the important landmarks in the child's understanding of emotion.

Children start to use emotion terms quite early – around the beginning of their second year (Bretherton *et al.*, 1986; Smiley & Huttenlocher, 1989). Words like 'laugh' and 'cry' are understood earlier than words like 'happy' and 'sad' (Honkavaara, 1961), indicating that the overt elements of the emotional process are easier to grasp than the internal states. By 2 to 3 years, children realise that there can be a variety of personal reasons for an emotional reaction and they start asking spontaneously for these reasons (Cairns & Hsu, 1977; Bretherton & Beeghly, 1982). Connections between emotional states and emotional determinants are sought. Around 4 years, there is a fair consensus among children about the kind of situations that will provoke the basic emotions: happiness, fear, sadness and anger (Barden et al., 1980).

Other emotions will follow in a fairly stable order, determined by a number of factors. The early understanding of basic emotions is probably related to the fact that these emotions are characterised by a unique facial expression, that makes them easy to identify (Reichenbach & Masters, 1983). The order of acquisition is also determined by the simple opportunity to learn. For example, disgust is often considered one of the basic emotions (e.g. Ekman & Friesen, 1974), but, unlike the labels of the other basic emotions, the word is not frequently used in children's immediate environment. Therefore, its understanding comes relatively late. However, the concept of 'shyness' is understood not much later than happiness, fear, sadness and anger (Harris et al., 1987). Shyness is not accompanied by a unique expression (at least not a unique facial expression) but the concept is used quite frequently in the presence of children. The third and probably most influential factor that determines the order of acquisition is the complexity of the emotions involved (Harris et al., 1987). For example, the understanding of 'social emotions' such as shame, guilt or pride requires an appreciation of social standards or rules, the ability to recognise violations of those standards or rules, and the ability to anticipate other people's reactions to such violations. It is often argued that we cannot be sure that children even at the age of 10 have acquired an adult concept of these emotions (Colby et al.,1983).

TIME-COURSE OF EMOTIONS AND AMBIVALENCE

Knowledge of the antecedents of emotion is a substantial part of the emotion concept. However, the internal emotional state is often prolonged for quite some time after the eliciting situation is over. The connection with its cause is not important any more and may even be completely lost. In this case, Izard et al. (1965) talk about 'free-floating emotion' in everyday life better known as *mood*.

We know of only one study that addresses the question of whether or not children appreciate the typical time-course of emotions. Harris

(1983) asked 6- and 10-year-olds about their immediate and later reactions to a sad situation (for instance, the death of a pet). Both age-groups gave a consistent picture of emotions as gradually waning over time, although in general the younger children indicated a faster decline. The older children were somewhat more outspoken in their acknowledgement of the irregularities in this pattern. 'During dinner daddy talks mainly about my school work, and then I probably think less of Blacky. But later on, when I'm alone in my bed, I become sad again'.

Statements like this one illustrate that 10-year-olds seem to appreciate the ambivalence of some situations: 'talking with daddy' has an emotional impact different from 'thinking of Blacky'. As we will see, the explicit recognition of ambivalence is difficult for children. At a behavioural level, ambivalence can be observed in early childhood. Older siblings often vacillate between tenderness and hostility in their approach to a younger sibling (Dunn, 1984). Yet, if we ask them to tell us how they feel in these situations, they are likely to acknowledge only one of these feelings (Harter, 1983; Harter & Buddin, 1987). Around the age of 6, children accept that you can experience two different emotions immediately after one another, although they still find it hard to accept that those emotions can be completely opposite, such as happiness and sadness (Olthof et al., 1987). The acceptance of the co-occurrence of conflicting emotions is hardly to be expected before the age of 10 (Harter & Buddin, 1987; Meerum Terwogt et al., 1986a).

Why are mixed feelings so hard to understand? Once children have acquired a firm grasp of each separate concept, it might be that they come to the logical conclusion that *happy* and *sad* are mutually exclusive opposites, just as a brick cannot be described both as *big* and *little* (Harris, Morris & Meerum Terwogt, 1986). They simply 'don't go together'. Young children do not understand that it is possible to look at the same situation or the same object from different perspectives. 'The brick is little as compared to the whole house, but big as compared to that pebble', and likewise 'I'm sad because Blacky is ill, but happy since he seems to recover quite well'.

Harris (1989) provides an alternative explanation for the young child's problems. He argues that the initial appraisal system and the explanatory system might be operating quite differently. Initial appraisal operates in an exhaustive fashion, and includes both the positive and negative elements of the situation, but reflection might stop as soon as the first feeling is detected (see also the dissertation by Meerum Terwogt, 1984). The link between emotion and situation is then stored

39

accordingly. Therefore, it is possible to express ambivalence without being consciously aware of the fact that ambivalence is felt (Meerum Terwogt, 1987). Only if both conflicting elements are very salient, the child realises that more than one emotion is experienced. And even then, he or she will try to hold on to the initial model of a one-to-one relationship between situations and emotions. The child will be inclined to regard the different feelings as successive reactions to successive situations before finally acknowledging the possibility of simultaneously experiencing more than one emotion in one and the same situation. This need for a progressive reconceptualisation of the link between situation and emotion offers an explanation for the huge time-lag between the expression of ambivalence and its recognition on a conscious level.

In emotionally disturbed children, the acknowledgement of experiencing conflicting feelings at the same time seems to be delayed (Meerum Terwogt, 1990). This is particularly the case if we ask them for self-evaluative statements. Like young children, they are inclined to look at themselves as 'all smart' or 'all dumb', 'all good' or 'all bad', which makes it hard for them to acquire a realistic self-image (Harter, 1977).

THE SUBJECTIVE CHARACTER OF EMOTION: BELIEFS AND DESIRES

Although an understanding of the common causal relations between particular situations and particular emotions is very important, it is not sufficient for a full understanding of emotion. In addition, children must have the ability to go beyond the objective characteristics of a situation. The fact is, the emotional impact of an event is determined by a person's subjective appraisal of the situation, an appraisal (de)formed by personal beliefs, expectations, and desires (Harris, 1989). A gift will not elicit happiness if the recipient does not want it or suspects the motive of the donor.

One way of understanding other people's emotions is to take ourselves as a frame of reference: 'What would I feel under these circumstances?' But this information does not guarantee an accurate prediction. No two people are the same. We have to realise that our own reaction pattern may be somewhat peculiar: 'I'm afraid of guinea pigs, but most people think they are cute'. However, it's possible that information on the personal history of the other suggests that that person holds an opinion different from our own: 'I like to see my grandma, but he never visits his. So maybe he doesn't like her very much'. The child has to make adjustments to his or her own frame of reference in the light of this kind of knowledge.

Even very young children acknowledge the fact that other people may have desires or beliefs different from their own. This can be observed in *pretend play* (Piaget, 1962; Leslie, 1987). In most children, the first signs of pretend play emerge somewhere in their second year of life. A young girl acts as if her doll is a genuine person (Wolf, Rygh & Altshuler, 1984). At first, the young 'mother' treats her 'child' as a passive recipient of her own actions, but later on she makes the doll talk and act independently and eventually supplies it with desires, sensations and emotions. Around $3\frac{1}{2}$ to 4 years of age, we can hear the child use a different voice if she talks for the doll.

The child clearly acknowledges that her make-believe companion is not simply an extension of herself. The 'other person' has distinct qualities, can do things that the child pretends not to know about. When playing 'hide and seek' the child puts her doll in the closet, and shouts directly afterwards 'Where are you?'. Preferences and feelings of the doll might be different from the preferences and feelings of her 'creator'. The doll likes spinach, while the child herself does not.

Despite occasional confusion between the rules of play and the rules of reality (DiLalla & Watson, 1988; Harris *et al.,* 1991), even 3-year-olds can make a systematic distinction between the real world and the world of their imagination (Wellman & Estes, 1986). This capacity for imaginative projection helps children to put themselves in place of another person and to experience the world through the eyes of the other. In this way, children learn to take into account other people's particular desires and beliefs.

The perspective of another person might differ from that of the child. This can be nicely demonstrated in the kind of experiments in which the child knows that somebody else is misled (e.g. Wimmer & Perner, 1983; Harris *et al.,* 1989). For example, in a short puppet play children observe that one of the puppets puts away a can of coke to drink it later. But then another puppet secretly replaces the coke with milk. The children are asked for the reactions of the first character *before* and *after* he discovers the deceit. Even 3-year-olds realise that this person will be sad on discovering the trick if he or she prefers coke to milk, or pleased if he or she prefers milk to coke. However, the 3-year-olds were quite poor at working out that the person's initial feelings (i.e. before discovering the trick) must be based on the subjective situation (i.e. this

41

person's beliefs about the contents of the can) instead of the objective situation (the actual content of the can). Five-year-olds and some 4-year-olds were much better in acknowledging that the critical factor in eliciting the emotion is the person's mistaken belief, i.e. his or her subjective appraisal of the situation.

SOCIAL EMOTIONS: NORMS AND VALUES

In the previous sections we have shown how young children begin to understand simple emotions like anger, happiness or sadness in terms of private mental states. We will now extend this analysis to some of the more complex emotions: guilt, shame and pride. Although the terms 'guilt' and 'shame' are often used interchangeably, it is now generally acknowledged that the two terms refer to phenomenologically different experiences (Tangney, 1990; Ferguson, Stegge & Damhuis, 1991; Ferguson & Stegge, 1994). Guilt is a self-critical reaction to a specific act of wrongdoing, that is perceived immoral in nature. The person feels responsible for the resulting consequences, ruminates about what he or she has done, wants to confess and to make reparations. Shame, in contrast, involves a negative evaluation of the entire self which conveys a sense of fundamental defectiveness. The person feels weak and isolated. Since there is a fear of being ridiculed and rejected, the person who feels ashamed reveals a strong desire to hide from other people.

Guilt, shame and pride are so-called social emotions, due to the fact that social norms and values play a critical role in their experience. Young children do not yet acknowledge the importance of this kind of social information. They simply pursue their goals and analyse a situation in terms of the outcome (Thompson, 1989). Getting what you want leads to happiness, while not getting it results in feelings of sadness or frustration. A young boy, who completes a jigsaw puzzle for the twentieth time, is as happy as he was after completing it for the first time. Being successful is all that counts. If he were a few years older, his appreciating that 'some tasks are easy' and 'some tasks are difficult' (in relation to his own norms and skills) would make a difference. The first time he would experience pride, whereas this emotion would no longer be felt if the job is considered easy.

In the course of development, children also begin to realise that some behaviours are approved of by other people, while others are reacted to with disapproval. Gaining other people's approval becomes an important goal that guides children's behaviour. Normative standards for behaviour become more and more important. As children also start to causally analyse their own behaviour and the behaviour of others in more depth, personal responsibility becomes an important determinant of affective experience. In the achievement domain, children realise, for example, that there is a difference between failure that is due to controllable causes (such as the amount of effort), and failure that is caused by uncontrollable factors (such as a lack of ability). The former attribution results in feelings of guilt, while the latter causes feelings of shame (Stipek & DeCotis, 1988). Likewise, in the moral domain, blaming others for harm becomes increasingly dependent on the other's intentions and the avoidability of the event. Intentional and avoidable harm results in more anger and aggression towards the perpetrator than accidental and unavoidable harm (Ferguson & Rule, 1983; Olthof, Ferguson & Luiten, 1989).

Between the ages of 5 and 10, the relevance of personal responsibility and normative standards is more and more acknowledged and taken into account (Graham, Doubleday & Guarino, 1984; Ferguson Stegge & Damhuis, 1991). Again, we observe a developmental time-lag between children's actual knowledge in a certain domain and their judgement of the relevance of this knowledge on an emotional and a behavioural level. Although 5- and 6-year-old children know the difference between accidental success and success that is the result of hard work, they do not include that information in their evaluation of the situation (Graham, 1988). The same goes for knowledge in the moral domain. Young children do have a fair sense of right and wrong. Even 3-year-olds provide differentiated judgements about 'very bad things' like 'stealing' and 'killing', and things that are only 'a little bad', like 'not saying your prayers before you go to sleep' and 'not tidying your room in time' (Smetana, 1981). However, this knowledge does not have an impact on their course of action (Harris, 1989).

Why is it that young children do not acknowledge the relevance of this information? Firstly, they may not yet possess the *cognitive capacities* that are needed to effectively combine all the different kinds of perspectives in their emotional evaluation. Secondly, the fact that young children know the difference between good and bad does not tell us anything about the question of whether or not they have *internalised* the rules they express. Clearly, there is a big difference between knowing the rule and really subscribing to it and behaving accordingly. For instance, we all know that we have to pay taxes. However, many of us see no

43

harm in trying to dodge them if we can. We know the rule, but it is not an effective guideline for behaviour. No feelings of guilt are elicited to stop us from breaking the rule. Thirdly, children initially need an actual *audience* to make them realise that norms and values are important. The child with the jigsaw puzzle, in our earlier example, can probably count on his mother's approval when he finishes the puzzle for the first few times. Later on, his accomplishment gets less and less admiration. If the child were a bit older, the mother would probably even openly react with annoyance if the child tried to attract her attention for the twentieth time. Reissland (1988) argues that the onset of pride is marked by the fact that it is exactly this social approval rather than the personal experience of success itself that elicits the pleasure in the child. In fact, this is what Cooley refers to as the 'looking glass self' (Cooley, 1902; see also Harris, 1989). At first, feeling pride or shame is dependent on the close proximity of another person and his or her approval or disapproval. Later on, the child will experience these emotions with greater autonomy. Internalisation of norms and values is completed and the proximity of the audience is no longer critical. The child is able to judge his or her own actions with respect to his or her own normative standards of conduct. This is also reflected in the child's language. Whereas young children refer to other people when talking about pride and shame, 8-year-olds speak about feeling proud or ashamed of *themselves* (Harter & Whitesell, 1989).

Social emotions become mechanisms of (spontaneous) self control provided that several prerequisites are fulfilled, including an awareness of standards of conduct, a felt obligation to regulate behaviour with respect to these standards and an ability to recognise discrepancies between one's own behaviour and these internalised values (Ausubel, 1955). As they grow older, children become more vulnerable to the experience of discrepancies, since they are increasingly able to detect them. Moreover, these experienced discrepancies have longer-lasting implications for the child's self-esteem and his or her future expectations and motivation, since children begin to describe themselves as well as other peoples' ideas about them in more stable terms (Ruble & Rholes, 1981; Moretti & Higgins, 1990). They start to do so in behavioural terms (4 to 6 years), but later on (9 to 11 years) they are inclined to use more generalised trait-like descriptions. As a consequence, it becomes more and more difficult for the child to reduce a certain discrepancy, since not only the actual behaviour must be changed, but also certain features of the self. Hence, children might be increasingly vulnerable to the feelings of helplessness and hopelessness that are so characteristic of depression (Moretti & Higgins, 1990).

DISPLAY-RULES

We have seen that emotions can be a powerful instrument in the socialisation of behaviour. Emotional behaviour itself, i.e. the display of emotion, is also governed by all kinds of social rules. Earlier on, for instance, we mentioned that a great number of 3- to 4-year-old children already spontaneously concealed their disappointment in reaction to a disappointing gift (Cole, 1986). These children probably have been told over and over again to smile and say 'thank you' whenever they get a present. They have learned a simple rule of politeness and are able to apply it if the situation calls for it. Probably, they are hardly aware of the fact that they were showing an emotion that did not correspond to what they felt, let alone appreciate the potentially misleading impact of this action on other people. In fact, all the 3-year-olds, whether they were able to conceal their disappointment or not, claimed that the experimenter would know how they really felt. This was quite different in 6-year-olds. At that age children know that facial expressions can be misleading. As a person's internal state is not necessarily visible on his or her face, the real emotion experienced might be quite different from the emotion that is displayed (Saarni, 1979; 1984; Harris *et al.*, 1986).

The notion of being able to hide an emotion is very important. 'It offers the child a barricade between the private world of experience known only to the self, and the public world in which behaviour and facial expression are visible to others' (Harris, 1989, p. 141). It can be proved that this barricade provides effective shelter; the difference between genuine and faked emotions is hard to detect, by children as well as adults (DePaulo & Jordan, 1982). Once the child acknowledges the possible advantages of hiding an emotion, we might expect deliberate attempts to disguise vulnerability by misleading actions. Harris & Guz (1986) illustrated this in a nice field study. They interviewed a group of 8-year-old boys soon after their arrival at preparatory boarding school. For most of them, this is a stressful situation. However, the children acknowledge that showing fear and worry is not appropriate and will have social repercussions. Deceptive behaviour is the only way out: 'Well, you'd have to act cheerfully (irrespective of how you feel) and try and make friends with everybody'.

45

Emotionally disturbed children also appreciate that you can hide your feelings from others, i.e. manipulate the expression (Meerum Terwogt, Schene & Koops, 1990). However, their strategic use of this knowledge shows an important limitation. Between 7 and 11 years of age, normal children use the option of hiding or pretending emotions for two reasons: for self-protection and out of consideration for others ('I didn't want my sister to know that I felt sad on her birthday'). Emotionally disturbed children of the same age-group claim to adopt display rules just for selfish reasons (Taylor & Harris, 1984; Adlam-Hill & Harris, 1988). This can be interpreted in terms of a general developmental delay. The notion of deception to protect the feelings of others takes an extra cognitive step: a change of perspective. Alternatively, we can argue that emotionally disturbed children have grown up in an environment that gave them little opportunity to learn the rules governing the emotional dialogue that normally takes place between people. How can you learn the subtle rules of mutual influence when the reactions of your caregivers bear almost no relation to your own behaviour, as seems to be the case both with neglective and overprotective parents.

CONCLUSIONS

Although it is tempting to assume that the child's emotional development is largely dependent on the level of cognitive maturity, we have to look at this conclusion with caution. Indeed, the development from a rigid to a more flexible emotional life can be described as a function of the child's cognitive capacities and limitations. Also, the child's (cognitive) representation of the emotional process has a major impact on the development of his or her emotional behaviour. But both of these conclusions are only part of the story. Cognitive abilities are necessary to discover the linkages between different elements of the emotional process and the relation between our own and other people's emotional behaviour, but they are not sufficient. Besides, the environment must provide the child with the opportunity to learn all those connections.

In this respect, it is important to realise that to a large extent the social community regulates the information that reaches the child. People's reactions are strongly determined by the child's age. Sometimes we just help the child by making certain pieces of information more salient than we usually do in adult life. Otherwise, we also anticipate on the child's perspective of the world by withholding information. We do not want the child's world to be 'more complex than necessary'. Also, we do not expect young children to follow social norms and values to the same extent as adults do. Therefore, we do not let them suffer the consequences if they violate these rules. But, as long as we do not appeal to the child's feelings of guilt, we cannot expect him or her to find out what it means to feel guilty and how this feeling can be avoided.

Socialisation has a lot to do with the distribution of information and the opportunity to learn. The gradual release of information and the systematic confrontation with social constraints goes on much longer than the process of cognitive maturation. A 12-year-old child's cognitive functions closely resemble those of adults (Flavell, 1985). Basically, there are no limitations anymore. None the less, the 12-year-old can still count on a lot of allowances. Social development still has an important stretch to go.

Within one and the same culture, there usually is a fair consensus about what to expect from a child; the children have to 'act their age'. However, we must realise that important deviations from this norm are possible, dependent on the individual history of a child. A study in which hospitalised children were compared to healthy children shows the possibility of fluctuations in children's conceptualisation of emotion. Harris & Lipian (1989) showed that under conditions of strong emotion (i.e. being hospitalised), children are inclined to doubt that emotions can be mixed, masked or changed, notwithstanding their cognitive maturity. They all claim that mentally there is no way to redirect the course of their illness. Since no follow-up study is available, we do not know whether this helpless state is temporary or not. However, in many ways their ideas have a strong resemblance to the ideas of emotionally disturbed children.

Within this emotionally disturbed group the deviating conceptions seem to have a more permanent and generalised influence on everyday behaviour. Earlier in this chapter, we mentioned that they too have difficulties in accepting mixed feelings. In their case this results in self-evaluations that are all positive or all negative. Probably even more important is the observation that emotionally disturbed children also express the opinion that one can not effectively change emotions. As in hospitalised children, these ideas can be (partly) explained in terms of environmental factors. A large fraction of this emotional disturbance is raised by neglective *or* overprotective parents (Meerum Terwogt *et al.*, 1990). In these circumstances, we may assume that these children have a difficult job to establish a comprehensible relationship between their

47

own emotional behaviour and the reactions from their near environment. They lose their 'perception of control' (Watson, 1977) and may adopt a helpless attitude (Abramson et al., 1978). Consequently, they claim that there is no sense in paying attention to one's own emotions or those of others (Meerum Terwogt et al., 1990).

Emotionally disturbed children also put great trust in hiding emotions. As observed earlier, they use this possibility mainly for self-protective reasons. They probably seldom experience an adequate reaction to their display of feelings. Hiding is their way to stay out of trouble. This also makes it difficult for a therapist to give them a renewed sense of control by facilitating the contingency between emotional display and social experiences.

REFERENCES

Abelson, R. P. (1963). Computer simulation of 'hot cognition's'. In *Computer simulation of personality* (ed. S. Tomkins & S. Messick), pp. 224–43. Wiley, New York.

Abramson, L., Seligman, M. & Teasdale, J. (1978). Learned helplessness in humans: Critique and reformulation. *Journal of Abnormal Psychology*, **87**, 49–74.

Adlam-Hill, S. & Harris, P. L. (1988). Understanding of display rules for emotion by normal and maladjusted children. Unpublished paper, Department of Experimental Psychology, University of Oxford.

Arnold, M. B. (1960). *Emotion and personality,* Vol.1. Columbia University Press, New York.

Astington, J. W. & Gopnik, A. (1991). Theoretical explanations of children's understanding of the mind. *British Journal of Developmental Psychology* **9**, 7–31.

Ausubel, D. P. (1955). Relationships between shame and guilt in the socialisation process. *Psychological Review*, **62**, 378-90.

Barden, R. C., Zelko, F. A., Duncan, S. W. & Masters, J. C. (1980). Children's consensual knowledge about the experiential determinants of emotion. *Journal of Personality and Social Psychology*, **39**, 368–76.

Bretherton, I. & Beeghly, M. (1982). Talking about internal states of mind: The acquisition of an explicit theory of mind. *Developmental Psychology*, **18**, 906–21.

Bretherton, I., Fritz, J., Zahnwaxler, C. & Ridgeway, D. (1986). Learning to talk about emotions: A functionalist perspective. *Child Development*, **57**, 529–48.

Cairns, H. & Hsu, J. (1977). Who, why, when, and how: A developmental study. *Journal of Child Language*, **5**, 477–88.

Colby, A., Kohlberg, L., Gibbs, J. & Lieberman, M. (1983). A longitudinal study of moral judgement. *Monographs of the Society for Research in Child Development*, **200**.

Cole, P. M. (1986). Children's spontaneous control of facial expression. *Child Development*, **57**, 1309–21.

Cooley, C. H. (1902). *Human nature and the social order*. Charles Scribner Sons, New York.

Darwin, C. (1872). *The expression of emotions in man and animals*. John Murray, London.

DePaulo, B. M., & Jordan, A. (1982). Age changes in deceiving and detecting deceit. In *Development of non-verbal behaviour in children* (ed. R.S. Feldman). Springer Verlag, New York.

DiLalla, L. F. & Watson, M. W. (1988). Differentiation of fantasy and reality: Preschoolers' reactions to interruptions in their play. *Developmental Psychology*, **24**, 286–91.

Duffy, E. (1934). An explanation of 'emotional' phenomena without the use of the concept 'emotion'. *Journal of General Psychology*, **25**, 283–93.

Dunn, J. (1984). *Sisters and brothers*. Fontana, London.

Ekman, P. & Friesen, W. V. (1974). Detecting deception from body and face. *Journal of Personality and Social Psychology*, **29**, 288–298.

Ferguson, T. J. & Rule, B. G. (1983). An attributional perspective on anger and aggression. In *Aggression: Theoretical and empirical reviews*, Vol. I (ed. R. G. Green & E. I. Donnerstein). Academic Press, New York.

Ferguson, T. J. & Stegge, H. (1994) Emotional states and traits in children: The case of guilt and shame. In *The psychology of guilt and shame* (ed. J. P. Tangney & K. Fischer), Guilford, in press.

Ferguson, T. J., Stegge, H. & Damhuis, I. (1991) Children's understanding of guilt and shame. *Child Development*, **62**, 827–39.

Flavell, J. H. (1985). *Cognitive development* (edn 2) Prentice Hall, Englewood Cliffs, NJ.

Folkman, S., Schaefer, C. & Lazarus, R. S. (1979). Cognitive processes as mediators of stress and coping. In *Human stress and cognition: An information processing approach* (ed. V. Hamilton & D.M. Warburton). Wiley, New York.

Frijda, N.H. (1986). *The emotions*. Cambridge University Press, Cambridge.

Graham, S. (1988). Children's developing understanding of the motivational role of affect: An attributional analysis. *Cognitive Development*, **3**, 71–88.

Graham, S., Doubleday, C. & Guarino, P. A. (1984). The development of relations between perceived controllability and the emotions of pity, anger, and guilt. *Child Development*, **55**, 561–65.

Harris, P. L. (1983). Children's understanding of the link between situation and emotion. *Journal of Experimental Child Psychology*, **33**, 1–20.

Harris, P. L. (1989). *Children and emotion. The development of psychological understanding*. Blackwell, Oxford.

Harris, P. L., Brown, E., Marriott, C. (1991). Monsters, ghosts and witches: Testing the limits of the fantasy–reality distinction in young children. *British Journal of Developmental Psychology*, **9**, 105–23.

Harris, P. L., Donnelly, K., Guz, G. R. & Pitt-Watson, R. (1986). Children's understanding of the distinction between real and apparent emotion. *Child Development*, **57**, 895–909.

Harris, P. L., & Guz, G. R. (1986). Models of emotion: How boys report their emotional reactions upon entering an English boarding school. Unpublished paper, Department of Experimental Psychology, University of Oxford.

Harris, P. L., Johnson, C. N., Hutton, D., Andrews, G. & Cooke, T. (1989). Young children's theory of mind and emotion. *Cognition and Emotion*, **3**, 379–400.

Harris, P. L. & Lipian, M. S. (1989). Understanding emotion and experiencing emotion. In *Children's understanding of emotion* (ed. C. Saarni & P. L. Harris), pp. 241–58. Cambridge University Press, New York.

Harris, P. L., Morris, J. E. & Meerum Terwogt, M. (1986). The early acquisition of spatial adjectives: a cross-linguistic study. *Journal of Child Language*, **13**, 335–52.

Harris, P. L. & Olthof, T. (1982). The child's concept of emotion. In *Social cognition; Studies of the development of understanding* (ed. G. Butterworth & P. Light), pp. 188–209. Harvester Press, Brighton.

Harris, P. L., Olthof, T. & Meerum Terwogt, M. (1981). Children's knowledge of emotion. *Journal of Child Psychology and Psychiatry*, **22**, 247–61.

Harris, P. L., Olthof, T., Meerum Terwogt, M. & Hardman, C. E. (1987). Children's knowledge of situations that provoke emotion. *International Journal of Behavioural Development*, **10**, 319–43.

Harter, S. (1977) A cognitive-developmental approach to children's expression of conflicting feelings and a technique to facilitate such expression in play therapy. *Journal of Consulting and Clinical Psychology*, **45**, 417–32.

Harter, S. (1983). Children's understanding of multiple emotions: A cognitive-developmental approach. In *The relationship between social and cognitive development*. (ed. W.F. Overton), pp. 147–94. Erlbaum, Hillsdale, NJ.

Harter, S. & Buddin, B. (1987). Children's understanding of the simultaneity of two emotions: A five-stage acquisition sequence. *Developmental Psychology*, **23**, 388–99.

Harter, S. & Whitesell, N. (1989). Developmental changes in children's emotion concepts. In *Children's understanding of emotions* (ed. C. Saarni & P. L. Harris) pp. 81–116. Cambridge University Press, New York.

Honkavaara, S. (1961). The psychology of expression. *British Journal of Psychology Monograph Supplements*, **32**.

Izard, C. E. (1977). *Human emotions*. Plenum Press, New York.

Izard, C. E. (1991). *The psychology of emotions*. Plenum Press, New York .

Izard, C. E., Wehmer, G. M., Livsey, W. L. & Jennings, J. R. (1965). Affect, awareness and performance. In *Affect, cognition and personality* (ed. S.S. Tomkins & C.E. Izard), pp. 2–41. Tavistock Publishers, London.

Kagan, J. (1978). On emotion and its development: A working paper. In *The development of affect* (ed. M. Lewis & L.A. Rosenblum). Plenum, New York.

Lazarus, R. S. (1975). The self-regulation of emotion. In *Emotions; Their parameters and measurement* (ed. L. Levi), pp. 47–67. Raven Press, New York.

Lazarus, R. S., Averill, J. R. & Opton, E. M., Jr. (1970). Towards a cognitive theory of emotions. In *Feelings and emotions* (ed. M. Arnold), pp. 207–32. Academic Press, New York.

Lazarus, R. S., Coyne, J. C. & Folkman, S. (1982). Cognition, emotion and motivation: The doctoring of Humpty-Dumpty. In *Psychological stress and psychopathology* (ed. R.W. Neufield), pp. 218–39. McGraw-Hill, New York.

Leslie, A. M. (1987). Pretence and representation: The origins of 'theory of mind'. *Psychological Review*, **94**, 412–26.

Lewis, M. & Michalson, L. (1983). *Children's emotions and moods*. Plenum Press, New York.

MacLean, P. D. (1970). The limbic brain in relation to the psychosis. In *Pysiological correlates of emotion* (ed. P.D. Black). Academic Press, New York.

Meerum Terwogt, M. (1984). Emotional development in middle childhood: A cognitive view. Unpublished dissertation. Free University Amsterdam.

Meerum Terwogt, M. (1986). Affective states and task performance in naive and prompted children. *European Journal of Psychology of Education*, **1**, 31–40.

Meerum Terwogt, M (1987). Children's behavioural reactions in situations with a dual emotional impact. *Psychological Reports*, **61**, 100–2.

Meerum Terwogt, M. (1990). Disordered children's acknowledgement of multiple emotions. *Journal of General Psychology*, **117**, 59–69.

Meerum Terwogt, M., Koops, W., Oosterhoff, T. & Olthof, T. (1986a). Development in processing of multiple emotional situations. *Journal of General Psychology*, **113**, 109–19.

Meerum Terwogt, M. & Olthof, T. (1989). Awareness and self-regulation of emotion in young children. In *Children's understanding of emotion* (ed. C. Saarni & P.L. Harris), pp. 209–37. Cambridge University Press, New York.

Meerum Terwogt, M., Schene, J. & Harris, P. L. (1986*b*). Self-control of emotional reactions by young children. *Journal of Child Psychology and Psychiatry*, **27**, 357–66.

Meerum Terwogt, M., Schene, J. & Koops, W. (1990) Concepts of emotion in institutionalised children. *Journal of Child Psychology and Psychiatry*, **31**, 1131–43.

Moretti, M. M. & Higgins, E. T. (1990). The development of self-esteem vulnerabilities: Social and cognitive factors in developmental psychopathology. In *Competence considered* (ed. R. J. Sternberg & J. Kolligian, Jr), pp. 286–314. Yale University Press, New Haven, CT.

Neisser, U. (1963) The multiplicity of thought. *British Journal of Psychology*, **54**, 1–14.

Nisbett, R. E., & Wilson, T. D. (1977). Telling more than we can know: Verbal reports on mental processes. *Psychological Review*, **84**, 231–59.

Olthof, T., Ferguson, T. J. & Luiten, A. (1989). Personal responsibility antecedents of anger and blame reactions in children. *Child Development*, **60**, 1328–66.

Olthof, T., Meerum Terwogt, M., van Panthaleon van Eck, O. & Koops, W. (1987). Children's knowledge of the integration of successive emotions. *Perceptual and Motor Skills*, **65**, 407–14.

Piaget, J. (1962). *Play dreams and imitation* . Norton, New York.

Plutchik, R. (1980). *Emotion, a psycho-evolutionary synthesis*. Harper & Row, New York.

Reichenbach, L. & Masters, J. (1983). Children's use of expressive and contextual cues in judgements of emotion. *Child Development*, **54**, 993–1004.

Reissland, N. (1988). Neonatal imitation in the first hour of life: Observations in rural Nepal. *Developmental Psychology*, **24**, 464–9.

Rholes, W.S., Blackwell, J., Jordan, C. & Walters, C. (1980). A developmental study of learned helplessness. *Developmental Psychology*, **16**, 616–24.

Rozin, P. (1975). The evolution of intelligence and access to the cognitive unconscious. In *Progress in psychobiology and physiological psychology*, Vol. 6 (ed. J. Sprague & A. N. Epstein), pp. 245–80, Academic Press, New York.

Ruble, D. & Rholes, W. (1981). The development of children's perceptions and attributions about their social world. In *New directions in attribution research* Vol. 3, (ed. J. Harvey, W. Ickes & R. Kidd), pp. 3–36. Lawrence Erlbaum, Hillsdale, NJ.

Saarni, C. (1978). Cognitive and communicative features of emotional experience, or do you show what you think you feel? In *The development of affect* (ed. M. Lewis & L.A. Rosenblum). Plenum, New York.

Saarni, C. (1979). Children's understanding of display rules for expressive behaviour. *Developmental Psychology*, **15**, 424–9.

Saarni, C. (1984). Observing children's use of display rules: Age and sex differences. *Child Development*, **55**, 1504–13.

Selman, R. L., Lavin, D. R., & Brion-Meisels, S. (1982). Troubled children's use of self-reflection. In *Social cognitive development in context* (ed. F. C. Serafica). Guilford Press, New York.

Smetana, J. G. (1981). Preschool children's conception of moral and social rules. *Child Development*, **52**, 1333–6.

Smiley, P. & Huttenlocher, J. (1989). Young children's acquisition of emotion concepts. In *Children's understanding of emotion* (ed. C. Saarni & P. L. Harris), pp. 27–49. Cambridge University Press, New York.

Stipek, D. J. & DeCotis, K. M. (1988). Children's understanding of the implications of causal attributions for emotional experiences. *Child Development*, **59**, 1601–16.

Tangney, J. P. (1990). Assessing individual differences in proneness to shame and guilt: Development of the Self-Conscious Affect and Attribution Inventory. *Journal of Personality and Social Psychology*, **59**, 102–11.

Taylor, D. A. & Harris, P. L. (1984). Knowledge of strategies for the expression of emotion among normal and maladjusted boys: A research note. *Journal of Child Psychology and Psychiatry*, **24**, 223–9.

Thompson, R. A. (1989). Causal attribution and children's emotional understanding. In *Children's understanding of emotion* (ed. C. Saarni & P. L. Harris), pp. 117–50. Cambridge University Press, New York.

Watson, J. S. (1977). Depression and the perception of control in early childhood. In *Depression in childhood: diagnosis, treatment and conceptual models.* (ed. J. G. Schulterbrandt & A. Raskin). Raven Press, New York.

Weiner, B. (1986). *An attributional theory of motivation and emotion.* Springer Verlag, New York.

Wellman, H. M. (1990) *The child's theory of mind.* MIT Press/Bradford, Cambridge, MA.

Wellman, H. M. & Estes, D. (1986). Early understanding of mental entities: a re-examination of childhood realism. *Child Development*, **57**, 910–23.

Wimmer, H. & Perner, J. (1983). Beliefs about beliefs: Representations and constraining function of wrong beliefs in young children's understanding of deception. *Cognition*, **13**, 103–28.

Wolf, D. P., Rygh, J. & Altshuler, J. (1984). Agency and experience: Actions and states in play narratives. In *Symbolic play* (ed. I. Bretherton). Academic Press, Orlando, FL.

Wundt, W. (1903). *Grundriss der psychologie.* Engelmann, Stuttgart.

Zajonc, R.B. (1980). Feeling and thinking: Preferences need no inferences. *American Psychologist*, **35**, 151–73.

3

The development of emotional regulation and emotional response

Elizabeth McCauley, Kim Kendall and Karen Pavlidis

INTRODUCTION

The task of understanding the underpinnings of depressive disorders in young people is complex and must take a multitude of factors into consideration. This task is made more challenging because depression is not a unitary phenomenon. Depression is a disorder that involves physiological and cognitive functioning as well as dysregulation of mood. Difficulties with moodiness and increased depression appear common among adolescents, while few of these youths develop full blown clinical symptomology. Moreover, depressive symptoms develop in some children with stable families and a highly competent track record, while in others depression presents following longstanding exposure to abuse or family dysfunction.

Onset of clinical depression during childhood or adolescence has been shown to have a negative impact on social, academic and family functioning, as well as being associated with an increased risk for recurrence (McCauley & Myers, 1992a) and impairment in social–emotional functioning that extends into adult life (Harrington et al., 1990). Efforts to identify effective prevention and treatment strategies for depression in children are ongoing (McCauley & Myers, 1993). Prevention and treatment approaches need to be informed by a developmentally sensitive understanding of the mechanisms that underlie the onset of depression in young people.

This chapter will explore the developmental variables that might contribute to, or constitute, a predisposition to onset of depression (unipolar) during childhood or adolescence. Developmental processes that are central

53

to the child's formation of a sense of self and view of the world will be reviewed. The ultimate goal is to present a working model of what areas of development, when compromised, might come together to lower a child's threshold for depression. Every effort will be made to present supporting data but the model can only be speculative since in many areas a definitive database does not exist. Proposed influential factors will be organised within a developmental framework and based on the assumption of a constructionistic or an organisational approach which posits that the child actively creates his or her own view of the world and that completion of each developmental task influences in turn how the child approaches the next developmental challenge (Cicchetti & Schneider-Rosen, 1986).

FAMILY STUDIES

Family studies of adults have consistently identified an increased prevalence of depressive disorders among first degree relatives of clinically depressed probands (Weissman et al., 1982, 1984; Andreasen et al., 1987). An increased prevalence of depressive disorder has also been observed in relatives of depressed youth in comparison to relatives of youth with no psychiatric disturbance (Puig-Antich et al., 1989). Furthermore, offspring of depressed parents have a 6-fold increase in risk for depression, with additional risk conferred if both parents are affected (Weissman et al., 1987; Mitchell et al 1989; Downey & Coyne, 1990). Thus it has been generally held that a familial or genetic predisposition for depression exists.

In addition, considerable research has been done on the impact of mother's depression on psychosocial functioning of her children. In these studies, maternal depression is associated with increased prevalence of a wide variety of behavioural and emotional problems in offspring, rather than being a specific predictor of depression (Downey & Coyne, 1990; McCauley & Myers, 1992b). These studies, however, also document that depressed mothers interact with their children differently from non-depressed mothers, introducing environmental and learning variables as confounds within the biological, hereditary model. Furthermore, when parents of depressed youth are contrasted with parents of children with psychiatric disorders other than depression, both groups of parents have elevated rates of depressive disorders (Mitchell et al., 1989). Thus, while there is support for a genetic factor in clinical depression, intervening environmental variables appear to be important in moderating the expression of this risk.

TEMPERAMENT

Factors such as health status, cognitive and physical attributes, maturational rate (e.g. timing of developmental milestones, puberty) and temperament may also play a role in the development of emotional disturbances such as depression. Temperament refers to the infant's characteristic way of interacting with the world. Researchers differ in the degree to which they propose that temperament is a genetically transmitted trait versus an initial response style that is then moulded by interactions with the environment (see review by Prior, 1992). Different constellations of traits have also been identified. Thomas & Chess' (1977) study of the longitudinal course of temperament originally investigated nine areas, whereas Buss & Plomin (1984) utilised a three factor (Sociability, Emotionality, and Activity) approach. These styles have been categorised into broad patterns that differ in terms of how 'easy' or 'difficult' a child is, with 'difficult' temperament constituting a risk factor for poorer outcome over the course of development.

To understand the nature of temperamental factors and their meaning in the developmental process, two central questions must be addressed. First, attention has been focused on evaluating the extent to which these traits are genetically determined by investigating the behavioural patterns of monozygotic and dizygotic twins. Results suggest modest heritability of traits such as activity level, behavioural inhibition, observed shyness, and expression of negative emotion, whereas expression of positive emotion appears more environmentally controlled (Emde et al., 1992; Prior, 1992).

Secondly, the importance of temperament in the developmental process depends on the continuity and stability of these traits over time. Prior's (1992) review of the temperament literature identified considerable variability in the data on continuity and stability depending on the specific trait studied, the details of the study design, and the sex of the child followed. Kagan and colleagues (Kagan, Reznick & Snidman, 1989) have tracked the course of socially inhibited children from 3 to 7 years of age, and found considerable stability. Moreover, these youngsters were more fearful than socially outgoing controls at age 7, and exhibited greater physiological reactivity. These findings led to speculation that children who are extremely socially inhibited may have a 'lower threshold for limbic–hypothalamic arousal to unexpected changes in the environment'. Temperamental differences in sensitivity to the environment and in reaction to arousal, such as those identified by

Kagan *et al.* (1989) may play a central role in shaping a child's coping responses well beyond infancy (Compas, 1987). If these research findings hold up, then risk factors for depression such as social inhibition and increased negative affect may be part of the child's initial, biologically programmed, make-up. There is no universally agreed definition of difficult temperament. Integral to all definitions, however, are the presence of negative emotions (easily upset and tearful) and adverse social interactions (Prior, 1992).

Children with difficult temperament are over-represented in clinical samples (Maziade *et al.*, 1990) and support exists for a relation between 'difficult' temperament and later externalising disorders (Maziade *et al.*, 1990; Prior, 1992). Data supporting a link between temperamental factors and depression are less prevalent. Shyness has been associated with later depression (Lazarus, 1982), as well as with anxiety disorders in Kagan's sample of behaviourally inhibited children (Hirschfeld *et al.*, 1992). Parental anxiety disorders have also been associated with increased behavioural inhibition in offspring (Rosenbaum *et al.*, 1988). Chess and colleagues (Chess, Thomas & Hassibi, 1983), however, found no early temperamental characteristics which differentiated the children in their longitudinal study who became clinically depressed in childhood or adolescence. More recently, Rende (1993) reported the results of a longitudinal study linking temperament measured during infancy and early childhood with behavioural patterns at age seven. Using Buss & Plomin's (1984) model, this study assessed the ability of the early temperamental dimensions of sociability, emotionality, and activity to predict later delinquency, depression, and hyperactivity. Temperamental traits were significantly associated with later behavioural profiles but the patterns of relations differed for boys and girls. Higher maternal ratings of anxiety/depression on the Child Behaviour Checklist at age 7 were related to early temperament ratings of greater emotionality and less sociability in girls. For boys, greater emotionality was related to later anxiety/depression, more activity to later attention problems, but sociability was not predictive of later behavioural profiles.

Few studies have directly explored temperamental characteristics of depressed children. In an epidemiologic study of children in an English secondary school, Goodyer and colleagues (1993) observed a significant association between the temperamental quality of increased emotionality and depression. However, as noted by the researchers, the number of children in this sample who met criteria for clinical depression was quite small (16 girls and 3 boys in a sample of 193). Furthermore, report of temperamental style might have been confounded by prodromal depressive symptomology or by depression itself.

Finally, and perhaps most importantly, temperament may contribute to risk for depression by impacting the child's relationships with others. Parental qualities and 'goodness of fit' between mother and child play a critical role in how a difficult temperament, such as social inhibition or hyperarousal, is expressed over-time (Prior, 1992). This is particularly important if temperamental factors impact the resolution of early developmental tasks, which in turn might contribute to the development of depression.

ATTACHMENT

Attachment formation

One central developmental task is the formation of early attachment (Bowlby, 1977, 1988a). Temperament may influence the quality of the attachment. Attachment refers to the infant and young child's relationship with her primary caregivers. Attachment theory posits that, from an evolutionary perspective, attachment to a primary caregiver is necessary for survival. This relationship protects the child and provides a 'secure base' from which the child can explore the environment (Bowlby, 1969/1982). Attachment is conceptualised in terms of the quality of the relationship, not its intensity.

Tools have been developed to assess the attachment relationship for use with subjects of all ages ranging from infancy to adulthood. Measurement of attachment during infancy consists primarily of the Ainsworth Strange Situation (Ainsworth et al., 1978), a paradigm in which the caregiver–infant relationship is assessed by coding behavioural reactions by the infant to two brief laboratory separation–reunion episodes. Initially, three main categories were identified to reflect the quality of the caregiver–infant relationship. Classifications of attachment are, for the most part, based on organisation of behaviour, rather than frequency counts or ratings of behaviour on a continuum. Infants who were classified as securely attached tended to show distress upon separation, but eagerly greeted their caregiver upon return, and were settled by the caregiver. Infants who were classified as insecurely attached fell into two categories, insecure-avoidant or insecure-ambivalent/resistant. Insecure-avoidant infants showed little distress upon separation and avoided or ignored the caregiver upon reunion. Insecure-ambivalent/resistant infants were highly distressed by the separation, but showed some resistance and ambivalence to the caregiver during reunion, and were not able to be settled. Since these initial classifications, each category has been subdivided and a fourth category, disorganised/disoriented, has been added to characterise the behaviour frequently seen in children who have been maltreated (Main & Solomon, 1990). Research on correlates of attachment classification has shown relationships between quality of attachment and adaptation during the pre-school years. For example, Greenberg, Speltz & DeKlyen (1993) found relationships between insecure attachments and behavioural problems in pre-school and early school aged boys.

A critical aspect of attachment theory is the notion of internal working models (Bowlby, 1980). These models constitute the child's mental representations of the attachment relationship that guide his or her reactions and expectations of others according to what his or her experience has been with the primary caregiver. This concept of representation has guided measures of the attachment relationship during early childhood, adolescence, and adulthood under the theoretical assumption that the representational organisation of attachment, or internal working model, can be captured using measures that are developmentally sensitive. Measures of attachment used with older children and adolescents include self-report scales such as the Inventory of Parent and Peer Attachment developed by Armsden & Greenberg (1987) to assess the positive and negative affective/cognitive dimensions of adolescents' relationships with their parents and close friends – particularly how well these figures serve as sources of psychological security. Three broad dimensions are assessed: degree of mutual trust, quality of communication, and extent of anger and alienation but discrete attachment categories are not identified. The Adult Attachment Interview (George, Kaplan & Main, 1984) is a semistructured interview used to assess early attachment relationships, and the individual's evaluation of the effects of these experiences on current functioning. Classifications of the Adult Attachment Interview are based not so much on the content of responses, but rather on the coherence and organisation of the entire transcript. Securely classified adults provide coherent and consistent descriptions, rich with memories of earlier attachments and how they contribute to their present relationships. Security in adulthood is the ability to integrate information that is relevant to attachment. A second category is Dismissive; these people tend to idealise early relationships, provide inconsistent information, and claim an inability to recall memories regarding their relationships. The third classification is Preoccupied; these adults provide irrelevant and overly long reports of their relationships (Main, Kaplan & Cassidy, 1985; Main, 1991). Studies that have investigated both parent and infant attachments have shown high correlations between securely attached mothers and securely attached infants, between dismissive mothers and avoidant infants, and between preoccupied mothers and anxious/resistant infants (Main et al., 1985).

The stage for two extremely important aspects of development, the establishment of an internal working model of the world based on the mental representation of the attachment relationship (Cassidy, 1988; Kobak & Sceery, 1988), and the initial phases of emotion regulation (Kobak & Sceery, 1988; Cohn & Tronick, 1989), is set during the attachment process. Quality of the parent–child relationship has been implicated as a contributing factor in the aetiology of depression (Bowlby, 1980; Cummings & Cicchetti, 1990; Hammen, 1992), and there is some evidence that insecure attachment is associated with depression in adolescents (Armsden et al., 1990; Kobak, Sudler & Gamble, 1991).

Attachment and temperament

Regarding the influence of temperament on the caregiver–child attachment bond, research findings have been mixed (Goldsmith & Alansky, 1987). While some researchers emphasise the importance of temperament in determining the security of the attachment relationship (Goldsmith, Bradshaw & Rieser-Danner, 1986), others view infant temperament as a relatively insignificant factor in attachment security outcome (Sroufe, 1985). Several studies have shown, however, that temperament does predict attachment status when considered as a factor interacting with various maternal characteristics. Mediating circumstances, such as low maternal social support (Crockenberg, 1981) and maternal personality characteristics (Mangelsdorf et al., 1990), appear to influence the outcome of the attachment security. In Mangelsdorf et al.'s (1990) study, high maternal 'constraint', a category reflecting greater rigidity, traditionalism, and low risk taking, was associated with insecure attachment in the high distress infants only. This study suggests that maternal characteristics are particularly important when the infant has a difficult temperament.

In addition, evidence suggests that while temperament may not predict traditional attachment classification status (Vaughn *et al.*, 1989; Mangelsdorf *et al.*, 1990), it may predict the way the attachment relationship is expressed (Belsky & Rovine, 1987). Fish & Belsky (1991) found that within a group of children with difficult temperaments, those with secure attachments tended to express negative affect more adaptively than those with insecure attachment. These findings suggest that while a difficult temperament does not predict the general quality of attachment, it has implications for the development of successful emotion regulation when viewed in conjunction with the child's relationship to the caregiver.

Attachment and parental characteristics

The child's temperament is only one of the factors that helps to shape the attachment process. Other equally important factors include characteristics of mother and of the child's larger environment. Parental characteristics including mental health, environmental resources, presence of other children in the home, stressors, and parental attitudes and values all impact what the parent brings to the parent–child interaction. Mothers' attitudes toward parenting and physiological responsiveness to the cries of both their own and other children have been found to predict attachment classification (Frodi, Bridges & Shonk, 1989). These factors, measured both pre- and postnatally, predict later mother–child attachment classification, suggesting that certain maternal characteristics which are determined prior to the birth of the infant are as influential in determining the quality of attachment as is the temperament of the infant.

Attachment, self-schema, and emotion regulation

Current thinking in the area of attachment theory has recently moved more toward viewing attachment theory as also a theory of emotion regulation (Sroufe & Waters, 1977; Kobak & Sceery, 1988). It is thought that the process of attachment is also the process through which children develop emotion regulation skills and expectations. The basic assumptions to this perspective include (Sroufe, 1983):

1. Individuals are innately disposed to form intimate (attachment) relationships, and development takes place within the context of these relationships.

2. It is within the earliest relationships that children learn about themselves as reflected by their caregivers. These early understandings of self and others will become the prototypes for later relationships.
3. Early prototypes are carried forward as the result of attitudes and expectations the child forms about the likely responses of others, and the likely result of the child's personal efforts to cope with stress (regulate their emotions and get their needs met).
4. The organisation of attachment and emotion-regulating styles should therefore be consistent across subsequent developmental stages.

More specifically, the type of responsiveness a child receives from its parents will determine the type of attachment that evolves. This attachment style will contain within it a set of feelings and specific strategies needed to regulate distress (Kobak & Sceery, 1988). Rules are developed within the relationship to the attachment figure that will guide how the child responds to distressing events. These rules about behaviour are accompanied by consistent expectations about oneself and others. A child with a secure attachment to its parents will develop rules that allow for the recognition of distress and the subsequent behaviour of seeking support. A child with avoidant attachment will adopt rules that restrict the recognition of distress and also restrict the seeking of support due to assumptions that support will not be forthcoming. A child with ambivalent attachment will have expectations that increase its anxiety about whether support will be available when needed, and if a response is forthcoming, anxiety about what form it will take (Kobak & Sceery, 1988).

The development of effective emotional regulation and coping skills, as well as a positive sense of the self, will depend on the caregiver's role in assisting the infant in controlling her emotional state through social interaction and routines established during the early years of life (Als, 1978; Kopp, 1982). Sroufe (1983) gives the example of a child that has been neglected by its caregivers and develops an expectation that in times of strong emotional distress others will not be available to provide soothing, reassurance, and attention to her needs. If parents are abusive the child may learn to avoid expressing needs and avoid close relationships in general. Children may cope with strong feelings by withdrawal, or outbursts of hostility. They may develop distorted or restricted ways of expressing needs, and therefore become less effective at coping with difficult situations. Emotion regulation is done poorly, if at all, and needs are met inconsistently as a result.

In fact, there is some good evidence now that certain attachment styles observed within the first year to year-and-a-half of age, are consistent with style of coping with stress at later ages. In 1978, Ainsworth *et al* . (1978) noted that caregiver's sensitivity to the infant's needs and respect for the infant's autonomy (parent responded promptly and effectively and avoided intrusive or interfering care) predicted the quality of attachment at 12 months of age. Waters (1978) showed that Ainsworth's attachment patterns were stable from 12 to 18 months. Matas, Arend & Sroufe (1978) found that there was consistency in attachment patterns at 24 months. Secure attachment correlated with a toddler that was more autonomous, approached problems with more energy, positive affect and persistence, and was more effective in using maternal assistance than anxiously attached infants. In 1979 these trends were again found in preschool age children, who were found to be more socially competent, flexible and self-reliant, more curious and involved than anxiously attached children (Arend, Gove & Sroufe, 1979; Waters, Wippman & Sroufe, 1979). In a pioneering longitudinal study, Main *et al.* (1985), also found continuity of attachment from 12 months to 6 years.

More recently, Kobak & Sceery (1988) looked at the correlates of attachment in first-year college students who completed the Adult Attachment Interview. They found that secure attachment was related to constructive affect regulation, low anxiety, low distress, low hostility, higher social competence and higher evidence of ongoing family support in late adolescence. Dismissive attachment was related to more loneliness, hostility with peers, peer ratings of low self-esteem and high anxiety, self-ratings of relationships with others as distant and unsupportive, less ongoing support from families. Interestingly, these people rated themselves as competent and low in distress, in contrast to their peer ratings. Preoccupied attachment led to peer ratings of high anxiety, self-ratings of low competence, high symptoms. These people viewed their families as supportive, but showed a preoccupation about the availability of others. Finally, youth self-report of less secure sense of attachment to parents differentiated depressed young adolescents from adolescents with other psychiatric disorders (Armsden *et al.*, 1990).

A very interesting line of work appears to be closing the intergenerational loop regarding the transmission of attachment and patterns of affect regulation from one generation to the next. Hall, Pawlby & Wolkind (1979) found mothers who had had disrupted families as children tended to engage less in close, stimulating, and contingent interaction with their infants. They responded less to the infants' fretful and positive vocalisations, and spent more time in a different room than the baby. In an intergenerational study of attachment, Ricks (1985), having used the strange situation paradigm to classify infants into secure and insecure attachment categories, found that mothers of securely attached infants reported more positive recollections of childhood relationships with their mothers, fathers, and peers than did mothers of insecurely attached infants. In a follow-up study (Ricks, 1985) found that mothers of infants classified as insecurely attached were more defensive and likely to idealise their parents. These mothers were also more likely to report that their own mothers were currently unhappy. When good child outcome was associated with a mother who had disruption or rejection in her family of origin, the mother lived in a stable marriage, reported positive self-esteem and often had very strong ties with her husband's family.

These studies show a consistency between attachment, emotion regulation and coping styles across developmental stages. Furthermore, these patterns appear to be transmitted across generations by primary caregivers. Clearly these findings from the study of attachment are of interest in understanding the aetiology of depression. Many of the characteristics associated with insecure attachment, such as low self-esteem, poor emotion regulation and ineffective coping styles are features related to depression when it presents in later life.

Coping and emotion regulation

We are speculating then that the abilities to regulate negative emotion, and to evolve coping skills, are important in protecting against the onset of depression. Positive coping skills refer to the child's ability to tolerate the negative emotion associated with life stresses and respond in a manner that will contribute to positive growth and development. Children develop, however, a wide variety of coping responses many of which are not constructive. Coping responses generally include cognitive techniques, such as self-talk, rationalisation, problem solving, behavioural strategies such as aggression, avoidance, withdrawal, support seeking, distraction. Coping strategies have also been classified as emotion focused versus problem focused. Few studies, however, have examined differences between depressed and non-depressed children's attempts to reduce the experience of, or regulate, negative emotions. Garber and colleagues (Garber, Braafladt & Zeman, 1991) asked depressed and non-depressed children, between the ages of 8 and 17, how they might try to reduce the experience of a negative (sad, mad, or scared) emotion. Non-depressed children offered more problem-focused and more active distraction strategies than did depressed children. Depressed children, on the other hand, tended to use more active avoidant strategies and negative behaviours (such as aggression) than did the non-depressed children. In addition, depressed children were more likely to use passive strategies to raise their mood from a neutral state to a positive state.

Similarly, Compas, Malcarne & Fondacaro (1988) found that for girls, the use of emotion-focused coping strategies was associated with higher depression scores. Emotion-focused coping included avoidant behaviours ('ignore the situation'), as well as aggressive behaviours ('throw things'). Use of problem-focused coping was negatively related to depression in girls. The use of emotion-focused coping and problem-focused coping had no relation to ratings of depression in boys. The findings of these two studies indicate that while distraction and active problem solving may be effective in reducing one's negative emotions, strategies used by depressed children, such as passive, avoidance and aggressive strategies may be less effective in mediating negative emotions.

Garber et al. (1991) also investigated whether depressed children differed from non-depressed children in their evaluation of the effectiveness of different coping strategies. Depressed children tended to have lower expectations of the effectiveness of various coping responses than did non-depressed children. These results suggest that, in addition to a tendency to use maladaptive coping strategies, depressed children may be less likely to utilise active coping due to the expectation that it may not make them feel better. This outcome is consistent with the expectations of self and others predicted by poor attachment quality. Indeed, Garber and colleagues (1991) suggest that the lower effectiveness ratings of coping strategies made by depressed children may be a reflection of their actual experiences with their parents, with whom their efforts at regulating their emotions were ineffective.

Gender differences in coping and emotion regulation

Given the sharp rise in the incidence of depression in females by adolescence it is important to consider differences in how males and females respond to stressors and negative emotions. Studies of coping in adolescents suggest that while boys tend to turn against others as a coping mechanism, girls are more likely to internalise and turn against themselves (Cramer, 1979). While these differences in coping mechanisms were not related specifically to depression, the findings for female coping are consistent with those in the adult literature on sex differences in depression where females tend to be more likely to focus on, and ruminate about, their emotional state than males (Nolen-Hoeksema, 1987).

In sum, it appears that girls, by adolescence, may be more likely to use emotion-focused coping strategies than boys. Emotion-focused strategies tend to be more passive and internalising, tend to be associated with depression, and may in part account for the increased incidence in female depression by adolescence. It is possible, in addition, that emotion-focused coping may not be as maladaptive for boys, and suggests a difference in aetiology and/or manifestation of depression in girls.

Attachment and cognitive styles

There has been a large focus in the depression literature on how particular cognitive styles are associated with, and predict, depression in both children and adults. Much of this focus has been on the study of Beck's (1967) cognitive model of depression. This model posits that people with depression exhibit a cognitive style whereby they have negative views about the world, the self, and the future. In addition, a model of depression has been proposed by Abramson, Metalsky & Alloy (1989), which stresses the importance of attributional style. Depressed individuals are described as attributing the occurrence of negative events in their lives to stable, integral characteristics of themselves, while positive events are seen as chance occurrences outside of the depressed person's control. This pattern of thinking contributes to feelings of hopelessness and helplessness. Several studies have found associations between cognitive styles and depression in children that are consistent with these models (Seligman et al., 1984; Haley et al., 1985; Bodiford et al., 1988; McCauley et al., 1988).

Although there has been a significant amount of research investigating the association between particular cognitive styles and depression, there has been little research examining the origins of these cognitive styles. Bowlby (1980) points out that although the models of depression described by Beck (1967) and Seligman (1975) acknowledge that these cognitive styles are a result of childhood experience, they do not address specific origins of these cognitions. Bowlby (1980) describes more specifically how these styles can emerge out of the individual's internal representations of her relationship with an attachment figure. If the attachment process has left the child insecure, the internal representation of the self is that he or she is a failure or unlovable, therefore there is the expectation of negative events, hostility or rejection by others.

More recently, other researchers have discussed the significance of the child's attachment relationship as contributing to the development of a depressogenic cognitive style (Cummings & Cicchetti, 1990; Hammen, 1992). A depressogenic cognitive style refers to the tendency to see the self and the environment in a negative light, as reflected in low self-esteem and a negative attributional style – the tendency to always see the cup as half empty rather than half full. A detailed model of the development of cognitive vulnerability to depression has been proposed by Rose & Abramson (1992). This model describes how children's social cognitive developmental level and environmental circumstances surrounding abusive (physically, sexually, or emotionally) events can contribute to the development of cognitive distortions. These processes (withdrawal, rage, dissociation), at the time when they originally occur, may represent an adaptive response to the environment by the child, but later become maladaptive as the social environment changes.

Also consistent with this notion of the child's internal representations of the self and others as contributing to depressogenic cognitions is the work of Hammen and colleagues (Hammen *et al.*, 1985; Zupen, Hammen & Jaenicke, 1987; Hammen & Goodman-Brown, 1990), who have shown associations between particular self-schemas and vulnerability to depression. Self-schema is the child's cognitions or beliefs about the self, how one views one's own traits such as worthiness, competency. Other-schema refers to the child's cognitions about the environment and events around her (Hammen, 1988). Hammen & Goodman-Brown (1990) investigated children's self-schemas via their patterns of recalled associations to a set of questions. They were able to classify the subjects into two groups based on the predominant patterns of recalled events. If the child recalled mostly events pertaining to interpersonal relationships they were classified as 'interpersonally vulnerable'; if recall focused on performance or achievement, they were classified as 'achievement vulnerable'. Next, Hammen & Goodman-Brown (1990) demonstrated that children who rated interpersonal events as particularly important to their sense of self were more likely to experience depression when faced with an interpersonal threat than were children with a self-efficacy or achievement type of self-schema classification. Harter and colleagues (Renouf & Harter, 1990; Harter, Marold & Whitesell, 1992) also provide support for an integral relation between self-schema as reflected in sense of self-worth and depressed affect in early adolescence. Sense of self-worth was highly correlated with depressed mood among their sample of middle school children, with almost one-to-one correspondence of depressed mood and low self-worth among the 'depressed' group (Renouf & Harter, 1990). Mood and self-worth ratings also changed in unison over a one-year follow-up period. Moreover, two clusters of self-concept features were found to be related to depression and hopelessness, as well as suicidal ideation, in young adolescents. One cluster included a sense of competency in terms of physical appearance, peer likeability and athletics, while the other cluster included scholastic competence and behavioural conduct. These findings are similar to those in the personality literature reviewed next.

SELF-SCHEMA AND THE NATURE OF PERSONALITY

As the child matures the various components of response style begin to form a more cohesive whole, which is frequently referred to as personality. Personality is used as a unifying construct or organising system which includes the emotional, behavioural, and cognitive components of an individual's characteristic style of interacting with the world as it has been shaped by experience. Self-system or schemata is also used to describe this organising construct. This system directs how the individual interprets the experiences he or she encounters but the system can also be modified by these experiences. Because it shapes choices as well, personality can also play a role in determining what kind of experiences an individual encounters. In the study of depression in adults considerable attention has been paid to personality characteristics as risk factors for subsequent depression. This literature initially grew out of the psychoanalytic tradition (Chodoff, 1972; Blatt et al., 1982) but has come to include cognitive behavioural perspectives as well (Beck, 1983). The underlying assumption is that certain individuals, because of unsuccessful resolution of earlier developmental tasks (e.g. attachment), form personality styles that put them at risk for depression.

Within the personality literature two clusters of characteristics are most consistently linked with depression. Although varied names for these clusters are proffered the characteristics are remarkably consistent across theoretical frameworks (Akiskal, Hirschfeld & Yerevanian, 1983; Blatt, et al., 1982; Beck, 1983). The first cluster includes helplessness, fears of abandonment, and a neediness for love or caring – the dependent personality. The second clusters focuses more on achievement themes with core characteristics including heightened guilt, sense of worthlessness and a feeling of not living up to standards. Individuals within these two groups might evidence the same depressive symptoms but have different internal models (or experiences of depression) which stem from their individual early experiences and resulting self-system. The two personality types parallel the outcomes hypothesised in anxious and avoidant attachment relationships as well as the self-concept clusters described by Harter and her co-workers (Harter et al., 1992). Blatt and colleagues (1982) propose that the issues of dependency and self-criticism are activated in the experience of normal, transistory depressed mood. Furthermore, individuals with dependent or self-critical personality styles are at increased risk for significant, clinical bouts of depression in times of stress. A number of theorists have suggested that it is the particular type of stress, loss in terms of either a personal relationship or personal status, that combines with these personality vulnerabilities to culminate in depression (Blatt et al , 1982; Hammen, 1992). Unfortunately, empirical support delineating the role of pre-existing personality features is scant. Although there has been long-standing interest in the question of predisposing personality factors, research in this area has faced a number of complex methodological barriers. The most central limitation is that few studies have looked prospectively at personality factors as precursors of clinical depression. The bulk of the research has been conducted on non-clinical samples or samples of individuals in the midst of, or recovering from, an episode of clinical depression. Both acute and resolving depressions have been found to impact on responses to personality assessments (Akiskal et al., 1983; Hirschfeld et al., 1989) making clear interpretation of what came first impossible. However, recently two prospective studies have become available. Hirschfeld and colleagues (1989) assessed the personality characteristics of 438 first-degree relatives and spouses of clinically depressed individuals as part of the NIMH collaborative study. The original personality assessments of those who became depressed (N = 29) reflected significantly less 'emotional strength', more introspection, increased emotional arousal, and greater need for attention, than the non-depressed group. The analyses also revealed some interesting age effects. Subjects were divided into two groups based on age at first evaluation; the younger group included those aged 17 to 30, the older group included subjects of 31 to 41. Within the younger group, the personality assessments of those who became depressed (N = 15) could not be differentiated from the never-depressed subjects, in part because of the marked variability of the personality measures demonstrated across the entire group of younger subjects. In the older subjects, measures of personality variables, among those who did not become depressed, reflected considerable emotional stability, which was not apparent in the subgroup of older subjects who became depressed. The failure to find predictive value of personality measures among younger subjects may reflect an overall immaturity in personality formation, with more stable emotional characteristics coming with age. However, cohort effects or the possibility that depression in the younger sample had a more dominant biological diathesis could not be ruled out.

The second study that looked at personality factors in a prospective way was done with a sample of older adolescents. As part of Block and Block's (Gjerde, Block & Block, 1988; Block, Gjerde, & Block, 1991) longitudinal study of development, a group of 87 young people, followed since age 3, completed a self-report depression scale at the time of their 18-year-old evaluation. All subjects had participated in detailed assessments of personality and cognitive development at ages 3–4, 7, 11, 14 and 18. Boys and girls differed significantly in the pattern of early characteristics related to later depressive symptoms (Block et al., 1991; Block & Gjerde, 1990). Girls who later endorsed greater depressive tendencies were described as 'oversocialised, intropunitive' and over-controlled, whereas later depression was associated with a more externalised pattern of behaviour in boys. For instance, items assessed at the 7-year-old evaluation associated with later depression in girls included shyness, liking to be alone, as well as greater ability to develop close and lasting relationships. By the 14-year-old evaluation concern over self-adequacy, increased vulnerability, anxiety and tendency to ruminate emerged as characteristics predictive of greater depression at age 18, in girls.

For the boys, a different pattern emerged. Depressive symptoms at age 18 were associated with more transient relationships with peers and a willingness to stretch limits observed even in early childhood years. By early adolescence, boys who later endorsed depressive symptoms were described as more negativistic, sensitive to criticism, and distrustful. Another important sex difference emerged: higher IQ scores at preschool assessment were related to greater chance of later depression in girls, while lower IQ was associated with later depression in boys.

Block and colleagues (Block et al., 1991; Block & Gjerde, 1992) view problems with accomplishment and hostility as central to the early presentation of boys who later endorse depressive features, while for girls self-esteem issues appear more critical. They place these gender differences in early trajectories within the larger context of differential socialisation of boys and girls within our society (Block et al., 1991). This research group also reported extensive data from personality assessments of the subjects obtained at the same time as the assessment of depressive tendencies (Gjerde *et al.*, 1988). The findings were quite consistent with earlier developmental patterns. The males with greater self-reported depression continued to have a more externalised pattern of behaviour with greater interpersonal antagonism, unrestraint, discontent with self, and unconventionality than less depressed 18-year-old males. Depression in girls was associated with increased rumination or introspection and sense of inadequacy.

In summary, there is considerable support for a developmental model of vulnerability to depression. Temperamental characteristics are viewed by some researchers as the 'foundation for later personality' (Goldsmith, *et al.*, 1987). Thus traits such as emotionality, expressed via shyness or increased negative emotion, might be the initial building blocks which lead to the development of a dependent or self-critical personality style. Mediating between early, biologically based temperamental characteristics and the emergence of a cohesive personality structure, are a host of critical interactions with the environment. We have suggested that these experiences, or more importantly how the child interprets these experiences, depends in great part on the attachment process which provides the child with her internalised models of both self and the world around her. Much more careful research is needed to determine the viability of this developmental model. There are some very compelling common threads which emerge from quite divergent research areas. It is, however, difficult to know if, for instance, shyness as identified in the temperament literature refers to the same behaviour profile as the shyness described in the studies by Block and colleagues of early personality characteristics of girls who become depressed. Careful definition of variables, plus attention to validity of measurements, especially those taken at very different periods in development, is needed. The difficulties with measurement can clearly be seen in the attachment literature. Although there is general acceptance of the strange situation as a means of assessing the relationship between mother and infant, it is much less clear if the measures of attachment used with adolescents and adults actually tap the same construct. Self-report scales and retrospective reports are influenced by many factors including selective memory and mood state. Of course as one becomes older, perception of early relationships may be more important to understanding the internalisation of attachment than a behavioural measure of interaction but any parallels between adult and infant attachment must be drawn cautiously.

ADOLESCENT CHALLENGES

The material presented so far has focused on factors which might constitute increased vulnerability to depression. The second part of the risk equation suggests that depression occurs when the vulnerable individual is faced with significant life stress. In studies of depression in adults, onset of episodes and severity of short-term clinical course has been associated with increased psychosocial stressors (Billings, Cronkite & Moos, 1983; Swindle, Cronkite & Moos, 1989). Certain types of life stressors, particularly those that involve personal loss such as death or divorce or loss of status as in a job loss have been found to be associated with onset of a depressive episode (Paykel & Tanner, 1976).

In samples of younger subjects the prevalence of depression increases significantly during the adolescent years. This factor suggests there may be something unique about adolescence, and the stresses encountered during this developmental period, which triggers the expression of depression. Adolescents begin to function as part of the larger world and the ongoing process of separation and individuation from family becomes more significant as the young person strives to establish her own independent identity. Resolution of these challenges builds on skills acquired throughout the developmental process. Thus the child with poorly resolved issues of attachment, poor affect regulation skills, and a negative coping and cognitive style, is highly vulnerable in the face of the multitude of adolescent challenges. Most young adolescents are faced with significant changes in every aspect of their lives: pubertal development, cognitive maturation, school transition, increased performance pressures in all arenas – academia, sports, social, family. Many researchers have hypothesised that the increase in depression during the adolescent period is secondary to the hormonal changes and brain maturation that accompany pubertal development (Susman et al., 1987; Brooks-Gunn & Warren, 1989; Petersen, Sarigiani, & Kennedy, 1991; Angold & Rutter, 1992). However, data on the impact of puberty and hormonal fluctuation on depression have not supported this hypothesis. Timing of puberty, as a single factor, was not related to onset of depression (Angold & Rutter, 1992) and hormonal fluctuation, although related to change in mood, was not as important in explaining depressed mood as other environmental stressors (Brooks-Gunn & Warren, 1989). Thus environmental and developmental demands, and the stressors associated with these demands, appear to play an important role in the onset of depression in adolescence.

Moreover, there is a greater increase in depression among girls than boys during the adolescent years. This may reflect something about the developmental process that distinguishes boys from girls or something unique about how girls, especially the vulnerable girl, experience the stresses of adolescence. As suggested in the work reviewed above by Block and colleagues (Block & Gjerde, 1992; Block *et al.*, 1991), there is growing evidence that boys and girls follow different developmental pathways before presenting with depressive symptomology. Petersen and colleagues (1991) also found problems throughout development in boys who became depressed during middle school years whereas the depressed girls in their sample were less likely to have histories of previous adjustment difficulties. Thus it may be that the stressors of adolescence have more of an impact on girls than boys. Pubertal development is one adolescent change that appears to impact boys and girls differently. Early puberty has been associated with increased self-esteem in boys while girls who develop early have lower self-esteem and more negative body image than those with later adolescent development. Pubertal changes per se do not appear to be critical in the onset of depression but may play a critical role in setting the stage for depression by influencing how the young adolescent girl feels about her body and her subsequent self-esteem (Petersen *et al.*, 1991; Harter *et al.*, 1992). Furthermore, it appears that the number of stressors faced at once is important (Garmezy, 1992). Simmons *et al.* (1987) found lowest self-esteem among young adolescent girls who experienced a change in school while going though their pubertal growth whereas both boys and girls whose growth spurt occurred after transitioning into a new school setting reported more positive self concept. Petersen also found this 'synchronicity of change' to be an important factor which had greater impact on girls because they were more likely, given the earlier time of their growth spurt, to experience pubertal and school changes simultaneously (Petersen *et al.*, 1991). Petersen and colleagues (1991) concluded from their study of 335 young adolescents 'that girls were at greater risk for developing depressed affect by 12th grade because they experienced more challenges in early adolescence than did boys'.

Furthermore, two important adolescent challenges appear to take a somewhat different form for girls than boys. The first has to do with friendship patterns. Whereas boys tend to have more stable, loosely knit friendship networks, friendships among early adolescent girls are frequently extremely intense and very stormy, with closeness with friends changing day to day. This pattern of relationships clearly taps the young adolescent girl's ability to regulate negative affect and maintain an internalised sense of positive self-esteem. Also, recent data on the development of adolescent girls suggests that the process of separation and individuation from family has a different sub-theme or flavour for girls, who place greater value on maintaining a sense of connectedness, especially to their mothers, than has been traditionally acknowledged in studies looking at the individuation process in groups of boys and girls together (Rich, 1990). Furthermore, the separation–individuation process must reactivate poorly resolved issues for the young adolescent whose early attachment process was compromised. Without an internalised schema of a competent self and a responsive world, individuation becomes a much more daunting challenge. It appears that the developmental tasks of early adolescence test the very skills, such as emotion regulation, and representational models, such as internalised schema of self and the world, that the early attachment process establishes.

CONCLUSIONS

This chapter has attempted to pull together multiple research areas to explore the factors that currently appear to be the developmental underpinnings of depression in adolescence and perhaps adulthood as well. We found remarkable consistency between various research areas, a consistency that continually reinforces the notion that attachment begins the developmental processes that later affect one's ability to cope effectively with both stressful internal process, such as individuation, and external stressors, such as adverse life events. Each area of research has built upon the other, exposing various aspects of the complex developmental process that underlies good coping and vulnerability to depression. Figure 3.1 illustrates how various aspects of development affect the onset of depression.

Our model is similar to one suggested by Hammen (1992) in its emphasis on viewing unsuccessful resolution of the attachment process as the precursor to the development of a negative self-schema and a subsequent compromised ability to regulate negative affect. The model presented in this chapter further elaborates on factors that may lead to compromised attachment, incorporates the role of emotion regulation, and focuses on a more holistic view of the development of depression. Hammen's model places more emphasis on cognitive components in isolation from other factors. In addition, our model allows for the specifi-

E. McCauley, K. Kendall & K. Pavlidis

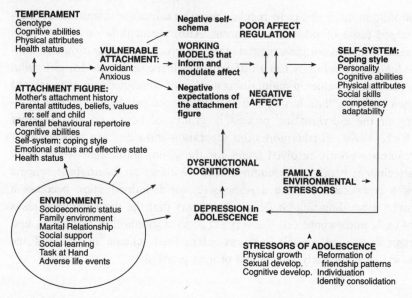

Figure 3.1. Factors affecting vulnerability to depression in adolescence.

cation of stressors unique to any developmental state across the life cycle, as well as the delineation of broader environmental factors that interact with these stressors. In this case the stressors unique to adolescence have been highlighted in terms of their likely contribution to the onset of depression in adolescence.

REFERENCES

Abramson, L. Y., Metalsky, G. I. & Alloy, L. B. (1989). The hopelessness theory of depression: Does the research test the theory? In *Social cognition and clinical psychology: A synthesis* (ed. L. Y. Abramson), pp. 33–65. Guilford Press, New York

Ainsworth, M. D. S., Blehar, M. C., Waters, E. & Wall, S. (1978). *Patterns of attachment: A psychological study of the strange situation.* Lawrence Erlbaum Associates, Inc., Hillsdale, N.J.

Akiskal, H. S., Hirschfeld, R. M. A. & Yerevanian, B. I. (1983). The relationship of personality to affective disorders. *Archives of General Psychiatry*, **40**, 801–10.

Als, H. (1978). Assessing an assessment: conceptual considerations, methodological issues, and a perspective on the future of the Neonatal Behavioural Assessment Scale. In *Organisation and stability: A commentary on the Brazelton Neonatal Behavioural Assessment Scale. Monographs of the Society for Research in Child Development* (ed. A.J. Sameroff), 43 (5–6 Serial No. 177).

Andreasen, N. C., Rice, J., Endicott, J. *et al.* (1987). Familial rates of affective disorder: A report from the NIMH collaborative study. *Archives of General Psychiatry*, **44**, 461–9.

Angold, A. & Rutter, M. (1992). Effects of age and pubertal status on depression in a large clinical sample. *Development and Psychopathology*, **4**, 5–28.

Arend, R., Gove, F. & Sroufe, L.A. (1979). Continuity of individual adaptation from infancy to kindergarten. A predictive study of ego-resiliency and curiosity in preschoolers. *Child Development*, **50**, 950–9.

Armsden, G. C. & Greenberg, M. T. (1987). The Inventory of Parent and Peer Attachment: Individual differences and their relationship to psychological well-being in adolescence. *Journal of Youth and Adolescence*, **16**, 427–54.

Armsden, G. C., McCauley, E., Greenberg, M. *et al.* (1990). Parent and peer attachment in early adolescent depression. *Journal of Abnormal Child Psychology*, **18**, 683–97.

Beck, A. T. (1967). *Depression: Causes and treatment*. University of Pennsylvania, Philadelphia

Beck, A. T. (1983). Cognitive therapy of depression: New perspectives. In *Treatment of depression: Old controversies and new approaches* (ed. P. Clayton & J. Barrett), pp. 265–90. Raven Press, New York

Belsky, J. & Rovine, M. (1987). Temperament and attachment security in the strange situation: An empirical rapprochement. *Child Development*, **58**, 787–95.

Billings, A., Cronkite, R. & Moos, R. H. (1983). Social environmental factors in unipolar depression: Comparisons of depressed patients and non depressed controls. *Journal of Abnormal Psychology*, **92**, 119–33.

Blatt, S. J., Quinlan, D. M., Chevron, E. S. & McDonald, C. (1982). Dependency and self-criticism: Psychological dimensions of depression. *Journal of Consulting and Clinical Psychology*, **50**, 113–24.

Block, J. & Gjerde, P.F. (1990). Depressive symptoms in late adolescence: A longitudinal perspective on personality antecedents. In *Risk and protective factors in the development of psychopathology* (ed. J. Rolf, A.S. Masten, D. Cicchetti, K. H. Nuechterlein & S. Weintraub), pp. 334–60. Cambridge University Press, Cambridge.

Block, J., Gjerde, P. F. & Block, J. H. (1991). Personality antecedents of depressive tendencies in 18-year-olds: A prospective study. *Journal of Personality and Social Psychology*, **60,** 726–38.

Bodiford, C. A., Eisenstadt, T. H., Johnson, J. H. & Bradlyn, A. S. (1988). *Journal of Clinical Child Psychology*, **17**, 152–8.

Bowlby, J (1969/1982). *Attachment and loss: Vol. I. Attachment*. Basic Books, New York.

Bowlby, J. (1977). The making and breaking of affectional bonds: I. Aetiology and psychopathology in light of attachment theory. *British Journal of Psychiatry*, **130**, 201–10.

Bowlby, J. (1980). *Attachment and loss, Vol. III: Loss, sadness and depression*. Basic Books, New York

Bowlby, J. (1988a). *A secure base: Parent–child attachment and healthy human development*. Basic Books, Inc., New York.

Bowlby, J. (1988b) Developmental psychiatry comes of age. *American Journal of Psychiatry*, **145**, 1–10.

Brooks-Gunn, J. & Warren, M. P. (1989). Biological and social contributions to negative affect in young adolescent girls. *Child Development*, **60**, 40–55.

Buss, A. H. & Plomin, R. (1984). *Temperament: Early-developing personality traits*. Erlbaum, Hillsdale, NJ.

Cassidy, J. F. (1988). Child–mother attachment and the self in six-year-olds. *Child Development*, **59**, 121–34.

Chess, S., Thomas, A. & Hassibi, M. (1983). Depression in childhood and adolescence: A prospective study of six cases. *Journal of Nervous and Mental Disease*, **171**, 411–20.

Chodoff, P. (1972). The depressive personality: A critical review. *Archives of General Psychiatry*, **27**, 666–73.

Cicchetti, D. & Schneider-Rosen, J. (1986). An organizational approach to childhood depression. In *Depression in young people: Clinical and developmental perspectives* (ed. M. Rutter, C. Izard & P. Read), pp. 71–134. Guilford, New York.

Cohen, L. B. & Salapatek, P. (ed.) (1978). *Infant perception: from sensation to cognition: Vol. 1. Basic visual processes.* Academic Press, New York.

Cohn, J. E. & Tronick, E. (1989). Specificity of infants' response to mothers' affective behaviour. *Journal of the American Academy of Child and Adolescent Psychiatry*, **28**, 242–8.

Compas, B. E. (1987). Coping with stress during childhood and adolescence. *Psychological Bulletin*, **101**, 393–403.

Compas, B. E., Malcarne, V. L. & Fondacaro, K. M. (1988). Coping with stressful events in older children and young adolescents. *Journal of Consulting and Clinical Psychology*, **56**, 405–11.

Cramer, P. (1979). Defence mechanisms in adolescence. *Developmental Psychology*, **15**, 476–7.

Crockenberg, S. B. (1981). Infant irritability, mother responsiveness, and social support influences on the security of infant–mother attachment. *Child Development*, **52**, 857–65.

Cummings, E. M. & Cicchetti, D. (1990). Toward a transactional model of relations between attachment and depression. In *Attachment in the preschool years, theory, research, and intervention* (ed. M. T. Greenberg, D. Cicchetti & E. M. Cummings), pp. 339–74. The University of Chicago Press, Chicago.

Downey, G. & Coyne, J.C. (1990). Children of depressed parents: An integrative review. *Psychological Bulletin*, **108**, 50–76.

Emde, R. N., Plomin, R., Robinson, J. *et al.* (1992). Temperament, emotion, and cognition at fourteen months: The MacArthur longitudinal twin study. *Child Development*, **63**, 1437–55.

Fish, M. & Belsky, J. (1991). Temperament and attachment revisited: Origin and meaning of separation intolerance at age three. *American Journal of Orthopsychiatry*, **61**, 418–27.

Frodi, A., Bridges, L. & Shonk, S. (1989). Maternal correlates of infant temperament ratings and of infant–mother attachment: A longitudinal study. *The Infant–Maternal Health Journal*, **10**, 273–89.

Garber, J., Braafladt, N. & Zeman, J. (1991). The regulation of sad affect: An information-processing perspective. In *The development of emotion regulation and dysregulation* (ed. J. Garber & K.A. Dodge), pp. 208–42. Cambridge University Press, New York.

Garmezy, N. (1992). Stress and developmental psycho-pathology. Paper presented at the NIMH. Developmental Approaches to the Assessment of Psychopathology meeting, Rockville, MD.

George, C., Kaplan, N. & Main, M. (1984). Attachment interview for adults. Unpublished manuscript, University of California, Berkeley.

Gjerde, P.F., Block, J. & Block, J.H. (1988). Depressive symptoms and personality during late adolescence: Generic differences in the externalization-internalization of symptom expression. *Journal of Abnormal Psychology*, **97**, 475–86.

Goldsmith, H. H. & Alansky, J.A. (1987). Maternal and infant temperament predictors of attachment: A meta-analytic review. *Journal of Consulting and Clinical Psychology*, **55**, 805–16.

Goldsmith, H. H., Bradshaw, D. L. & Rieser-Danner, L. (1986). Temperament as a potential developmental influence on attachment. In *'Temperament and social interaction in infancy and childhood. New directions for child development* (ed. J. V. Lerner & R. J. Lerner), no. 31 (March). pp. 5–34. Jossey-Bass, San Francisco.

Goldsmith, H. H., Buss, A. H., Plomin, R. *et al.* (1987). Roundtable: What is temperament? Four approaches. *Child Development*, **58**, 505–29.

Goodyer, I. M., Ashby, L., Altham, P. M. E. *et al.* (1993). Temperament and major depression in 11 to 16 year olds, *Journal of Child Psychology and Psychiatry*, **34**, 1409–23.

Greenberg, M. T., Speltz, M. L. & DeKlyen, M. (1993). The role of attachment in the early development of disruptive behaviour problems. *Development and Psychopathology*, **5**, 191–214.

Haley, G. M., Fine, S., Marriage, K, *et al.* (1985). Cognitive bias and depression in psychiatrically disturbed children and adolescents. *Journal of Consulting and Clinical Psychology*, **53**, 535–7.

Hall, F., Pawlby, S. & Wolkind, S. (1979). Early life experiences and later mothering behaviours: a study of mothers and their 20-week-old babies. In *The first year of life* (ed. D. Shaffer & J. Dunn), pp. 153–74. Wiley, New York

Hammen, C. (1988). Self-cognitions, stressful events, and the prediction of depression in children of depressed mothers. *Journal of Abnormal Child Psychology*, **16**, 347–60.

Hammen, C. (1992). Cognitive, life stress, and interpersonal approaches to a developmental psychopathology model of depression. *Development and Psychopathology*, **4**, 189–206.

Hammen, C. & Goodman-Brown, T. (1990). Self-schemas and vulnerability to specific life stress in children at risk for depression. *Cognitive Therapy and Research*, **14**, 215–27.

Hammen, C., Marks, T., Mayol, A. & deMayo, R. (1985). Depressive self-schemas, life stress, and vulnerability to depression. *Journal of Abnormal Psychology*, **94**, 308–19.

Harrington, R., Fudge, H., Rutter, M. *et al.* (1990). Adult outcomes of childhood and adolescent depression: I. Psychiatric status. *Archives of General Psychiatry*, **47**, 465–73.

Harter, S., Marold, D.B. & Whitesell, N.R. (1992). Model of psychosocial risk factors leading to suicidal ideation in young adolescents. *Development and Psychopathology*, **4**, 167–88.

Hirschfeld, R. M. A., Klerman, G. L., Lavori, P. *et al.* (1989). Premorbid personality assessments of first onset of major depression. *Archives of General Psychiatry*, **46**, 345–50.

Hirschfeld, D. R., Rosenbaum, J. F., Biederman, J. *et al.* (1992). Stable behavioural inhibition and its association with anxiety disorder. *Journal of the American Academy of Child and Adolescent Psychiatry*, **31**, 103–11.

Kagan, J., Reznick, S. & Snidman, N. (1989). Biological bases of childhood shyness. *Science*, **240**, 167–71.

Kobak, R. & Sceery, A. (1988). Attachment in late adolescence: working models, affect regulation, and representations of self and others. *Child Development*, **59**, 135–46.

Kobak, R. R., Sudler, N. & Gamble, W. (1991). Attachment and depressive symptoms during adolescence: A developmental pathways analysis. *Development and Psychopathology*, **3**, 461–74.

Kopp, C. B. (1982). Antecedents of self-regulation: a developmental perspective. *Developmental Psychology*, **18**, 199–214.

Lazarus, P. J. (1982). Incidence of shyness in elementary school age children. *Psychological Reports*, **51**, 904–6.

Main, M. (1991). Metacognitive knowledge, metacognitive monitoring, and singular (coherent) vs. multiple (incoherent) model of attachment. In *Attachment across the life-cycle* (ed. C. M. Parkes, J. Stevenson-Hinde & P. Marris), pp. 127–59. Routledge, New York.

Main, M., Kaplan, N. & Cassidy, J. (1985). Security in infancy, childhood and adulthood: a move to the level of representation. In *Growing points of attachment theory and research. Monographs of the Society for Research in Child Development*, **50** (1–2, Serial No. 209), (ed. I. Bretherton & E. Waters).

Main, M. & Solomon, J. (1990). Procedures for identifying infants as disorganised/disorientated during the Ainsworth strange situation. In *Attachment in the preschool years: theory, research and intervention* (ed. M. T. Greenberg, D. Cicchetti & E. M. Cummings), pp.121–60. University of Chicago Press, Chicago.

Manglesdorf, S., Gunnar, M., Kestenbaum, R. *et al.* (1990). Infant proneness-to-distress temperament, maternal personality, and mother-infant attachment: Associations and goodness of fit. *Child Development*, **61**, 820–31.

Matas, L., Arend, R. & Sroufe, L.A. (1978). Continuity of attachment in the second year: the relationship between quality of attachment and later competence. *Child Development*, **49**, 547–56.

Maziade, M., Caron, C., Cote, R. *et al.* (1990). Extreme temperament and diagnosis. *Archives of General Psychiatry*, **47**, 477–84.

McCauley, E., Mitchell, J.R., Burke, P., & Moss, S. (1988). Cognitive attributes of depression in children and adolescents. *Journal of Consulting and Clinical Psychology*, **56**, 903–8.

McCauley, E. & Myers, K. (1992*a*). The longitudinal clinical course of depression in children and adolescents. *Child and Adolescent Psychiatric Clinics of North America*, **1**, 183–96.

McCauley, E. & Myers, K. (1992*b*) Family interaction in mood-disordered youth. *Child and Adolescent Psychiatric Clinics of North America*, **1**, 111–27.

McCauley, E. & Myers, K. (1993). Treatment of depressive disorders in adolescence. In *Current psychiatric therapy* (ed. D. Dunner), pp. 432–40. W. B Saunders, Philadelphia.

Mitchell, J., McCauley, E., Burke, P. *et al.* (1989). Psychopathology in parents of depressed children and adolescents. *Journal of the American Academy of Child and Adolescent Psychiatry*, **28**, 352–7.

Nolen-Hoeksema, S. (1987). Sex differences in unipolar depression: Evidence and theory. *Psychological Bulletin*, **101**, 259–82.

Paykel, E. S. & Tanner, J. (1976). Life events, depressive relapse, and maintenance treatment. *Psychological Medicine*, **6**, 481–5.

Petersen, A.C., Sarigiani, P. A. & Kennedy, R.E. (1991). Adolescent depression: Why more girls? *Journal of Youth and Adolescence*, **20**, 247–71.

Prior, M. (1992). Childhood temperament. *Journal of Child Psychology and Psychiatry*, **33**, 249–79.

Puig-Antich, J., Goetz, D., Davies, M. *et al.* (1989). A controlled family history study of prepubertal major depressive disorder. *Archives of General Psychiatry*, **46**, 406–18.

Rende, R. (1993). Longitudinal relations between temperament traits and behavioural syndromes in middle childhood. *Journal of the American Academy of Child and Adolescent Psychiatry*, **32**, 287–90.

Renouf, A. G. & Harter, S. (1990). Low self-worth and anger as components of the depressive experience in young adolescents. *Development and Psychopathology*, **2**, 293–310.

Rich, S. (1990). Daughters' view of their relationships with their mothers. In *Making connections: The relational worlds of adolescent girls at the Emma Willard School*, (ed. C. Gilligan, N. P. Lyons, T. J. Hanmer), pp. 258–73. Harvard University Press, Cambridge.

Ricks, M. H. (1985). The social transmission of parental behaviour: attachment across generations. In *Growing points of attachment theory and research. Monographs of the Society for Research in Child Development*, (ed. I. Bretherton & E. Waters), **50** (1–2, Serial No. 209).

Rose, R.T. & Abramson, L.Y. (1992). Developmental predictors of depressive cognitive style: Research and theory. In *Developmental perspectives on depression. Rochester Symposium of Developmental Psychopathology*, Vol. 4 (ed. D. Cicchetti and S. L. Toth) pp. 323–50. University of Rochester Press, New York.

Rosenbaum, J. F., Biederman, J., Gersten, M.*et al.* (1988). Behavioural inhibition in children of parents with panic disorder and agoraphobia. *Archives of General Psychiatry*, **45**, 463–70.

Seligman, M.E.P. (1975). *Helplessness: On depression, development, and death.* Freeman, San Francisco.

Seligman, M.E.P., Peterson, C., Kaslow, N. *et al.* (1984). Attributional style and depressive symptoms among children. *Journal of Abnormal Psychology*, **93**, 235–8.

Simmons, R.G., Burgeson, R., Carlton-Ford, S. & Blyth, D.A. (1987). The impact of cumulative change in early adolescence. *Child Development*, **58**, 1220–34

Sroufe, L.A. & Waters, E. (1977). Attachment as an organizational construct. *Child Development*, **48**, 1184–99.

Sroufe, L.A. (1983). Infant–caregiver attachment and patterns of adaptation in preschool: the roots of maladaption and competence. In *Development and policy concerning children with special needs*: The Minnesota Symposia on Child Psychology, Vol. 16 (ed. M. Perimutter), pp. 42–79. Lawrence Erlbaum Associates, Inc., Hillsdale, NJ.

Sroufe, L. A. (1985). Attachment classification from the perspective of infant–caregiver relationships and infant temperament. *Child Development*, **56**, 1–10.

Susman, E.J., Inoff-Germain, G., Nottelmann, E. D. *et al.* (1987). Hormones, emotional dispositions, and aggressive attributes in young adolescents. *Child Development*, **48**, 1114–34.

Swindle, R. W., Cronkite, R.C. & Moos, R.H. (1989). Life stressors, social resources, coping, and the 4-year course of unipolar depression. *Journal of Abnormal Psychology*, **98**, 468–77.

Thomas, A. & Chess, S. (1977). *Temperament and Development.* Brunner-Mazel, New York.

Vaughn, B. E., Lefever, G. B., Seifer, R. & Barglow, P. (1989). Attachment behaviour, attachment security, and temperament during infancy. *Child Development*, **60**, 728–37.

Waters, E. (1978). The reliability and stability of individual differences in infant–mother attachment relationships. *Child Development*, **49**, 483–94.

Waters, E., Wippman, J. & Sroufe, L.A. (1979). Attachment, positive affect and competence in the peer group: Two studies in construct validation. *Child Development*, **50**, 821–9.

Weissman, M. M., Kidd, K. K. & Prusoff, B. A. (1982). Variability in rates of affective disorders in relatives of depressed and normal probands. *Archives of General Psychiatry*, **39**, 1397–403.

Weissman, M. M., Gammon, G. D., John. K. *et al.* (1987). Children of depressed parents: Increased psychopatholgy and early onset of depression. *Archives of General Psychiatry*, **44**, 847–53.

Weissman, M. M., Wickramaratne, P., Merikangas, K. R. *et al.* (1984). Onset of

E. McCauley, K. Kendall & K. Pavlidis

major depression in early adulthood: Increased familial loading and specificity. *Archives of General Psychiatry*, **41**, 1136–43.

Zupen, B., Hammen, C. & Jaenicke, C. (1987). The effects of current mood and prior depressive history of self-schematic processing in children. *Journal of Experimental Child Psychology*, **43**, 149–58.

4

Physiological processes and the development of childhood and adolescent depression

Jeanne Brooks-Gunn, Anne C. Petersen and Bruce E. Compas

INTRODUCTION

Recent conceptualisations of developmental psychopathology provide a useful framework for studying depression in childhood and adolescence (Sroufe & Rutter, 1984; Cicchetti & Schneider-Rosen, 1984, 1986; Rutter, 1986). Developmental psychopathology offers a framework within which to see how depressed mood and clinical depression develop within sociocultural, biogenetic, personality, and family domains, and how both types of depression change over time as a function of these domains. A developmental perspective focuses on the continuities and discontinuities between normal growth and psychopathology, age-related and gender-related alterations in coping and in symptom expression, behavioural reorganisations that occur around salient developmental transitions, internal and external sources of competence and vulnerability, and the effects of development on pathology and of pathology on development (Attie & Brooks-Gunn, 1992, p. 35). More work has been conducted on depression using such a framework than on other forms of psychopathology (Cicchetti & Schneider-Rosen, 1984; Cicchetti & Toth, 1991; Rutter, Izard, & Read, 1986; Goodyer, 1990; Brooks-Gunn & Petersen, 1991; Cicchetti, Nucombe, & Garber, 1992).

In this chapter, we take a look at childhood and adolescent depression by examining five issues, all of which consider the interplay between continuity and risk. The first focuses on the rate of various forms of depression in the childhood and adolescence years, to see whether, and at what ages, discontinuities in the prevalence of depression exist. Since children and adolescents do differ in their rates of depressed mood and clinical depression, we go on to ask about the factors that might account for these discontinuities. The second issue, then, tracks the physiological concomitants and possibly predictors of depression, since adolescence is marked by physiological changes. However, adolescence is not just characterised by physical growth, but also by social, emotional, cognitive, and academic changes, as well (Brooks-Gunn & Petersen, 1983, 1991; Lerner & Foch, 1987; Gunnar & Collins, 1988; McAnarney & Levine, 1988; Feldman & Elliot, 1990). It has been hypothesised that rises in emotional problems generally, and depression specifically, are due to the confluence of events with which the adolescent must cope. Physiological change becomes only one set of a series of challenges (Brooks-Gunn & Petersen, 1984; Brooks-Gunn & Reiter, 1990). Third, the timing and sequencing of biopsychosocial changes in the first half of adolescence are discussed as they shed light on increases in depression seen at this time. The fourth issue is perhaps the greatest risk factor in the development of depression – family history and rearing environment. Familial history combines both possible physiological and environmental pathways to clinical depression. Finally, we take a brief look at what is known about continuity between clinical depression and less severe forms of depressed affect, especially as the study of physiological processes might shed light on this most important aspect of continuity.

CONTINUITY OF RATES OF DEPRESSION ACROSS AGE AND GENDER

Following others such as Kazdin (1990), we distinguish between depressed affect and symptomatology on the one hand, and clinical depression, on the other (ignoring for the moment various forms of clinical depression as defined by DSM-III-R). Depressive affect refers to periods of sadness, unhappiness, or dysphoric mood that most individuals experience at some point in their lives. Depressed affect may co-occur with other negative emotions, such as fear, guilt, anger, and disgust (Watson & Kendall, 1989). It also represents, in part, one of two broad affective dimensions identified by Watson & Tellegen (1985) – the two being negative and positive affect. Depressed affect is distinguishable from anxiety, in part because depressed mood is inversely correlated with positive affect while anxiety generally is not associated with positive mood (Watson & Kendall, 1989). Depressed affect occurs in about one-third of all youth at any point in time (range across studies is 15% to 45%: Roberts, Lewinsohn & Seeley, 1991; Compas, Petersen & Brooks-Gunn, 1994). There is little research charting age trends over the adolescent years, although a few studies suggest that it peaks in the middle adolescent years (see Brooks-Gunn, 1991; Petersen, Kennedy, & Sullivan, 1991). Girls are more likely to report depressed mood than boys. Fewer children report experiencing depressed mood, and reliable gender differences do not exist until adolescence (Rutter et al., 1976).[1]

A diagnosis of clinical depression is based on DSM-III-R criteria, and unlike mood and symptomatology, must be derived from clinical interviews, not just self-report scales. Clinical depression is much more severe and lengthy; it has a major impact on the activities of daily life. Epidemiological studies suggest that the point prevalence is around 4% to 5% for adults, with the figures being about 1% to 3% for adolescents (Blazer, George, & Lauderman, 1985; Rutter et al., 1976; Weissman et al., 1987; Fendrich, Warner, & Weissman, 1990)[2] (see also chapter 6). Rates are lower for children (Rutter et al, 1976). Additionally, large sex differences are seen following the transition to adolescence. Increases are much more rapid for girls than boys so that by the middle of adolescence, girls have rates that are twice those of boys (Cohen & Brook, 1987; Bird et al., 1988; Angold & Rutter, 1992).

In summary, depressed mood and clinical depression increase during the adolescent years, as compared to the childhood years, with adolescent girls being at much more risk for both aspects of depression than adolescent boys.

CONTINUITY IN PHYSIOLOGICAL BASES OF DEPRESSION ACROSS DEVELOPMENTAL STAGES

Physiological bases of clinical depression and other forms of psychopathology have long been postulated, and research continues at a rapid pace. Even environmentally focused theories must take into account physiological change, because environmental events are mediated by the brain. Regardless of the contribution of environmental and physiological events to its onset, biological dysregulation occurs once a depressive episode is triggered. Akiskal & McKinney (1973) have termed this the 'final common pathway' model. Shelton et al. (1991) describe biological dysregulation following the onset of depression as

83

taking 'a life of its own' (Shelton *et al.*, 1991, p. 212), which further influences behaviour, thought, mood, and physiological patterns.

Theories differ in the amount of weight they place on the centrality of physiological processes in the emergence of depression and in the recovery from an episode. Physiological processes may be: (a) a response to environmental events, with biological dysregulation a result of psychosocial factors, (b) different prior to the occurrence of any environmental event for those individuals who go on to have a depressive episode, or (c) a reflection of a genetic susceptibility to experiencing the biological dysregulation associated with depression. To further complicate matters, different subtypes of depression probably have some common and some different physiological precursors and concomitants. The same is true for disorders that often co-occur with depression.

In this section, evidence is reviewed for children, adolescents, and adults in several areas: biological dysregulation in the hypothalamic–pituitary axes, neurotransmitter deficits and links with the hypothalamic–pituitary axes, and other possible physiological influences. Data on children are included since any differences seen in physiological responses of children and adolescents might be due to the dramatic changes in the hypothalamic–pituitary–gonadal (HPG) and hypothalamic–pituitary–adrenal (HPA) axes which are a part of puberty. Whenever possible, reference is made to whether younger or older adolescents were studied. If changes in the neuroendocrine system at puberty influence the patterning of biological dysregulation associated with puberty, it is likely that older adolescents, having completed the pubertal process to a large extent, will evidence physiological patterns more similar to adults than will younger adolescents in the midst of puberty. As yet, however, no unique mechanisms have been delineated for adolescent onset depression.

All of this physiologically oriented research focuses on individuals with clinical depression; in contrast, research on psychological mechanisms considers both clinical depression and depressed affect.

PHYSIOLOGICAL MARKERS OF DEPRESSION

Biological studies have the potential to provide information on the aetiology of various subtypes of depression, but can do so only with the use of specific comparative and longitudinal methodologies. Much of the current research is not designed to address aetiology; rather, it is concentrated on demonstrating associations between depression and neuroendocrine dysregulation. Consequently, even though literally hundreds of studies have been published on the physiological concomitants of depression and affective disorder, little evidence has been found for the existence of physiological markers for depression (Gold, Goodwin & Chrousos, 1988). No physiological test exists that provides a reliable diagnosis of depression. Consequently, the term 'marker' must be interpreted with caution.

However, the concept of physiological markers is a useful way to think about physiological influences upon psychopathology in general and depression in particular. Distinguishing between state and trait physiological markers allows for a separation of instances of biological dysregulation that are concomitant versus predictive. State markers are those that occur during a depressive episode but not at other times. Trait markers are those that differentiate individuals who are depressed from those who are not across depressive episodes, recovery, and illness-free phases.

Several possible explanations for a continuing abnormality in a physiological marker after recovery from a depressive episode must be ruled out before assuming that a true trait marker has been demonstrated (Puig-Antich, 1986). First, the timing of assessment is critical, since recovery in a physiological marker might continue during and past the recovery period of the episode. Second, a physiological marker might appear in the first depressive episode, and remain different thereafter. This would not be an example of a true trait marker because the abnormality was not present *prior* to the onset of any depressive episode. Third, a physiological marker may be generally associated with psychopathology or affective disorder, not depression per se.

Additionally, studies need to follow individuals for a long enough time, using repeated clinical and physiological assessment, in order to rule out the possibility that physiological markers are not due to lags and leads in biological dysregulation, which no doubt occur. At the very minimum, studies of individuals who are depressed and those who are not must be conducted, seeing the depressed individuals during recovery as well as during the depressive episode. The majority of studies do not meet this minimal requirement. Additionally, given the expense of obtaining a sample prior to the onset of any depressive episode, a factor necessary to rule out the second factor above, prospective studies of offspring of depressed parents are recommended.

Finally, studies should compare not only individuals who are depressed and those who are not, but also those individuals who have another disorder. This is particularly important given the high degree of comorbidity that occurs between depression and other forms of psychopathology (Maser & Cloninger, 1990). Similar arguments could be made for the study of different subtypes of depression, although the lack of agreement on what symptoms constitute a subtype and the historical changes in definitions of what symptoms constitute a subtype make it difficult to review the extant literature. However, given the variability in response to different treatment modalities and the often observed lack of response in adolescents, the possibility that physiological markers might differ for depressed individuals who are suicidal and those who are not, and the speculation that physiological abnormalities may be more likely for those with a greater genetic risk for depression (i.e. offspring of depressed parents who exhibit their first depressive episode as children or adolescents, or bipolar versus unipolar depressed individuals), future research on physiological mechanisms must pay more attention to subtypes and the timing of depressive episodes (Puig-Antich, 1986). Such approaches might allow for the identification of individuals at risk for depression (especially in families with a history of affective disorder) and for specifying treatment, if true physiological markers are discovered.

DYSREGULATION IN HYPOTHALAMIC–ENDOCRINE SYSTEMS

The bulk of the literature on physiological bases of depression focuses on the limbic system, specifically the hypothalamus–pituitary axes. Those involving the adrenal (HPA), the thyroid (HPT), the gonadal (HPG), and the somatotropic (HPS) axes have been studied, with all systems exhibiting varying degrees of dysregulation in association with depression. Additionally, sleep architecture changes and melatonin secretion have been the subject of study, with alterations occurring in many depressed individuals. All of this research supports the general notion that biological dysregulation occurs during episodes of depression and, in a few cases, during recovery periods as well. But research is needed that examines the correlations among biological indicators during episodes of depression and subsequent recovery. In addition, the identification of links between behavioural manifestations and types of biological dysregulation would be valuable.

Several endocrine systems are involved in depression. In all cases, a releasing hormone in the hypothalamus moves to the pituitary gland and influences the release there of a stimulating hormone. This hormone then stimulates the release of a hormone by the particular gland in question (thyroid, adrenal, gonad). This hormone is secreted into the circulation, where it acts to inhibit the production of the releasing and stimulating hormone at the hypothalamic and pituitary levels (Shelton *et al.*, 1991).

During the foetal period, gonads develop. In males, androgens are secreted by the gonads, initiating a process that results in male internal and external sex organs and the HPG axis. In the absence of androgens the sex organs are female (Money and Erhardt, 1972). In the first few months of life, the levels of circulating hormones increase for what appears to be a short period of time (in males and probably in females as well). For the rest of the pre-school period, levels of sex steroid hormones are quite low (Reiter, 1987). Sex steroids are due to the suppression of GnRH production and secretion (Reiter & Grumbach, 1982).

During middle childhood, sex steroid levels begin to increase (Kaplan, Grumbach & Aubert, 1976). The process that triggers these increases is not well understood. Two different processes occur; they are relatively independent. The first is adrenarche, which occurs when the adrenal gland in both boys and girls begins producing androgens. The second is gonadarche, which occurs a few years after adrenarche. The HPG axis is reactivated. A release of inhibition by the increase in steroid hormones, which is probably mediated by the central nervous system, accounts for the increase in gonadotropin secretion. Large increases in gonadal and adrenal sex steroids occur for both boys and girls (Brooks-Gunn & Reiter, 1990).

These changes occur prior to the onset of secondary sexual characteristics. Increases in gonadotropins (luteinising hormone and follicle-stimulating hormone) occur as the HPG axis is reactivated. Additionally, the pituitary secretes these gonadtropins in pulsatile patterns, such that 'bursts' seems to influence the gonads, which then increase production of androgens and oestrogens (Boyar *et al*, 1972). Physical changes associated with puberty follow, as does the maturation of the gonads (ova in females, sperm in males). The pulsatile secretion of the gonadtropins occurs during sleep.

Two questions are relevant to our focus on depression in adolescents. The first has to do with whether the early physiological changes of adrenarche and gonadarche have any effect on children's behaviour, in this case depressed affect. To our knowledge, research has not looked at physiological changes and behaviour in middle childhood, either in terms of overall levels of sex steroid activity or the onset of pulsatile secretions. The second question has to do with children diagnosed with clinical depression. No work has looked at the association between childhood episodes and early physiological pubertal changes, nor whether children who are not diagnosed have major depressive disorders. Interestingly, research with young women who have anorexia nervosa suggests that gonadtropin output often reverts to prepubertal patterns, i.e. night-time pulsatile secretions; cortisol secretion also is affected (Boyar *et al.*, 1977; Katz *et al.*, 1978). With weight gain and recovery gonadtropin secretions return to post-pubertal secretory patterns. Given the fact that sleep architecture seems to be affected in some youth with depressive disorders, and that gonadtropin secretion changes are first seen at night, comparable research with clinically depressed children and young adolescents might prove fruitful.

Hypothalamic–pituitary–adrenal axis (HPA)

Proportionately more research has focused on the HPA axis than other hypothalamic–pituitary axes. Generally, dysregulation in the HPA axis occurs during depressive episodes in adults, as evidenced by cortisol hypersecretion and responses of challenges of cortisol secretion in some but not all depressed adults.

Adults who are depressed are more likely to secrete more cortisol over 24 hours, to have more secretory sessions, and to secrete in the late evening and early morning, thus having the usually diurnal secretory pattern broken (Sachar, 1975; Asnis *et al.*, 1985; Pepper & Krieger, 1985; Sachar, Puig-Antich & Ryan, 1985). It has been estimated that 30% to 50% of adults with endogenous depression hypersecrete (Sachar *et al.*, 1973; Jarrett, Coble & Kupfer, 1983). Hypersecretion tends to disappear with recovery (Greden *et al.*, 1983). Within the adult age range, depressed individuals who are older may be more likely to hypersecrete, whereas this is not true in non-depressed individuals (Asnis *et al.*, 1981).

In contrast, depressed children and adolescents are less likely to hypersecrete cortisol (Klee & Garfinkel, 1984; Puig-Antich, 1987; Kutcher & Marton, 1989; Dahl,, *et al.*, 1991). However, cortisol secretion is higher at the beginning of sleep for depressed than non-depressed adolescents, with this elevation being most pronounced for depressed adolescents who are suicidal (Dahl *et al.*, 1991). Indeed, recent evidence suggests these effects may only be seen for a subsample of depressed youth, specifically those who are suicidal (Dahl *et al.*, 1991; Kutcher *et al.*, 1991).

The provocative test most often used involves giving a dose of dexamethasone to see whether cortisol is suppressed. Non-suppression may be more likely to occur in depressed adults than non-depressed adults. The estimates of non-suppression vary greatly, however. Most studies report that between 30% to 70% of adults during an episode of depression do not suppress cortisol, as compared to less than 15% of adults who have not been depressed (Amsterdam *et al.*, 1982; Rabkin *et al.*, 1983; Kutcher & Marton, 1989). Non-suppression rates are lower during recovery periods; dexamethasone escape during recovery may be predictive of the onset of another depressive episode (Greden *et al.*, 1983).

Estimates for dexamethasone non-suppression are similar or, more likely, lower for adolescents, with most studies falling within the 30% to 50% range for depressed in-patients (Crumley *et al.*, 1982; Extein *et al.*, 1982; Robins, Alessi, & Yanchyschyn, 1982; Targum & Capodanno, 1983). Examining the dexamethasone suppression test (DST) results from four adolescent studies yielded a sensitivity estimate of 32% and a specificity of 67% (Kutcher & Marton, 1989), not high enough for use as a diagnosis but similar to what is reported for adults. Little evidence is available on dexamethasone suppression during recovery in adolescents.

Studies using DST for children report mixed findings (Klee & Garfinkel, 1984; Livingston, Reis, & Ringdahl, 1984; Weller *et al.*, 1984; Puig-Antich, 1987; Pfeffer *et al.*, 1989; Naylor, Greden & Alessi, 1990). Some studies report evidence of dexamethasone non-suppression in depressed children (Puig-Antich, 1987; Pfeffer *et al.*, 1989; however, see the paper by Birmaher *et al.*, 1992, who found no evidence of 24 hour cortisol or DST responses discriminating among several groups of 6 to 12-yearolds – outpatients with MDD, non-affectively disturbed psychiatric controls and normal controls). Mixed findings may be due in part to initial plasma dexamethasone levels for DST suppressors and non-suppressors and possibly DST dose by weight differences across studies (Naylor *et al.*, 1990).

Hypothalamic–pituitary–somatotropic axis (HPS)

Most of the studies of secretion of the growth hormone (GH) have focused on children, because that GH is highly age-related. GH is secreted mostly at night in children prior to puberty. After puberty, GH secretion occurs more evenly during the day and night (Finkelstein *et al.*, 1972). It has been suggested that daytime and night-time secretion might be under the control of different neurotransmitter systems (Mendelson, 1982). Studies to date differ as to whether at night-time secretion of growth hormone is elevated (Dahl *et al.*, 1991) or blunted (Kutcher *et al.*, 1991).

Hypothalamic–pituitary–thyroid axis (HPT)

There is some evidence that thyroid-stimulating hormone (TSH) may be lower in depressed than non-depressed adult patients (Amsterdam *et al.*, 1979; Extein, Pottash, & Gold, 1980). However, the response to thyroid stimulating hormone seems to be similar for depressed and non-depressed children and adolescents (Khan, 1987; Puig-Antich, 1987). (Chapter 11 provides an extensive account of the association between alterations in neuroendocrine physiology and depression).

Hypothalamic–pituitary–gonadal axis (HPG)

Little research has focused on the HPG axis and its role in depression, given the cyclic release of these hormones in women. However, it has been hypothesised that low levels of oestrogen are associated with depressive symptoms in adult women (Benedek, 1952; Melges & Hamburg, 1977; Buchanan, Eccles, & Becker, 1992). Studies have focused on menarche, menstruation, pregnancy, and menopause, typically with respect to depressive symptoms, not clinical depression per se.

Pubertal studies using menarche as a marker usually do not report an increase in depressive affect or negative affect (Brooks-Gunn & Ruble, 1983; Brooks-Gunn, 1984). However, increases in oestrogen, specifically during the most rapid period of increase during puberty, have been associated with non-linear increases in depressive symptoms in one study (Brooks-Gunn & Warren, 1989; Warren & Brooks-Gunn, 1989); the increases in depressive symptoms occurred with the most rapid increase in hormones. Nevertheless, the magnitude of these effects was small; oestradiol accounted for about 1% of the variance, while life events occurring in the past 6 months accounted for 8% of the variance in depressive symptoms. These increases were predictive of depressive affect a year later, even controlling for initial depressive symptom scores (Paikoff, Brooks-Gunn, & Warren, 1991). Another study, using levels of oestrogen rather than categories of oestrogen functioning, and only looking at non-linear effects, did not report associations between oestradiol and depressive symptoms (Susman *et al.*, 1987*a*, *b*).

Surprisingly, given the prevalence in the clinical literature of discussions of pre- and post-pubertal depression, few studies actually measure pubertal status relative to depression. Rutter (1980, 1986) found some evidence that boys were more likely to be diagnosed with depression if they were later in puberty compared to those prior to or just beginning the process.[3] More recent work (involving medical record review) does not confirm this hypothesis (Angold & Rutter, 1992).

Most studies have focused on the occurrence of negative moods and various phases of the menstrual cycle, with more negative moods being hypothesised during times of low oestrogen concentrations or falling oestrogen concentrations. Research does not support this hypothesis when cognitive and social attributions are controlled (Ruble & Brooks-Gunn, 1979, 1987). Another line of research actually measures oestrogen concentration. Two studies report that oestrogen levels and the ratio of oestrogen to progesterone were higher in the premenstrual phase for those women who reported premenstrual symptoms, including negative affect (Backstrom *et al.*, 1976; Munday, Brush & Taylor, 1981). At first glance, these findings do not fit with the prediction that cycles characterised by low oestrogen production are linked to negative moods. The effect could be due to an abnormality in hormonal functioning rather than actual levels in women who report premenstrual symptoms (see Dinnerstein *et al.*, 1984). The findings of increased depressive effect as hormone levels rise during puberty do not accord with beliefs about low oestrogen and depressed mood either.

Postpartum depression and depressive affect also have been thought to be associated with the rapid decreases in oestrogen and perhaps progesterone (Melges & Hamburg, 1977; Kumar & Robson, 1984). Few studies measuring actual hormone concentrations or changes in hormones around the time of birth have been conducted. Additionally, social and psychological factors as well as previous depression have been associated with negative affect at the time of birth (Parlee, 1978; Hopkins, Marcus & Campbell, 1984;).

Menopause brings with it a decline in oestrogen, follicle-stimulating hormone (FSH) and luteinising hormone (LH). Research results are mixed as to whether depressive symptoms increase at the time of menopause, similar to the findings on menstruation. However, some studies have reported positive effects of oestrogen replacement therapy upon depressive symptoms (see Buchanan *et al.*, 1992).

Dysregulation in sleep patterns

Diurnal rhythms are expressed in neuroendocrine activity, sleep–wake cycles, and body temperature (Wehr & Goodwin, 1981). These rhythms are regulated by two oscillators, which exhibit dysregulation during depressive episodes probably due to central nervous system hyper-arousal (Gold *et al.*, 1986; Sack *et al.*, 1987; Gold *et al.*, 1988). Depression appears to impair the sleep onset mechanism rendering sleep disturbance a possible physiological marker (e.g. Reynolds, Gillin & Kupfer, 1987).

Sleep architecture has been studied extensively in adults who are depressed, with the findings indicating disturbances such as decreased REM (rapid eye movement) latency, increased electrical activity during REM, and sleep onset delays (Reynolds *et al.*, 1987). During periods of recovery, sleep rhythms return to normal for some but not all patients. Continuation of sleep dysregulation is probably predictive of recurrence (Giles *et al.*, 1987).

Over the past decade, there has been significant research activity on the question of sleep regulation in depressed children and adolescents (e.g. Puig-Antich *et al.*, 1984a–d). It now appears that the sleep onset mechanism is impaired in a subgroup of depressed adolescents (those who are suicidal) – blunting GH, increasing cortisol, and increasing sleep latency (Dahl *et al.*, 1992). Further, normal age-related changes in sleep features appear to be accelerated in depressed patients at all ages (Knowles & MacLean, 1990). Dahl *et al* (1992) proposed the interesting hypothesis that sleep is protected in children (see e.g. Carskadon & Dement, 1987), with the developmental changes of puberty reducing this protection.

Dysregulation in the neurotransmitter systems

Focus has also been on the neurotransmitter systems, specifically the serotonergic, the cholinergic, and the noradrenergic systems. Activity in all three has been implicated in depression, with current research testing the notion that patterns of dysregulation in different systems are associated with different subtypes of depression (Gold *et al.*, 1986; Shelton *et al.*, 1991). Simple notions of deficit theories have been abandoned, given the fact that interactions occur among neurotransmitter systems, among hypothalamic–pituitary systems, and between the two systems as well as between different substrates of the brain. Additionally, neurotransmitter activity is regulated at multiple levels, including synthesis, packaging and storage, release, reuptake, metabolism, and post-synaptic-receptor responsiveness (Gold *et al.*, 1988). Thus, current studies attempt to determine the level at which neurotransmitter dysregulation associated with depression occurs. For example, post-synaptic receptor responsiveness has been implicated in depression, which was suspected given the lag time between pharmacological treatment and response in adults.

Links between all hypothalamic–pituitary axes and neurotransmitter systems are being demonstrated at an ever increasing pace. These studies will provide much needed specific information on which neurotransmitter systems are affected in different subtypes of depression. This new generation of studies should result in more effective treatment, since specification of dysregulation in particular neurotransmitter systems provides the information necessary to determine which pharmacological agent, or mix of agents, will be effective for an individual. This is particularly important given the fact that the literature on adolescents to date does not find much evidence for the efficacy of antidepressant drugs (specifically tricyclic drugs see: Petersen *et al.*, 1993; Jensen, Prien & Ryan, 1994). Presently, it is very difficult if not impossible to know *a priori* how any individual will respond to a particular antidepressant drug (Joyce & Paykel, 1989).

Neurotransmitter systems have been implicated in depression for over 40 years. Current research has moved away from deficiency hypotheses to more complex models involving both pre-synaptic and post-synaptic events (down regulation and effects on 'second messenger' systems), rather than a focus on the former exclusively (Shelton *et al.*, 1991, p. 205; Vetulani & Sulser, 1975). Additionally, the complexity may be characterised as an unstable or dysregulated system, rather than a deficient one (Siever & Davis, 1985).

Maturational changes in neurotransmitter activity and regulation occur, although less research has traced these changes compared to those in the hypothalamic–endocrine systems. Catecholamine systems take until adulthood to become fully functional in primates (Goldman-Rakic & Brown, 1982). In humans, short attention spans in children

93

and the infrequency of mania in depressed children also may be indicative of an immature catecholamine system (Wender, 1971; Puig-Antich, 1987). In contrast, the serotonergic and cholinergic systems are functional prior to adulthood, at least in rats (Lidor & Molliver, 1982; Shelton et al., 1991).[4]

Generally, depression may be associated with an activated locus coeruleus-noradrenaline system. Besides the noradrenergic system, the cholinergic system may be hyper-responsive in depressed patients while gamma-aminobutyric acid (GABA) and serotonin may be low (Gold et al., 1988).

A number of studies are linking neurotransmitter functioning to hypothalamic-endocrine dysregulation, typically through the study of pharmacological substances with different neurotransmitter effects. In the HPA axis, non-suppression of cortisol to the dexamethasone test may be associated with cholinergic overactivity in some depressed individuals (Carroll et al., 1980). Noradrenergic system deficits have also been implicated, as seen in studies of administration of d-amphetamine, desmethylimipramine (DMI), and clonidine. All three tend to stimulate cortisol secretion, or result in a smaller increase in cortisol secretion, in non-depressed controls but not in depressed individuals (Sachar et al., 1973, 1985; Siever et al., 1984; Asnis et al., 1985; however, see the findings in the study of two samples by Waterman et al. (1991), with adolescents). The serotonergic system may also be involved, because when given 5-hydroxy-tryptophan (L-5-HP), depressed children show a blunted cortisol response relative to non-depressed controls (Ryan et al., 1990; Dahl et al., 1991).

In the HPS axis, dysregulation in GH in depressed individuals probably involves a functional noradrenergic deficit, as seen in studies using clonidine, desmethylimipramine, and d-amphetamine (Sachar, 1975; Langer et al., 1976; Checkley, Slade, & Shur, 1981; Siever et al., 1982). Similar findings have been reported for a sample of adolescents with major depressive disorder and those who are suicidal compared to non-depressed controls using DMI (Ryan et al., 1994). However, no differences were found in GH response using amphetamine with the exception of one finding in one of two samples examined (Waterman et al., 1991). As Ryan et al. (1988) point out, the serotonergic system is probably also involved (most likely in a decrease in pre-synaptic serotonergic activity), just as was seen in dysregulation of the HPA axis.

Possible physiological concomitants of depression

Work is beginning to focus on brain function other than the neuroendocrine systems. A particularly intriguing hypothesis involves the notion of kindling which 'refers to the eventual development of motor seizures to repeated electrical stimulation of the brain with current which was originally insufficient to produce overt behavioural effects' (Muñoz, 1993, pp. 35–36, see also Muñoz et al., 1993). The fact that subsequent depressive episodes often occur with shorter and shorter latencies might be due to such a kindling phenomenon (Post, Rubinow & Ballenger, 1984). The physiological changes that occur during the first few episodes might sensitise the organism to experience biological dysregulation more easily (i.e. in the face of a less potent environmental and/or physiological event). Consequently, early depressive episodes may predispose the individual to be more susceptible to subsequent episodes.

TIMING AND SEQUENCING OF PUBERTAL EVENTS

Generally, the evidence to date is not clear as to whether the biological underpinnings, or at least concomitants, of clinical depression differ dramatically across the life span. The next generation of neuroendocrinological studies may yield more age-related differences.

Adolescents differ from children cognitively, socially and emotionally, not just physiologically as indicated by their acquisition of a reproductively mature body. However, we believe that the more physiological approaches to the study of depression during adolescence would be enhanced by a consideration of the context in which physiological change occurs. As stated in the introduction, the transition towards adolescence brings with it a plethora of challenges in every realm of development. It has been hypothesised that the confluence of events, many of them novel, accounts in part for the rise in rates of clinical depression and depressed mood. Several studies have documented that the number of potentially stressful life events (in the peer, school and family realms) is higher during the young adolescent period than earlier or later (Compas, 1987; Brooks-Gunn, 1991; Paikoff & Brooks-Gunn, 1991). These events probably influence depressive symptoms via their effect on daily stress levels (Compas et al., 1989). The increase in life events over time is the strongest predictor of depressed symptom scores, and *changes* in these scores, as seen in one study measuring life events and girls' depression over four years (Brooks-Gunn, 1991; see also Simmons, Burgeson & Carlton-Ford, 1987, for a similar finding looking at life events cross-sectionally). Interestingly, timing of puberty, but not tempo or current status, was associated with depressive symptoms, such that being an early maturer was a risk factor.[5] However, like the findings using hormonal levels rather than pubertal timing, social life events accounted for much more of the variance than pubertal timing (Brooks-Gunn, 1991). [6]

The occurrence of life events also helps explain the gender differentials emerging during the middle of adolescence; girls experience more stressful events than boys in the first half of adolescence, which is directly associated with their higher depressed affect scores (Petersen, Sarigiani & Kennedy, 1991).[7] Girls may also perceive and even experience a particular event as more stressful than boys, adding further to the burden of multiple life events. For example, boys, being given more freedom at an earlier age than girls, may be able to manage stressful family events by relying on friends. Girls may be less likely to rely on peers as an 'arena of comfort' (Simmons *et al*, 1987). At the same time, girls (and boys) who have peers as an 'arena of comfort' when family relationships are strained, show less depressive symptoms (Colten & Gore, 1991). If puberty heralds an intensification of gender roles, as has been suggested (Hill & Lynch, 1983), then girls may experience certain gender-linked events differently, and more negatively, than boys (not dating, being perceived as unattractive: Faust, 1983; Duke-Duncan *et al.*, 1985; Gargiulo *et al.*, 1987; Attie, Brooks-Gunn & Petersen, 1990).

Boys' and girls' experiences and behavioural repertoires prior to adolescence may also play a role. For example, the Blocks have followed a cohort of children from the pre-school to the young adult years. Pre-school predictors of boys' depressive symptoms at age 18 years included being aggressive, self-aggrandising, and undercontrolled, while predictors for girls were being intropunitive, oversocialised, and overcontrolled (Block & Gjerde, 1990). These characteristics are reminiscent of early sex role stereotypes (Block, 1973; Brooks-Gunn & Matthews, 1979). Perhaps many of the negative effects of rigid role expectations and sex-role socialisation do not become evident until the young adolescent years, when pubertal changes, and society's responses to them, render gender and the different experiences and trajectories for males and females, highly salient. Such results suggest that continuities exist between early personality and emotional state, but that the creation of developmental trajectories may be quite gender-specific. Whether the same is true for children reared in different social and economic contexts is not known, although highly probable (Spencer & Dornbusch, 1990).

The point here is that research needs to consider physiological, social, and emotional changes of the pubertal period simultaneously. Additionally, potential interactions among these domains must be modelled if we are to understand the increase in depressive affect and clinical depression during the adolescent years. Focusing on physiological change in the absence of other changes or without considering the ecosystems in which the youth resides will probably yield little understanding of the onset of both types of depression, or of the developmental trajectories of children or youth who experience depression.

CONTINUITY IN DEPRESSION ACROSS GENERATIONS: A PHYSIOLOGICAL AND ENVIRONMENTAL PROCESS

Family aggregation of affective disorders has been demonstrated in studies of children, adolescents, and adults (Andreasen *et al.*, 1977; Gershon *et al.*, 1982; Weissman *et al.*, 1984; Hammen, 1991). Estimates of lifetime morbidity risks in first-degree relatives of probands with major depression, for adults, range from 0.18 to 0.30 (Gershon *et al.*, 1982; Puig-Antich, 1986). Twin studies suggest that monozygotic twins are four to five times more likely to exhibit concordance for major depression than dizygotic twins (Kendler *et al.*, 1986; Wender *et al.*, 1986).

Family aggregation is higher for bipolar than unipolar depression (Mendlewicz, 1988), which might be indicative of different biological substrates being involved or different temporal patterns of biological influence. For unipolar depression, family aggregation is higher for those individuals with more severe and frequent episodes (Nurnberger & Gershon, 1984). At the same time, it is possible that even less severe depressions have a genetic loading. A tantalising hypothesis has been put forth by Kendler and colleagues (Kendler *et al.*, 1986). They believe that there may be genetic transmission for 'distress' broadly construed, with the form this distress takes being influenced by the precipitation of environmental events expressed by an individual. The two types of distress considered are anxiety and depression, which are not only often present in the same individuals, but both may be characterised by dysregulation in the HPA axis (Butler & Nemeroff, 1990; Maser & Cloninger, 1990).

97

Generally, aggregation is higher in children than in adolescents, and higher in adolescents than in adults. Comparing age-corrected lifetime morbidity risks across studies in first-degree relatives of probands with major depression (since most studies do not include children, adolescents, and adults), rough estimates are about 0.50 for children, 0.35 for adolescents, and 0.18 to 0.30 for adults (Gershon *et al.*, 1982; Puig-Antich, 1987; Strober *et al.*, 1994; Weissman *et al.*, 1984). Thus, the genetic loading for childhood and adolescent depression may be higher than that for depression which first occurs in adulthood.

In addition, current longitudinal studies of childhood and adolescent onset of depression suggest that early onset may be associated with more frequent and severe depressive episodes (Strober, 1983; Kovacs *et al.*, 1984*a*, *b*). Looking at the timing of onset of depression within one study, Weissman *et al.* (1987) reported that individuals with an onset prior to age 20 were more likely to have family members who were depressed than those whose first episode was reported to occur after age 20.

Parental psychopathology itself is also accompanied by negative familial conditions – marital conflict, family conflict, other aspects of psychopathology, and possibly other life stressors (Downey & Coyne, 1990). Consequently, what might at first glance seem to be heritable might also be environmental. An elegant study was conducted on the children of parents with psychiatric diagnoses of schizophrenia or major affective disorder, a history of child abuse or neglect (reported to Child Protective Services), or both (Downey & Walker, 1992). Problem behaviours, both depression and aggression, were highest in children whose parents had a history of both abuse/neglect and psychopathology, and lowest in those whose parents had no history of abuse/neglect but had a clinical diagnosis of psychopathology. Using child-level variables to classify children into high, average and low risk groups (based on self-esteem, interpersonal problem solving, early developmental difficulties and intelligence) explains a significant amount of the variance in behaviour problems (more so for depression than aggression). Children at double jeopardy (high risk in child and family characteristics) were much more likely to exhibit depressed symptomatology.

Findings such as these show the importance of examining other characteristics of the family environment and, more specifically, other aspects of parental behaviour and psychopathology than just the existence of affective disorders (see also Hammen, 1991). For example, Mitchell and colleagues (1989) found that depressed children (ages 7 to 12) of affectively disordered mothers had mothers who reported more drug abuse and suicide attempts than a comparable sample of adolescents. And, in a study of children of unipolar, bipolar, medically ill, and non-ill mothers, chronic strain and current depressive symptoms of the mother were more predictive of the children's depressive symptomatology than maternal history of affective disorder (Hammen *et al.*, 1987). The early onset of clinical depression in childhood, therefore, may be due to the co-occurrence of other forms of psychopathology in conjunction with an affective disorder.[8]

The negative influence of a depressed parent is not specific to depression. Children and adolescents of parents with an affective disorder show symptoms beyond the depressive spectrum, including neurotic illness, neurotic behaviour disturbance, sociopathy, and criminal activities (Beardslee *et al.*, 1983; Beardslee, Keller & Klerman, 1985*a*; Hammen, 1991).

In summary, continuity across generations is seen. However, it is often more general to psychopathology than to depression, and it may be due to more than parental psychopathology per se, rather than depression. Whether familial aggregation is more generally associated with psychopathology or with clinical depression would possibly alter the part which physiological processes are hypothesised to play in the aetiology of childhood and adolescent depression.

CONCLUSIONS: PHYSIOLOGICAL AND ENVIRONMENTAL PATHWAYS TO DEPRESSION

Perhaps the largest unanswered question in the childhood and adolescent depression literature has to do with whether continuity exists between more and less severe forms of depression. While excellent prospective work has been conducted, most of it focuses on charting the developmental course of depressive symptomatology in a non-clinical sample of adolescents, following a sample of offspring of affectively disordered parents (and perhaps comparison groups of abusing or medically ill parents), or watching a sample of clinical patients *vis-à-vis* relapse. Little work considers what predisposes some youth or children who exhibit depressive symptomatology to go on to have a clinical episode while others do not. Who is vulnerable and who is not? What are the family-level and child-level factors that protect children and youth from depression? We do not even know if a history of depressed mood is a risk factor for the onset of a major affective disorder.

99

Perhaps the best samples in which to look for links between depressed mood and clinical depression are those focusing on children of affectively disordered parents. Several investigators are following families for a decade or more (Weissman *et al* 1987; Hammen, 1991).

Almost no work has explored possible similarities and differences in the onset and course of clinical depression and depressed mood *vis-à-vis* physiological processes. Additionally, the more biologically oriented research has focused on the clinically depressed. Little research has focused on those with less severe forms of depression.

Whether biological dysregulation occurs in adolescents without a clinical condition but with severe depressive symptoms is unexplored. Of particular interest is whether a subset of youth with depressed mood may exhibit physiological concomitants and if so, whether such youth are more likely to go on to experience a clinical episode. Until normative studies of adolescents include physiological measures, this potentially fruitful approach to identifying youth at risk for clinical depression and depressed youth who go on to have a clinical episode will not be realised.

NOTES

1. Depressed symptoms are often distinguished from depressive mood in terms of duration, severity, and number of symptoms. From a methodological point of view, behaviour problem checklists are the main source of research information on depressive symptomatology. These scales include a large number of symptoms, with either severity or duration ratings (or sometimes a combination of the two), and include behaviours representing internalising and externalising dimensions. Symptoms include sad, crying, moody, low appetite, sleep disturbances, feelings of worthlessness, guilt and loneliness. Estimates of the number of youth with depressive symptomatology are variable, in part because of the lack of a consensus about criteria. However, based on the review by Angold (1988), about one-sixth of youth at any point of time might be characterised as having depressed symptomatology (Petersen *et al.*, 1993). It is important to note that studies of risk factors do not differentiate between depressed mood and symptomatology. Consequently, the distinction is not made in the rest of this chapter.
2. However, a review of ten recent studies suggests that the rate for teenagers might be higher (Petersen *et al.*, 1993).
3. Pubertal timing, that is, whether or not one develops earlier or later than one's peers, is more likely to be associated with depressive symptoms in girls, than pubertal status. Early developing girls report more depressed affect than those who are average or late developers (Brooks-Gunn, 1988, 1991; Petersen *et al.*, 1991*a*).
4. Brain cell growth also occurs during childhood and adolescence (Greenough, Black & Wallace, 1987).
5. Timing of maternal reproductive status also may be associated with adolescent girls' depressive symptoms (Paikoff, Brooks-Gunn & Carlton-Ford, 1991).
6. Additionally, in a recent record review study of over 3000 psychiatric in-patients, pubertal status was not associated with the clinical diagnosis of depression, once age was controlled (Angold & Rutter, 1992). This finding also points to the importance of

other, possibly socially-mediated factors in explaining the rise of depression during adolescence (although it does not address the role of other biological factors).

7. There is some discrepancy in the life event literature on the issue of sex differences. The method of event recording and the measurement of the degree of undesirability are probably responsible for much of this difference. Thus self reports of the negative impact of recent events show greater sex differences – with girls reporting higher negative scores and more negative events than boys – than life event interviews using rater assessment of quality of recent life events occurring prior to the onset of disorder. See Chapter 8 for further discussion of interview procedures and findings.

8. On a more general level, low family cohesion and expression seems to be associated with depressive symptoms (Reinherz et al., 1989; Friedrich, Reams & Jacobs, 1982). Parents in such families tend to show a low degree of commitment and support for their children as well as low communication. Low parental commitment is associated with depressive symptoms and low self-esteem (Harter, Marold & Whitesell, 1992). Low family cohesion, when accompanied by stress, results in pronounced depressive symptoms among children (Friedrich et al., 1982; Seiffge-Krenke, 1991).

REFERENCES

Akiskal, H. S. & McKinney, W. T., Jr (1973). Depressive disorders: Toward a unified hypothesis. *Science*, **182**, 20–9.

Amsterdam, J. D., Winokur, A., Caroff, S. N. & Conn, J. (1982). The dexamethasone suppression test in outpatients with primary affective disorder and healthy control subjects. *American Journal of Psychiatry*, **139**, 287–91.

Amsterdam, J. D., Winokur, A., Mendels, J. et al. (1979). Distinguishing depressive subtypes of thyrotropin response to TRJ testing. *Lancet*, **2**, 904–5.

Andreasen, N. C., Endicott, J., Spitzer, R. L. & Winokur, G. (1977). Family history method using diagnostic criteria. *Archives of General Psychiatry*, **34**, 1223–9.

Angold, A. (1988). Childhood and adolescent depression: I. Epidemiological aspects. *British Journal of Psychiatry*, **152**, 601–17.

Angold, A. & Rutter, M. (1992). Effects of age and pubertal status on depression in a large clinical sample. *Development and Psychopathology*, **4**, 5–28.

Asnis, G. M. & Halbreich, R. (1985). Cortisol responses to desipramine in endogenous depressives and normal controls. Preliminary findings. *Psychiatry Research*, **14**, 225–32.

Asnis, G. M., Sachar, E. L., Halbreich, R. et al. (1981). Cortisol secretion in relation to age in major depression. *Psychosomatic Medicine*, **43**, 235–42.

Attie, I. & Brooks-Gunn, J. (1992). Developmental issues in the study of eating problems and disorders. In *The etiology of bulimia: The individual and familial context* (ed. J. H. Crowther, S. E. Hobfoll, M. A. P. Stephens, & D. L. Tennenbaum), pp. 35–58. Hemisphere Publishers, Washington, DC.

Attie, I., Brooks-Gunn, J. & Petersen, A. C. (1990). The emergence of eating problems: A developmental perspective. In *Handbook of developmental psychopathology* (ed. M. Lewis & S. Miller), pp. 409–20. Plenum Press, New York.

Backstrom, T., Wide, V., Sodergard, R. & Carstensen, H. (1976). FSH, LH, TeBG-capacity, oestrogen, and progesterone in women with pre-menstrual tension during the luteal phase. *Journal of Steroid Biochemistry*, **7**, 473–6.

Beardslee, W. R., Bemporad, J., Keller, M. B., & Klerman, G. L. (1983). Children of parents with major affective disorder: A review. *American Journal of Psychiatry*, **140**, 825–32.

Beardslee, W. R., Keller, M. B. & Klerman, G. L. (1985). Children of parents with affective disorder. *Paediatrics in Review*, **10**, 313–19.

Benedek, T. (1952). *Psychosexual functions in women*. Ronald Press, New York.

Bird, H. R., Canino, G., Rubio-Stipec, M. *et al.* (1988). Estimates of the prevalence of childhood maladjustment in a community survey in Puerto Rico. *Archives of General Psychiatry*, **45**, 1120–6.

Birmaher, B., Ryan, N. D., Dahl, R. *et al.* (1992). Dexamethasone suppression test in children with major depressive disorder. *Journal of the American Academy of Child Adolescent Psychiatry*, **31**, 291–6.

Blazer, D., George, L. K. & Lauderman, R. (1985). Psychiatric disorders: A rural/urban comparison. *Archives of General Psychiatry*, **42**, 651–6.

Block, J. H. (1973). Conceptions of sex role: Some cross-cultural and longitudinal perspectives. *American Psychologist*, **28**, 512–26.

Block, J. & Gjerde, P. F. (1990). Depressive symptomatology in late adolescence: A longitudinal perspective on personality antecedents. In *Risk and protective factors in the development of psychopathology* (ed. J. E. Rolf, A. Masten, D. Cicchetti, K. Neuchtstein, & S. Weintraub), pp. 334–60. Cambridge University Press, New York.

Boyar, R. M., Finklestein, J., Roffwarg, H. *et al.* (1972). Synchronization of augmented luteinizing hormone secretion with sleep during puberty. *New England Journal of Medicine*, **287**, 582–6.

Boyar, R. M., Hellman, L. D., Roffwarf, H. *et al.* (1977). Cortisol secretion and metabolism in anorexia nervosa. *New England Journal of Medicine*, **296**, 190–3.

Brooks-Gunn, J. (1984). The psychological significance of different pubertal events to young girls. *Journal of Early Adolescence*, **4**(4), 315–27.

Brooks-Gunn, J. (1988). Antecedents and consequences of variations in girls' maturational timing. *Journal of Adolescent Health Care*, **9** (5), 365–73.

Brooks-Gunn, J. (1991). How stressful is the transition to adolescence in girls? In *Adolescent stress: Causes and consequences* (ed. M. E. Colten & S. Gore), pp. 131–49. Aldine de Gruyter, Hawthorne, NY.

Brooks-Gunn, J. & Matthews, W. (1979). *He and she: How children develop their sex-role identity*. Prentice-Hall, Inc., Englewood Cliffs, NJ.

Brooks-Gunn, J. & Petersen, A.C. (ed.). (1983). *Girls at puberty: Biological and psychosocial perspectives*. Plenum Press, New York.

Brooks-Gunn, J. & Petersen, A. C. (1984). Problems in studying and defining pubertal events. *Journal of Youth and Adolescence*, **13**, 181–96.

Brooks-Gunn, J. & Petersen, A. C. (1991). Studying the emergence of depression and depressive symptoms during adolescence. *Journal of Youth and Adolescence*, **20**, 115–9.

Brooks-Gunn, J. & Reiter, E. O. (1990). The role of pubertal processes in the early adolescent transition. In *At the threshold: The developing adolescent* (ed. S. Feldman & G. Elliott), pp. 16–53. Harvard University Press, Cambridge.

Brooks-Gunn, J. & Ruble, D. N. (1983). The experience of menarche from a developmental perspective. In *Girls at puberty: Biological and psychosocial perspectives* (ed. J. Brooks-Gunn & A. C. Petersen), pp. 155–77. Plenum Press, New York.

Brooks-Gunn, J. Warren, M. P. (1989). Biological contributions to affective expression in young adolescent girls. *Child Development*, **60**, 372–85.

Buchanan, C. M., Eccles, J. & Becker, J. (1992). Are adolescents the victims of raging hormones? Evidence for activational effects of hormones on moods and behaviour at adolescence. *Psychological Bulletin*, **111**, 62–107.

Butler, P. D. & Nemeroff, C. B. (1990). Corticotropin-releasing factor as a possible cause of comorbidity in anxiety and depressive disorders. In *Comorbidity of mood and anxiety disorders* (ed. J. D. Maser & C. R. Cloninger), pp. 413–35. American Psychiatric Press, Washington, DC.

Carroll, B. J., Greden, J. F., Haskett, R. *et al.* (1980). Neurotransmitter studies of neuroendocrine pathology in depression. *Acta Psychiatrica Scandinavica*, **280**, 183–99.

Carskadon, M. A. & Dement, W. C. (1987). Daytime sleepiness: Quantification of a behavioural state. *Neuroscience & Biomedical Reviews*, **11**, 307–17.

Checkley, S. A., Slade, A. P. & Shur, E. (1981). Growth hormone and other responses to clonidine in patients with endogenous depression. *British Journal of Psychiatry*, **138**, 51–5.

Cicchetti, D., Nurcombe, B. & Garber, J. (1992). Developmental approaches to depression. *Development and Psychopathology*, **4**, 1–3.

Cicchetti, D. & Schneider-Rosen, K. (eds.). (1984). *Childhood depression: A developmental perspective*. Jossey-Bass, San Francisco, CA.

Cicchetti, D. & Schneider-Rosen, K. (1986). An organisational approach to childhood depression. In *Depression in young people: Clinical and developmental perspectives* (ed.M. Rutter, C. Izard, & P. Read), pp. 71–134. Guilford, New York.

Cicchetti, D. & Toth, S. (1991). The making of a developmental psychopathologist. In *Child behaviour and development: Training for diversity* (ed. J. H. Canter, C. C. Spiker, & L. P. Lipsitt), pp. 34–72. Ablex Publishing Corporation, Norwood, NJ.

Cohen, P. & Brook, J. S. (1987). Family factors related to the persistence of psychopathology in childhood and adolescence. *Psychiatry*, **50**, 332–45.

Colten, M. E. & Gore, S. (eds.) (1991). *Adolescent stress: causes and consequences*. Aldine de Grouyter, Hawthorne, NY.

Compas, B.E. (1987). Stress and life events during childhood and adolescence. *Clinical Psychology Review*, **7**, 275–302.

Compas, B. E., Howell, D. C., Phares, V. *et al.* (1989). Parent and child stress and symptoms: An integrative analysis. *Developmental Psychology*, **25**, 550–559.

Compas, B., Petersen, A. C., & Brooks-Gunn, J. (1994). *Depression in adolescence*. Sage, Newbury Park, CA.

Crumley, F., Clevenger, J., Steinfink, D. *et al.* (1982). Preliminary report on the dexamethasone suppression test for psychiatrically disturbed adolescents. *American Journal of Psychiatry*, **139**, 1062–4.

Dahl, R. E., Ryan, N. D., Puig-Antich, J. *et al.* (1991). 24-hour cortisol measures in adolescents with major depression: A controlled study. *Biological Psychiatry*, **30**, 25–36.

Dahl, R. E., Ryan, N. D., Williamson, D. E. *et al.* (1992). Regulation of sleep and growth hormone in adolescent depression. *Journal of the American Academy of Child and Adolescent Psychiatry*, **31**, 615–21.

Dinnerstein, L., Spencer-Gardner, C., Brown, J. B. *et al.* (1984). Pre-menstrual tension – hormonal profiles. *Journal of Psychosomatic Obstetrics and Gynecology*, **3**, 37–51.

Downey, G. & Coyne, J. C. (1990). Children of depressed parents: An integrative review. *Psychological Bulletin*, **108**, 50–76.

Downey, G. & Walker, E. (1992). distinguishing family-level and child-level influences on the development of depression and aggression in children at risk. *Development and Psychopathology*, **4**, 83–97.

Duke-Duncan, D., Ritter, P. L., Dornbusch, S. M. *et al.* (1985). The effects of pubertal timing on body image, school behaviour, and deviance. *Journal of Youth and Adolescence*, **14**, 227–35.

Extein, I., Gold, M. S., Pottash, A. L. C. & Sternback, H. (1982). The TRH and dexamethasone suppression tests in the diagnosis of major unipolar depression. In *Abstracts of the Collegium Internationale Neuro-Psychopharmacologicum*, 13th Congress, Jerusalem, Israel.

Extein, I., Pottash, A. L. C. & Gold, M. S. (1980). TRH test in depression. *New England Journal of Medicine*, **302**, 923–4.

Faust, M. S. (1983). Alternative constructions of adolescent growth. In *Girls at puberty: Biological and psychosocial perspectives* (ed. J. Brooks-Gunn & A. C. Petersen), pp. 105–25. Plenum Press, New York.

Feldman, S. S., & Elliott, G. (eds.) (1990). *At the threshold: The developing adolescent*. Harvard University Press, Cambridge, MA.

Fendrich, M., Warner, V. & Weissman, M. M. (1990). Family risk factors, parental depression, and psychopathology in offspring. *Developmental Psychology*, **26**, 40–50.

Finkelstein, J. W., Roffwarg, H. P., Boyar, R. M. *et al.* (1972). Age related change in the 24 hour spontaneous secretion of growth hormone. *Journal of Clinical Endocrinology*, **35**, 665–70.

Friedrich, W. M., Reams, R. & Jacobs, J. (1982). Depression and suicidal ideation in early adolescents. *Journal of Youth and Adolescence*, **11**, 403–7.

Gargiulo, J., Attie, I., Brooks-Gunn, J. & Warren, M. P. (1987). Girls' dating behaviour as a function of social context and maturation. *Developmental Psychology*, **23**, 730–7.

Gershon, E. S., Hanovit, J., Guroff, J. J. *et al.* (1982). A family study of schizoaffective, bipolar I, bipolar II, unipolar, and normal control probands. *Archives of General Psychiatry*, **39**, 1157–67.

Giles, D. E., Jarrett, R. B., Roffwarg, H. P. & Rush, A. J. (1987). Reduced REM latency: A predictor of recurrence in depression. *Neuropsychopharmacology*, **1**, 33–9.

Gold, P. W., Goodwin, F. K. & Chrousos, G. P. (1988). Clinical and biochemical manifestations of depression: Relation to the neurobiology of stress, part 1. *New England Journal of Medicine*, **319**, 348–53.

Gold, P. W., Loriauz, L., Roy, A. *et al.* (1986). Responses to corticotropin-releasing hormone in the hypercortisolism of depression and Cushing's disease. *New England Journal of Medicine*, **341**, 1329–35.

Goldman-Rakic, P. S. & Brown, R. M. (1982). Post-natal development of monoamine content and synthesis in the cerebral cortex of the rhesus monkey. *Brain Research Bulletin*, **256**, 339–49.

Goodyer, I. M. (1990). *Life experiences, development, and childhood psychopathology*. John Wiley, Chichester, New York.

Greden, J. F., Gardner, R., King, D. *et al.* (1983). Dexamethasone suppression tests in antidepressant treatment of melancholia. *Archives of General Psychiatry*, **40**, 493–500.

Greenough, W. T., Black, J. E. & Wallace, C. S. (1987). Experience and brain development. *Child Development*, **58**, 539–59.

Graber, J., Brooks-Gunn, J., Paikoff, R. L. & Warren, M. P. (1994). Prediction of eating problems and disorders: An eight year study of adolescent girls. *Developmental Psychology*, in press.

Graham J. & Brooks-Gunn, J. (1994). Reproductive Transitions: The experience of mothers and daughters. In *The parental experience in mid-life* (ed. C. D. Ryff & M. M. Seltzer). University of Chicago Press, Chicago, IL (in press).

Gunnar, M. R. Collins, W. A. (ed.) (1988). Transitions in adolescence: Minnesota Symposium on Child Psychology. Erlbaum, Hillsdale, NJ.

Hammen, C. (1991). *Depression runs in families*. Springer-Verlag, New York.

Hammen, C. L., Adrian, C., Fordon, D. & Jaenicke, C. (1987). Children of depressed mothers: Maternal strain and symptom predictors of dysfunction. *Journal of Abnormal Psychology*, **96**, 190–8.

Harter, S., Marold, D. B. & Whitesell, N. R. (1992). Model of psychosocial risk factors leading to suicidal ideation in young adolescents. *Development and Psychopathology*, **4**, 167–88.

Hill, J. P. & Lynch, M. E. (1983). The intensification of gender-related role expectations during early adolescence. In *Girls at puberty: Biological and psychosocial perspectives* (ed. J. Brooks-Gunn & A. C. Petersen), pp. 201–28. Plenum Press, New York.

Hopkins, J., Marcus, M. & Campbell, S. B. (1984). Postpartum depression: A critical review. *Psychological Bulletin*, **95**, 498–515.

Jarrett, D. B., Coble, P. A. & Kupfer, D. J. (1983). Reduced cortisol latency in depressive illness. *Archives of General Psychiatry*, **40**, 506–11.

Jensen, P.S., Prien, R. & Ryan, N. (1994). Psychopharmacology of child and adolescent depression: Present status and future directions. *Journal of the American Academy of Child and Adolescent Psychiatry*, in press.

Joyce, P. R. & Paykel, E. S. (1989). Predictors of drug response in depression. *Archives of General Psychiatry*, **46**, 89–99.

Kaplan, S. L., Grumbach, M. M. & Aubert, M. L. (1976). The ontogenesis of pituitary hormones and hypothalamic factors in the human foetus: Maturation of the central nervous system regulation of anterior pituitary function. *Recent Progress in Hormone Research*, **32**, 161–243.

Katz, J. L., Boyar, R. M., Roffwarg, H. *et al.* (1978). Weight and circadian luteinizing hormone secretory pattern in anorexia nervosa. *Psychosomatic Medicine*, **40**, 549–67.

Kazdin, A. (1990). Childhood depression. *Journal of Child Psychology and Psychiatry*, **31**, 121–60.

Kendler, K. S., Heath, A., Martin, N. G. & Eaves, L. J. (1986). Symptoms of anxiety and depression in a volunteer twin population. *Archives of General Psychiatry*, **43**, 213–221.

Khan, A. (1987). Heterogeneity of suicidal adolescents. *Journal of the American Academy of Child Adolescent Psychiatry*, **26**, 92–6.

Klee, S. H. & Garfinkel, B. D. (1984). Identification of depression in children and adolescents: The role of the dexamethasone suppression test. *Journal of the American Academy of Child Adolescent Psychiatry*, **23**, 410–15.

Knowles, J. B. & MacLean, A. W. (1990). Age-related changes in sleep in depressed and healthy subjects: A meta-analysis. *Journal of Neuropsychopharmacology*, **3**, 251–9.

Kovacs, M., Feinberg, T. L., Crouse-Novak, M. A. *et al.* (1984*a*). Depressive disorders in childhood. I. A longitudinal prospective study of characteristics and recovery. *Archives of General Psychiatry*, **41**, 229–37.

Kovacs, M., Feinberg, T. L., Crouse-Novak, M. A. *et al.* (1984*b*). Depressive disorders in childhood. II. A longitudinal study of the risk for a subsequent major depression. *Archives of General Psychiatry*, **41**, 643–9.

Kumar, R. & Robson, K. M. (1984). A prospective study of emotional disorders in childbearing women. *British Journal of Psychiatry*, **144**, 35–47.

Kutcher, S., Malkin, D., Silverberg, J. *et al.* (1991). Nocturnal cortisol, thyroid stimulating hormone, and growth hormone secretory profiles in depressed adolescents. *Journal of the American Academy of Child Adolescent Psychiatry*, **30**, 407–13.

Kutcher, S. P. & Marton, P. (1989). Parameters of adolescent depression, a review. *Psychiatric Clinics of North America*, **12**, 895–918.

Langer, G., Heinze, G., Rin, B. & Matussek, N. (1976). Reduced growth hormone response to amphetamine in endogenous depressive patients. *Archives of General Psychiatry*, **33**, 1471–5.

Lerner, R. M. Foch, T. T. (eds) (1987). *Biological-psychosocial interactions in early adolescence: A life-span perspective*. Lawrence Erlbaum Associates, Hillsdale, NJ.

Levine, M. & McAnarney, E. R. (1988). *Early adolescent transitions*. Health Publication, New York.

Lidor, H. G. & Molliver, M. E. (1982). An immunohistochemical study of serotonin neuron development in the rat: Ascending pathways and terminal fields. *Brain Research Bulletin*, **8**, 389–430.

Livingston, R., Reis, C. J., & Ringdahl, I. C. (1984). Abnormal dexamethasone suppression test results in depressed and non-depressed children. *American Journal of Psychiatry*, **141**, 106–7.

Maser, J. D. & Cloninger, C. R. (ed.) (1990). *Comorbidity of mood anxiety disorders*. American Psychiatric Press, Washington, DC.

Melges, F. T., Hamburg, D. A. (1977). Psychological effects of hormonal changes in women. In *Human sexuality in four perspectives* (ed. F. A. Beach), pp. 269–95. Johns Hopkins University Press, Baltimore.

Mendelson, M. (1982). Psychodynamics of depression. In *Handbook of affective disorders* (ed. E. Paykel), pp. 162–73. Guilford Press., New York.

Mendlewicz, J. (1988). Genetics of depression and mania. In *Depression and mania* (ed. A. Georgotas & R. Cancro), pp. 196–212. Elsevier, New York.

Mitchell, J., McCauley, E., Burke, P. *et al.* (1989). Psychopathology in parents of depressed children and adolescents. *Journal of the American Academy of Child and Adolescent Psychiatry*, **28**, 352–7.

Money, J. & Erhardt, A. A. (1972). *Man and woman, boy and girl*. John's Hopkins University Press, Baltimore.

Munday, M. R., Brush, M. G. & Taylor, R. W. (1981). Correlations between progesterone, estradiol, and aldosterone levels in the pre-menstrual syndrome. *Clinical Endocrinology*, **14**, 1–9.

Muñoz, R. F., Ying, Y. W., Perez-Stable, E. J. & Miranda, J. (1993). *The prevention of depression: Research and practice*. Johns Hopkins University Press, Baltimore.

Naylor, M. W., Greden, J. F. & Alessi, N. E. (1990). Plasma dexamethasone levels in children given the dexamethasone suppression test. *Biological Psychiatry*, **27**, 592–600.

Nurnberger, J. I. & Gershon, E. S. (1984). Genetics of affective disorders. In *Neurobiology of mood disorders* (eds. R. M. Post & J. C. Ballenger), (pp. 76–101). Williams & Wilkins, Baltimore.

Paikoff, R. & Brooks-Gunn, J. (1991). Do parent–child relationships change during puberty? *Psychological Bulletin*, **110**, 47–66.

Paikoff, R. L., Brooks-Gunn, J. & Carlton-Ford, S. (1991). Effect of reproductive status changes upon family functioning and well-being of mothers and daughters. *Journal of Early Adolescence*, **11**, 201–20.

Paikoff, R. L., Brooks-Gunn, J. & Warren, M. P. (1991). Effects of girls' hormonal status on depressive and aggressive symptoms over the course of one year. *Journal of Youth and Adolescence*, **20**, 191–215.

Parlee, M. B. (1978). Psychological aspects of menstruation, childbirth, and menopause: An overview with suggestions for further research. In *Psychology of women: Future directions of research* (eds. J. A. Sherman & F. L. Denmark), (pp. 181–238). Psychological Dimensions, New York.

Pepper, G. & Krieger, D. (1985). Hypothalamic-pituitary-adrenal abnormalities in depression: Their possible relation to central mechanisms regulating ACTH release. In *Neurobiology of Mood Disorders* (ed. R. M. Post & J. C. Ballanger), (pp. 245–270). Williams & Wilkins, Baltimore.

Petersen, A. C., Compas, B., Brooks-Gunn, J. *et al.* (1993). Depression in adolescence. *American Psychologist*, **48**, 155–68.

Petersen, A. C., Kennedy, R. E. & Sullivan, P. (1991*a*). Coping with adolescence. In *Adolescent stress: Causes and consequences* (ed. M. E. Colten & S. Gore), (pp. 93–110). Aldine de Gruyter, New York.

Petersen, A. C., Sarigiani, P. A. & Kennedy, R. E. (1991*b*). Adolescent depression:

Why more girls? *Journal of Youth and Adolescence*, **20**, 247–71.

Pfeffer, C. R., Stokes, P., Weiner, A. *et al.* (1989). Psychopathology and plasma cortisol responses to dexamethasone in prepubertal psychiatric in-patients. *Biological Psychiatry*, **267**, 677–89.

Post, R. M., Rubinow, D. R. & Ballenger, J. C. (1984). Conditioning, sensitisation, and kindling: Implications for the course of affective illness. In *Neurobiology of mood disorders* (ed. R. M. Post & J. C. Ballenger), (pp. 432–66). Williams & Wilkins, Baltimore.

Puig-Antich, J. (1986). Psychobiological markers: Effects of age and puberty. In *Depression in young people: Clinical and developmental perspectives* (ed. M. Rutter, C. E. Izard, & P. B. Read), (pp. 341–382), Guilford, New York.

Puig-Antich, J. (1987). Sleep and neuroendocrine correlates of affective illness in childhood and adolescence. *Journal of Adolescent Health Care*, **8**, 505–29.

Puig-Antich, J., Novacenko, H., Davies, M. *et al.* (1984*a*). Growth hormone secretion in prepubertal major depressive children. I. Sleep related plasma concentrations during a depressive episode. *Archives of General Psychiatry*, **41**, 455–60.

Puig-Antich, J., Goetz, R., Davies, M. *et al.* (1984*b*). Growth hormone secretion in prepubertal major depressive children. II. Sleep related plasma concentrations during a depressive episode. *Archives of General Psychiatry*, **41**, 463–6.

Puig-Antich, J., Davies, M., Novacenko, H. *et al.* (1984*c*). Growth hormone secretion in prepubertal major depressive children. III. Response to insulin induced hypoglycemia in a drug-free, fully recovered clinical state. *Archives of General Psychiatry*, **41**, 471–5.

Puig-Antich, J., Goetz, R., Davies, M. *et al.* (1984*d*). Growth hormone secretion in prepubertal major depressive children. IV. Sleep related plasma concentrations in a drug-free fully recovered clinical state. *Archives of General Psychiatry*, **41**, 479–83.

Rabkin, J., Quitkin, F., Stewart, J. *et al.* (1983). Dexamethasone suppression test with mild to moderately depressed outpatients. *American Journal of Psychiatry*, **140**, 926–8.

Reinherz, H. Z., Stewart-Berghauer, G., Pamkiz, B. *et al.* (1989). The relationship of early risk and current mediators to depressive symptomatology in adolescence. *Journal of the American Academy of Child and Adolescent Psychiatry*, **28**, 942–7.

Reiter, E. O. (1987). Neuroendocrine control processes: pubertal onset and depression. *Journal of Adolescent Health Care*, **8**, 479–91.

Reiter, E. O. & Grumbach, M. M. (1982). Neuroendocrine control mechanisms and the onset of puberty. *Annual Review of Physiology*, **44**, 595–613.

Reynolds, C. F., Gillen J. C. & Kupfer, D. J. (1987). Sleep and affective disorders. In *Psychopharmacology: The third generation of progress* (ed. H. Y. Meltzer), (pp. 647–54). Raven Press, New York.

Roberts, R. E., Lewinsohn, P. M. & Seeley, J. R. (1991). Screening for adolescent depression: A comparison of depression scales. *Journal of the American Academy of Child and Adolescent Psychiatry*, **30**, 58–66.

Robins, D. R., Alessi, N. E., Yanchyschyn, G. W. & Colfer, M. V. (1982). Preliminary report on the dexamethasone suppression test in adolescents. *American Journal of Psychiatry*, **14**, 1414–18.

Ruble, D. N. & Brooks-Gunn, J. (1979, June). Menstrual myths. *Medical Aspects of Human Sexuality*, 110–15.

Ruble, D. N. & Brooks-Gunn, J. (1987). Perceptions of menstrual and pre-menstrual symptoms: Self definitional processes at menarche. In *Pre-menstrual syndrome: Ethical and legal implications in a biomedical perspective* (ed. B. E. Ginsberg & B. F. Carter), (pp. 237–51). Plenum Press, New York.

Rutter, M. (1980). The long-term effects of early experience. *Developmental Medicine and Child Neurology*, **22**, 800–15.

Rutter, M. (1986). The developmental psychopathology of depression: Issues and perspectives. In *Depression in young people: Developmental and clinical perspectives* (ed. M. Rutter, C. E. Tizard & P. B. Read), (pp. 3–32). The Guilford Press, New York.

Rutter, M., Graham, P., Chadwick, O. F. D. & Yule, W. (1976). Adolescent turmoil: Fact or fiction? *Journal of Child Psychology and Psychiatry*, **17**, 35–56.

Rutter, M., Izard, C. E. & Read, P. B. (ed.). (1986). *Depression in young people: Developmental and clinical perspectives*. Guilford, New York.

Ryan, N. D., Birmaher, B., Perel, J. M. *et al.* (1990). Neuroendocrine response to L-5 hydroxytryptophan challenge in prepubertal major depression: Depressed versus normal children (unpublished manuscript).

Ryan, N. D., Dahl, R. E., Perel, J. M. *et al.* (1994). Three growth hormone tests in prepubertal depression: I: Depressed versus normal children. *Archives of General Psychiatry*, in press.

Ryan, N. D., Puig-Antich, J., Rabinovich, H. *et al.* (1988). Growth hormone response to desmethlimipramine in depressed and suicidal adolescents. *Journal of Affective Disorders*, **15**, 323–37.

Sachar, E. J. (1975). Neuroendocrine abnormalities in depressive illness. In *Topics in psychoendocrinology* (ed. E. J. Sachar), (pp. 182–201). Grune & Stratton, New York.

Sachar, E. J., Hellman, L., Roffwarg, H. P. *et al.* (1973). Disrupted 24-hour pattern of cortisol secretion in psychotic depression. *Archives of General Psychiatry*, **28**, 19–25.

Sachar, E., Puig-Antich, J. & Ryan, N. (1985). Three tests of cortisol secretion in adult endogenous depressives. *Acta Psychiatrica Scandinavica*, **71**, 1–8.

Sack, D. A., Rosenthal, N. E., Parry, B. L. & Wehr, T. A. (1987). Biological rhythms in psychiatry. In *Psychopharmacology: The third generation of progress* (ed. H. T. Meltzer), (pp. 669–85). Raven Press, New York.

Seiffe-Krenke, I. (1993*a*). Family climate and depressive mood in adolescence: The relative contribution of family and peer relationships.

Seiffe-Krenke, I. (1993*b*) Coping behaviour in normal and clinical samples: more similarities than differences. *Journal of Adolescence*, **16**, 285–303.

Shelton, R. C., Hollon, S. D., Purdon, S. E. & Loosen, P. T. (1991). Biological and psychological aspects of depression. *Behaviour Therapy*, **22**, 201–28.

Siever, L. J., & Davis, K. L. (1985). Overview: Toward a dysregulation hypothesis of depression. *American Journal of Psychiatry*, **142**, 1017–31.

Siever, L. J., Uhde, T. W., Jimerson, D. C. *et al.* (1984). Plasma cortisol responses to clonidine in depressed patients and controls. *Archives of General Psychiatry*, **41**, 63–71.

Siever, L. J., Uhde, T. W., Silberman, E. K. *et al.* (1982). The growth hormone response to clinidine as a probe of nonadrenergic receptor responsiveness in affective disorder patients and controls. *Psychiatry Research*, **6**, 171–83.

Simmons, R. G., Burgeson, R. & Carlton-Ford, S. (1987). The impact of cumulative change in early adolescence. *Child Development*, **58**, 1220–34.

Spencer, M. B. & Dornbusch, S. M. (1990). Challenges in studying minority youth. In *At the threshold: The developing adolescent* (ed. S. Feldman & G. Elliott), pp. 123–46. Harvard University Press, Cambridge.

Sroufe, A. & Rutter, M. (1984). The domain of developmental psychopathology. *Journal of Child Development*, **55**, 17–29.

Strober, M. (1983). *Follow-up of affective disorder patients*. Paper presented at the

Annual meetings of the American Psychiatric Association, New York.

Strober, M., Burroughs, J. & Salkin, B. *et al.* (1994). Ancestral secondary cases of psychiatric illness in adolescents with mania, depression, schizophrenia and conduct disorder. *Biological Psychiatry*, in press.

Susman, E. J., Inoff-Germain, G., Nottlemann, E. D. *et al.* (1987*a*). Hormones, emotional dispositions, and aggressive attributes in young adolescents. *Child Development*, **58**, 1114–34.

Susman, E. J., Nottelmann, E. D., Inoff-Germain, G. *et al.* (1987*b*). Hormonal influences on aspects of psychological development during adolescence. *Journal of Adolescent Health Care*, **8**, 492–504.

Targum, S. & Capodanno, A. (1983). The dexamethasone suppression test in adolescent psychiatric inpatients. *American Journal of Psychiatry*, **140**, 589–92.

Vetulani, J. & Sulser, F. (1975). Action of various antidepressant treatments reduces reactivity of nonadrenergic cyclic AMP-generating system in limbic forebrain. *Nature*, **257**, 495–6.

Warren, M. P. & Brooks-Gunn, J. (1989). Mood and behaviour at adolescence: Evidence for hormonal factors. *Journal of Clinical Endocrinology and Metabolism*, **69**, 77–83.

Waterman, G. S., Ryan, N. D., Puig-Antich, J. *et al.* (1991). Hormonal responses to dexamphetamine in depressed and normal adolescents. *Journal of the American Academy of Child and Adolescent Psychiatry*, **30**, 415–22.

Watson, D. & Kendall, P. C. (1989). Common differentiating features of anxiety and depression: Current findings and future directions. In *Anxiety and depression: Distinctive and overlapping features* (ed. P. C. Kendall & D. Watson), (pp. 493–508). Academic Press, New York.

Watson, D. & Tellegen, A. (1985). Toward a consensual structure of mood. *Psychological Bulletin*, **98**, 219–35.

Wehr, T. A. & Goodwin, F. K. (1981). Biological rhythms and psychiatry. In *The American Handbook of Psychiatry* (ed. S. H. Arieti & K. H. Brodie), (pp. 46–74). Basic Books, New York.

Weissman, M. M., Gammon, D., John, K. *et al.* (1987). Children of depressed parents: Increased psychopathology and early onset of major depression. *Archives of General Psychiatry*, **44**, 847–53.

Weissman, M. M., Gershon, E. S., Kidd, K. K. *et al.* (1984). Psychiatric disorders in the relatives of probands with affective disorders. *Archives of General Psychiatry*, **41**, 13–21.

Weller, E. B., Weller, B. Z., Fristad, M. A. & Preskorn, S. H. (1984). The dexamethasone suppression test in hospitalised prepubertal depressed children. *American Journal of Psychiatry*, **141**, 290–1.

Wender, P. H. (1971). *Minimal brain dysfunction in children*. Wiley-Interscience, New York.

Wender, P. H., Kety, S. S., Rosenthal, P. *et al.* (1986). Psychiatric disorders in the biological and adoptive families of adopted individuals with affective disorder. *Archives of General Psychiatry*, **43**, 923–9.

5

Childhood depression: Clinical phenomenology and classification

Israel Kolvin

THE CONCEPT OF DEPRESSION IN CHILDHOOD

The contribution of adult psychiatry to the concept of depression in childhood

In a clinical sense the term 'depression' denotes an illness characterised by a change in mood that is persistent and sufficiently severe for it to be labelled a disorder. The focus of this chapter is the clinical phenomenology and descriptive classification of unipolar disorders of childhood. Research into the nature and characteristics of depression in adults has however provided an important framework for much of the recent investigations into childhood depression.

In adult psychiatry, much research attention has focused on the classification of depression. Two major distinctions have emerged – first, between bipolar and unipolar affective disorders and second, between psychotic (or endogenous) and neurotic (or reactive) depression (Paykel & Priest, 1992; Ramana & Paykel, 1992).

Using multivariate analysis methods, the Newcastle school asserted that two separate depressive syndromes could be distinguished in adult patients – neurotic (reactive) and psychotic (endogenous) (Kiloh & Garside, 1963; Carney, Roth & Garside, 1965). This distinction within unipolar depression has not been replicated (Kendell, 1968, 1976). The term 'endogenous' has however come to reflect, clinically, a more severe and persistent depressive disorder possibly unrelated to environmental adversities (diagnostic criteria include somatic symptoms of anorexia or

111

weight loss, insomnia, early morning wakening and diurnal variation of mood, severe guilt, hopelessness and psychomotor retardation or agitation (Ramana & Paykel, 1992)). By contrast, neurotic or reactive depression is considered clinically, to be a milder disorder and possibly reactive to environmental adversities (accompanied by anxiety, initial insomnia, self-pity rather than self-blame, and complaints of anorexia rather than complaints of weight loss (Ramana & Paykel, 1992)).

A series of criteria for the classification of depression was subsequently proposed by Feighner and colleagues at St Louis (Feighner *et al.*, 1972). These criteria were not dependent on the presence or absence of environmental events. Spitzer and colleagues (Spitzer, Endicott & Robins, 1978) adopted and further refined these proposals when producing the Research Diagnostic Criteria for the diagnosis of depression. For these purposes 'a diagnostic category has to be supported by specific descriptive criteria that specify characteristics that lead to making the diagnosis (inclusion criteria) and characteristics that lead to not making the diagnosis (exclusion criteria)' (Ramana & Paykel, 1992). The above are the bases of the DSM-III-R Classification, which offers strict diagnostic criteria that depend primarily on symptoms and course of the disease; it is a system with a satisfactory inter-observer reliability. In addition to major depressive disorders, which are either single or recurrent, this classification includes dysthymia, which is a persistent, but fluctuating mild form of depression.

In ICD-10 there are similarly strict operationally defined diagnostic criteria. The main features have been described by Ramana & Paykel (1992) as follows: the single episode is distinguished from recurrent disorders and there is also a group of persistent affective disorders; three grades of severity are noted – mild, moderate and severe. The term 'somatic syndrome' indicates the presence of endogenous or biological symptoms; the term 'psychotic' the presence of delusions, hallucinations or depressive stupor; finally, dysthymia has been included as a persistent affective disorder.

Thus, in adulthood the clinical picture of a unipolar depressive syndrome or disorder is likely to vary (Gelder, Gath & Mayou, 1990). The core features are many and include: low mood (dysphoria), lack of interest, lack of enjoyment (anhedonia), reduced energy, psychomotor retardation, irritability and agitation, negative cognitions such as thoughts of helplessness and worthlessness, sleep disturbance, diurnal variation of mood, loss of appetite, loss of weight, and hypochondriacal complaints (Gelder *et al.*, 1990). Other psychiatric symptoms include depersonalisation, obsessional symptoms, phobias and also complaints of poor memory.

Developmental influences

In contrast to adults, children may not be capable of *experiencing* and/or *reporting* the symptoms thought to be representative of major depressive disorders (Kovacs, 1986). These include not only such characteristics as dysphoric mood and anhedonia, but especially negative cognitions of hopelessness, worthlessness and self-denigration, and feelings of guilt and self-blame. Kovacs (1986) has argued that many children may be unable to differentiate between basic emotions, neither have they an ability to give an account of their presence and duration. Indeed some authorities argue that it is only in the later primary school years that children begin to reveal thoughts of self-denigration and feelings of shame (Kovacs, 1986). It is probable that despair and a sense of hopelessness do not fully surface before adolescence – a stage when formal operational thinking emerges (Verhulst, 1989). Thus the pattern of depressive symptoms is likely to vary according to age and stage of development of the child or young adolescent. This indicates that there may be a difference in the clinical expression of depression at different ages. (An alternative possibility, that there are independent depressive syndromes or disorders at different ages and/or stages of development appears unlikely, but has yet to be adequately investigated.) Finally, it is now well known that by school-age children are reliable and valid informants of their own current mental state. They are therefore more able than their parents, to provide an account of their depressive symptoms (Barrett *et al.*, 1991).

Misery and sadness can occur as symptoms in children of all ages. It is only over the last 20 years however that the concepts of depressive syndromes in childhood have evolved (Carlson & Cantwell, 1980*a*, *b*). The diagnosis of a major depressive disorder as a prolonged condition associated with impairment of function has been particularly prominent. In addition to the topic of masked depression, other fundamental current issues include the validity of diagnostic criteria, developmental and age issues, how best classifying depression in childhood should proceed and the importance of psychiatric comorbidity.

Masked depression

The theme of one disorder masking or concealing another is not new in child psychiatry and dates from the writings of Glaser (1968), Cytryn & McKnew (1972) and Cytryn, McKnew & Bunney (1980). These incorporate two allied concepts, the first of which is **masked depression**. This is depression without mood change where a wide range of symptoms, including hyperactivity, delinquency, aggressive behaviour and learning disorders are the presenting clinical features. The second concept is that of **depressive equivalents**. Here the characteristic features are somatic complaints, such as aches and pains which can occur in 'school phobia', also considered by some as a depressive equivalent. It has been demonstrated that school-age children with so-called 'masked ' depression do, in fact, show overt depressive signs and may report depressed symptoms (Carlson & Cantwell, 1980a,b). The clinical features of depression may however be more covert or primitive in younger children (McConville, Boag & Purohit, 1973; Zeitlin, 1986). (This theme is addressed in the next section.) More recently, the Newcastle group have asserted that Cytryn et al. (1980) and Glaser (1968) were correct in suggesting that depression was often undetected (Kolvin et al., 1991). The Newcastle group did not, however, find any evidence to support the notion that depressive conditions may manifest in a different way. This group also asserted that depression remains undetected and poorly delineated, because of inadequate techniques of clinical assessment. Some consider it possible to diagnose major depression in childhood using criteria identical to those used in adults (Spitzer et al., 1978; Puig-Antich, 1980); others feel that different considerations should apply to children – particularly in those under 8 years old. Again, aspects of this theme are tackled in the next section.

DEPRESSION AS A SYMPTOM, SYNDROME OR DISORDER

Several authors have previously distinguished between symptoms and syndromes of depression in childhood (Carlson & Cantwell, 1980; Hamilton, 1982; Kolvin, Berney & Bhate, 1984; Kolvin et al., 1991). In other words sadness is not synonymous with depression. Thus, while dysphoria is commonly viewed as a necessary characteristic of depression, it is not a sufficient criterion in itself; for instance, sadness and misery are commonly observed both in clinical and non-clinical child populations. Verhulst, Akkerhuis & Althaus (1985) report that parents of clinically referred children describe a high rate of depressive affect, ranging from over 20% in pre-school children and over 40% of those in primary schools to 50% in those in secondary schools, with the rates for boys being marginally lower. The respective rates in the non-referred population were 5%, 6% and 9%, for girls; again, the rates for boys were marginally lower. Much higher rates are recorded in school population surveys in the United States.

There is some confusion about the distinction between syndromes and disorders. Nurcombe *et al.* (1989) have pointed out that the term depression may be used to refer to a symptom of affect or mood, a syndrome consisting of a cluster of depressive symptoms, or a disorder reflecting a category of individuals with a set of clinical features associated with impairment of function. Carlson & Cantwell (1980*b*), assert that the status of a depressive disorder should be distinguished from other depressive states by differences in environmental factors, family patterns of illness, natural history, biological factors and response to treatment.

Sub-classification of depression

A crucial issue, from both a clinical and a theoretical viewpoint, is how depression in childhood should be sub-classified. In adult psychiatry, this is a notoriously complex area and, even if depression in childhood is clinically similar, classification problems would be compounded by issues of child development.

There are two ways of defining depressive sub-syndromes in childhood. The first is the classical clinical approach where clinical pictures are drawn, utilising an inductive method combined with clinical judgement. In this way new sub-categories of depression can be defined and complement the general profile of depression. This necessary first step needs to be validated by empirical research. For example, it has not yet been established that depression in childhood is a homogeneous syndrome or disorder. The second method is a statistical approach using multivariate procedures such as exploratory factor analysis. In the latter it is hypothesised that a set of variates exist that account substantially for any interrelationships between symptoms (Maxwell, 1977). Hence, theoretically, exploratory factor analysis is capable of identifying those symptoms (and perhaps other features) with greatest validity because they will be grouped in characteristic patterns. This view is consistent with the hypothesis that there is one general factor representing *all the symptoms, as well as additional differentiating bipolar factors.* More often, Principal Component Analysis (PCA) is widely used for exploring a co-variance structure; it is a useful technique in non-standard situations where the data may not fit classical assumptions of multi-normality (Taylor, 1979). It is hoped that the derived components will represent more basic variability in the data than in the observed variates (Maxwell, 1977). Using PCA, the first few rotated components 'often give a robust identification of major trends in the data' (Taylor, 1979). For classification purposes, varimax rotation may help to clarify which symptoms are related to particular factors or components. It is possible, however, that in the process their variances may be greatly inflated by error (Maxwell, 1977).

If the sample is of sufficient size, PCA can be complemented with a further technique, cluster analysis. Cluster procedures are a way of identifying those subsets of individuals whose behavioural features cluster together, (i.e. which have much in common within each cluster, but little in common between the clusters (Aldenderfer & Blashfield, 1984)). Although the cluster analysis approach is theoretically sound there is still debate about the variability and meaning of the number of clusters identified (Kolvin *et al.*, 1991).

Kolvin and colleagues (1991) factor-analysed mental state data obtained from interviews using a modified version of the Kiddie-SADS. The subjects were clinically referred children, aged 9 to 16. Data from interviews carried out independently with both the child and their parents were used for the analysis. A number of components emerged, but only results concerning depressive syndromes are given here. The PCA revealed an '**endogenous**'-type depression component composed of the features of feeling depressed, anhedonia, increased fatigue and psychomotor retardation, and a **depressive cognitions** component accompanied by thoughts of suicide. The two emergent components overlapped extensively those identified by Ryan *et al.* (1987) in their Pittsburgh study.

A further cluster analysis also identified two clusters, negative cognitions and endogenous depression, with features markedly similar to the PCA findings. The depressive cognitions cluster consisted of self-denigration, hopelessness and guilt, irritability, suicide and a sense of anxiety, fear and anger; the endogenous depression cluster consisted of anhedonia, hopelessness, withdrawal, dysphoric mood, worrying, insomnia, loss of appetite, lack of energy, suicidal ideation, somatic complaints, slowing of thoughts, anxiety and school refusal (details of these analyses are available in Kolvin *et al.*, 1991).

Verhulst and colleagues carried out a similar factor analysis using data from the Child Behaviour Check List completed by samples of boys and girls aged 6 to 11 and 12 to 16 in a province of Holland (Verhulst *et al.*, 1985). These authors reported the presence of an empirically derived depressive syndrome in 6 to 11-year-olds, the main features that emerged being those of feeling unloved, unhappy sad depressed mood, feelings of worthlessness, feeling persecuted, feeling lonely, worrying, fears of schools, suicidal talk, suspiciousness, feelings of guilt and obsessions. However, in the 12 to 16-year-old sample the symptoms of depression seemed to vary and no distinctive depressive syndrome emerged. It would seem, therefore, that the findings from multivariate data analysis are influenced to some extent by the method by which data were obtained (such as self-rating compared with direct interview), the age and sex of the subjects, the population under scrutiny and the type of multivariate analysis that is employed.

It is important to note the similarities between cross-national studies and also with adult studies. For instance, Ryan *et al.* (1987) at Pittsburgh reported meaningful components (factors) that proved to be similar for both children and adolescents and that included 'endogenous' depression and depression with negative cognitions. This pattern proved to be the case in the Newcastle studies also. However, the Dutch study (Verhulst *et al.*, 1985) did not replicate the presence of a depressive syndrome in the senior school sample. Further, the Pittsburgh research cluster analysis was rather inconclusive, with the clusters not indicating any precise pattern of symptoms. However, as the Newcastle workers identified symptom clusters that proved to be discrete, it is likely that the basis of the discrepancy across these studies resides in the methods that have been employed.

The distinction between negative cognitions and endogenous depressive factors in the Pittsburgh (Ryan *et al.*, 1987) and Newcastle studies (Kolvin *et al.*, 1991) suggests that depression syndromes in childhood may differ in their nature and characteristics from those in adults (Kiloh & Garside 1963; Carney *et al.*, 1965). Thus both the Dutch and UK child studies support the notion that a number of the depressive symptoms considered to be 'characteristic' in adults emerge as less so in childhood: for instance, loss of weight, diurnal variation of mood and psychomotor retardation are less pronounced in childhood than in

117

adulthood (Verhulst, 1989; Kolvin *et al.*, 1991); further, whereas initial insomnia is frequently reported in childhood, terminal insomnia is reported less often (Ryan *et al.*, 1987; Carlson & Kashani, 1988; Kolvin *et al.*, 1991). In contrast, somatic symptoms are often reported by younger children with depression (Carlson & Kashani, 1988). It is essential that more is known about the origins, nature, duration and course of these sub-syndromes in child populations.

Mixed depression – comorbidity

Comorbidity is the concurrent presence of two or more disorders greater than would be expected by chance alone. As already indicated, the pattern of non-depressive comorbid disorders (such as phobic anxiety or conduct disorder) varies between depressed children and adolescents. These comorbid conditions suggest that depression in childhood is a clinically heterogeneous phenomenon (Ryan *et al.*, 1987, Kolvin *et al.*, 1992).

For example, Puig-Antich & Gittelman (1982) reported that one-third of boys who are diagnosed as having a major depressive disorder could also be diagnosed as having a conduct disorder. Similarly, Carlson & Cantwell (1980*a*) found that 50% of children diagnosed in their clinical survey as having affective disorders had another diagnosis, most commonly hyperactivity (25%) and anorexia (11%). In the Newcastle Child Depression project, which assessed 275 successive clinic referrals, some 25% had a depressive disorder (Kolvin *et al.*, 1991); while a major depressive disorder was common in this clinical population it presented *alone* in only 11%; the remainder presented with one or more comorbid disorders (Kolvin *et al.*, 1991). Thus about one-third of the depressed group proved to be phobic, one-half had a neurotic disorder and one-fifth a conduct disorder.

A high rate of comorbid depression in children presenting with school phobia has also been described (Kolvin *et al.*, 1984).

Kolvin and colleagues (Kolvin *et al.*, 1991) have argued that these findings do not support a single major category of classification for major depression in childhood and adolescence. Indeed such a classification may merely obscure the wider psychopathological picture of depressive disorders in this age group. This may be true even where the diagnosis is that of a conduct or phobic disorder. Hence, it is essential that whatever the predominant disorder, the assessor should check for associated disorders. In particular depression should be looked for in non-depressive presentations. Kolvin *et al.*, (1991) argued that, if such an assessment is omitted, depression may simply remain undetected because of diagnostic ideology, or may be concealed by other symptoms through an inadequate technique of clinical diagnosis. Cytryn *et al.* (1980) were therefore correct when suggesting that depression may be hidden but concluded erroneously that depressive disorders could manifest in a different form. So-called 'masked' depressive disorders do show overt depression (Carlson & Cantwell, 1980*a,b*; Rutter, 1988). All the above research underlines the importance of assessing for depression accurately, regardless of the presenting complaint (Kolvin *et al.*, 1991).

Diagnostic schemas

A range of diagnostic schemas have emerged from the different centres, all to a greater or lesser extent addressing the above issues. Recent work provides some information about the validity of these schemas and the extent to which they agree, or disagree, with each other. The main schemas so far are those developed in the United States by Puig-Antich & Chambers (1978) and by Weinberg *et al.* (1973), and in the UK by Kolvin *et al.* (1991).

The diagnostic schemas incorporate different criteria. For instance, in a recent study the Newcastle group used the **Standard Psychiatric Assessment** (SPI) (Goldberg *et al.*, 1970), which is a semi-structured schedule designed to study psychiatric disorders in adults in a community setting. It has a number of precise probes as well as clear-cut definition of symptoms and can provide ratings on a range of clinical disorders. For these purposes it was appropriately modified by the inclusion of an introductory interview; interviewers were encouraged to use phraseology and concepts appropriate to the child's cognitive level and stage of psychological development, and in this way accommodating the different abilities of children to give accounts about themselves. These workers reported that the instrument showed satisfactory reliability over both the pre-pubertal and adolescent periods, provided that it was administered by experienced child psychiatrists. In summary, Kolvin *et al.* (1991) reported that the SPI can be employed, using concepts and definitions of disorders more usually geared to adults, allowing both a clinical diagnosis of depression and rating of severity of disorder. Thus, major depressive episodes can be identified that are relatively discrete and associated with a specified number of symptoms of the depressive syndrome.

However, the most commonly used and validated schedule in assessing depression in children is the **Kiddie-SADS**. It is essentially a modification of the Schedule for Affective Disorders and Schizophrenia (Spitzer *et al.*, 1978) and has been employed with children between 6- and 17 years of age (Orvaschel *et al.*, 1982; Chambers *et al.*, 1985). This is a reliable instrument for measuring symptoms of depression and conduct disorders, although ratings of anxiety disorders have not been as consistent.

The schema devised by Weinberg *et al.* (1973) is one of the better-known of the earlier schemas; it offers a list of primary and secondary symptoms, based on the criteria for diagnosis of depression in adulthood (Feighner *et al.*, 1972). To be diagnosed as depressed, children need to display primary symptoms of dysphoric mood and self deprecation, plus two of a further eight symptoms. In the original version there was no guideline as to duration or severity of symptomatology. This gave rise to problems of broadness of the inclusion criteria and hence high rates of depression in the populations in which it was used.

One of the newer instruments is the Newcastle Depression Inventory (Kolvin *et al.*, 1984, 1989, 1991, 1992), which has been upgraded and modified. The inventory has themes borrowed from the Kiddie-SADS but with the ratings of symptoms reorganised so that they are scored on an ordinal scale to reflect severity (1, 2, 3 and 4), with subsequent recoding on a binary scale (0, 0, 1, 1). The technique allows either categorical rating of depression, based on a clinical algorithm, or a dimension of severity of depression, based on the summation of the specified criteria. Alternatively, it can be used for diagnosis, primarily being guided by DSM-III diagnostic categories.

Kolvin *et al.* (1991) have reported that, once the severity of diagnostic criteria had been taken into account, substantial agreement was found between such different schemas as the Weinberg and the Newcastle, each being equally valid in relation to an independent clinical assessment. Further, as all the diagnostic criteria are rated on ordinal scales, summation allows the emergence of quantitative variations within qualitatively distinct disorders (Rutter, 1986; Kolvin *et al.*, 1991).

Diagnostic algorithms

The distinction between symptoms and syndromes of depression in adulthood has been complemented by the specification of diagnostic criteria for depressive disorders by Feighner *et al.* (1972) and Spitzer *et al.* (1978). In a similar way, over the last decade clinicians in the child and adolescent psychiatric field have explored the distinction between symptoms and syndromes and such work has facilitated the development of diagnostic interviews or checklists. One such checklist that has emerged is that of Kolvin *et al.* (1992); its utility is that it not only allows a discrimination between depressed and non-depressed children attending a consulting child psychiatric clinic, but also it includes features of the two sub-types of childhood depression – 'endogenous' and 'negative cognitions'. The latter work focused on a brief inventory that had been developed previously in relation to distinction between school phobics who were depressed and not depressed (Kolvin *et al.*, 1984). It has been used as a research instrument and was intended to provide a reasonably rapid assessment of the presence of depression with a satisfactory degree of reliability and validity.

The questionnaire was intended primarily as a clinical interview instrument and the updated version also provides an algorithm for diagnosis of depressive syndromes of varying severity. These authors (Kolvin *et al.*, 1992) have provided evidence that dysphoria is not a mandatory criterion for childhood depression; this supports the view, previously mentioned, that although dysphoria is commonly viewed as a necessary characteristic of depression, it is not a sufficient criterion in itself (Hamilton, 1982; Rutter, 1988).

The extended questionnaire consists of 13 items and, although only slightly longer than the original, has many advantages. First, the constituent items offer a better representation of the different factors or clusters than the original scale; this is especially true of those reflecting depressive cognitions on the one hand and endogenous depression on the other. Second, there is good evidence of validity, although it could be argued that the validation levels may have been inflated by the methods used to select items. The items that have been identified and selected include the following:

1. dysphoric mood
2. anhedonia
3. feeling unloved
4. weeping
5. loss of energy
6. loss of interest
7. loss of appetite
8. lack of concentration
9. sense of emptiness

10. depersonalisation
11. suicidal ideation
12. depressive thoughts
13. sense of hopelessness

This brief scale is likely to make a useful contribution to symptomatic diagnosis of either marked or moderate depression, utilising a diagnostic algorithm, especially when used by a less experienced clinician. In the circumstances the inventory is used with a cut-off of 5 on a binary scale, for symptomatic diagnosis of marked depression, or with a cut-off of 4, for moderate depression, including endogenous depression.

The use of binary and ordinal scales in diagnosing depression merits further comment. It is essential that the clinician bears in mind the distinction between substantial and marginal symptomatology, to avoid giving equal importance to a large number of symptoms, some of which may have little diagnostic significance. For instance, when using a 4-point ordinal scale, a subject scoring 2 on each of the 13 items would score 26 but is unlikely to be depressed, whereas a subject scoring 4 on 4 items and only 1 on each of the other nine items will have a total of 25 points, and could well be depressed. Thus, the simple summation of scores when using an ordinal scale provides a good representation of overall severity, but it could be misleading diagnostically; hence, a binary system of re-coding is recommended as an essential supplement to the use of an ordinal scale, as it is likely to contribute to the valid discrimination of depression.

Finally, a fundamental drawback of the algorithm approach (and this is true for self-rating scales also) is the inability to incorporate criteria of impairment or of psychosocial or behavioural handicap. Such features may contribute to improving the reliability and validity of diagnosis (Weissmann, 1990).

SUMMARY AND CONCLUSIONS

The advent of reliable and valid measures of present mental state has greatly advanced our understanding of the phenomenology major (unipolar) depression. It is clear that children as young as 8 years (and perhaps somewhat younger) are capable of reporting their feelings and thoughts. It is also clear that in some cases of depression parents are unaware of their child's symptoms. Direct interviewing of the child provides a more accurate assessment of the child's mental state than interviewing of a parent. Parental information may be informative, especially for the less subjective and more externalising symptoms. The features of depression are similar to those found in adults. There are, however, important differences that suggest developmental influences on the nature and characteristics of depression in young people. Further research into the meaning of these developmental influences on the expression of depressive syndromes is required. Finally much more needs to be discovered about the natural history and outcome of depression. Exactly how the clinical features alter with clinical course and outcome remains unknown.

REFERENCES

Aldenderfer, M. S. & Blashfield, R. K. (1984). *Cluster analysis.* Sage Publications, London.

Barrett, L. M., Berney, T. P., Bhate, S. *et al.* (1991). Diagnosing childhood depression. Who should be interviewed – parent or child? *British Journal of Psychiatry,* **159** (Suppl. 11), 22–7.

Carney, M. W. P., Roth, M. & Garside, R. F. (1965). The diagnosis of depressive syndromes and prediction of ECT response. *British Journal of Psychiatry,* **111**, 659–74.

Carlson, G. A. & Cantwell, D. P. (1980a). Unmasking masked depression in children and adolescents. *American Journal of Psychiatry,* **137**, 445–9.

Carlson, G. A. & Cantwell, D. P. (1980b). A survey of depressive symptoms and disorder in a child psychiatric population. *Journal of Child Psychology and Psychiatry,* **21**, 19–25.

Carlson G. A. & Kashani, J.H . (1988). Phenomenology of major depressive disorder from childhood through adulthood: Analysis of three studies. *American Journal of Psychiatry,* **145**, 1222–5.

Chambers, W. J., Puig-Antich, J., Hirsch, M. *et al.* (1985). The assessment of affective disorders in children and adolescents by semi-structured interview. *Archives of General Psychiatry,* **42**, 696–702.

Cytryn, L. & McKnew, D. H. (1972). Proposed classification of childhood depression. *American Journal of Psychiatry,* **129**, 149–55.

Cytryn, L., McKnew, D. H. & Bunney, W. E. (1980) Diagnosis of depression in children: a reassessment. *American Journal of Psychiatry,* **137**, 22–5.

Feighner, J. P., Robins, E, Guze, S. B. *et al.* (1972). Diagnostic criteria for use in psychiatric research. *Archives of General Psychiatry,* **26**, 57–63.

Gelder, M. G., Gath D. & Mayou, R (1990). *Oxford text book of psychiatry.* Oxford University Press, Oxford.

Glaser, K. (1968). Masked depression in children and adolescents. *Annual Progress in Child Psychiatry and Child Development,* **1**, 345–55.

Goldberg, D. P., Cooper, B., Eastwood, M. R. *et al.* (1970). A standardised psychiatric interview suitable for use in community surveys. *British Journal of Preventative Social Medicine,* **24**, 18–27.

Hamilton, M. (1982). Symptoms and assessment of depression. In *Handbook of affective disorders* (ed. E. S. Paykel), pp. 3–11. Churchill-Livingstone, Edinburgh.

Kendell R. E. (1968). *The classification of depressive illnesses.* Oxford University Press, London.

Kendell R. E. (1976). The classification of depressions: a review of contemporary confusion. *British Journal Psychiatry* **129**, 15–28.

Kiloh, L. & Garside, R. F. (1963). The independence of neurotic depression and endogenous depression. *British Journal of Psychiatry*, **109**, 451–63.

Kolvin, I., Barrett, L., Berney, T. P. *et al.* (1989). The Newcastle child depression project: studies in the diagnosis and classification of childhood depression. In *Contemporary themes in psychiatry* – A tribute to Sir Martin Roth (ed. K. Davison & A. Kerr), pp. 149–55. Gaskell, London.

Kolvin, I., Berney, T. P. & Bhate, S. (1984). Classification and diagnosis of depression in school phobia. *British Journal of Psychiatry*, **145**, 347–57.

Kolvin, I., Berney, T. P., Barrett, L. M. & Bhate S. (1992). Development and evaluation of a diagnostic algorithm for depression in childhood. *European Child and Adolescent Psychiatry*, **1** (2), 1–13.

Kolvin, I., Barrett, L. M., Bhate, S. R., *et al.* (1991) Issues in the diagnosis and classification of childhood depression. *British Journal of Psychiatry*, **159** (suppl. 11), 9–21.

Kovacs, M. (1986). A developmental perspective on methods and measures in the assessment of depressive disorders: the clinical interview. In *Depression in young people: Developmental and clinical perspectives* (ed. M. Rutter, C. Izard & P. Read), pp. 435–65. Guilford Press, New York.

McConville, B. J., Boag, L. C. & Purohit, A. (1973). Three types of childhood depression. *Canadian Psychiatric Association Journal*, **18**, 133–8.

Maxwell, A. E. (1977). *Multivariate analysis in behavioural research*. Chapman & Hall, London.

Nurcombe, B., Seifer, R., Scioli, A. *et al.* (1989). Is major depressive disorder in adolescence a distinct diagnostic entity? *Journal of the American Academy of Childhood & Adolescent Psychiatry*, **22**, 333–42.

Orvaschel, H., Thompson, W. D., Belanger, A. *et al.* (1982). Comparison of the family history method to direct interview. *Journal of Affective Disorders*, **4**, 49–59.

Paykel E. S. & Priest, R. G. (1992). Recognition and Management of Expression in General Practice: Consensus Statement. *British Medical Journal*, **305**, 1192–202.

Puig-Antich, J. (1980). Affective disorders in childhood. *Psychiatric Clinics of North America*, **3**, 403–23.

Puig-Antich, J. & Chambers, W. (1978). *The schedule for affective disorders and schizophrenia for school-aged children*. New York State Psychiatric Institute, New York.

Puig-Antich, J. & Gittelman, R. (1982). Depression in childhood and adolescence. In *Handbook of Affective Disorders* (ed. E. S. Paykel), pp. 379–92. Churchill Livingstone, Edinburgh and London.

Ramana R. & Paykel, E. S. (1992). Classification of affective disorders. In *British Journal of Hospital Medicine*, **47**, 831–5.

Rutter, M. (1986). The developmental psychopathology of depression: issues and perspectives. In *Depression in young people: Developmental and clinical perspectives* (ed M. Rutter, C. E. Izard & P. V. Read), pp.3–30. Guilford Press, New York and London.

Rutter, M. (1988). Epidemiological approaches to developmental psychopathology. *Archives of General Psychiatry*, **45**, 486–95.

Ryan, N. D., Puig-Antich, J., Ambrosini, P. *et al.* (1987). The clinical picture of major depression in children and adolescents. *Archives of General Psychiatry*, **44**, 854–61.

Spitzer, T., Endicott, J. & Robins, E. (1978). Research diagnostic criteria: rationale and reliability. *Archives of General Psychiatry*, **35**, 773–82.

Taylor, C. C. (1979). *Principal component analysis and factor analysis of survey data.*

Vol. 1. Exploring data structures (ed. C. A. O'Muirchaertaigh & C. Payne). Wiley, London.

Verhulst, F. C. (1989). Childhood depression: Problems of definition. *Israel Journal of Psychiatry and Related Sciences.* **26**, 3–11.

Verhulst, F. C., Akkerhuis G. W. & Althaus M. (1985). Mental health in Dutch children: (I) a cross-cultural comparison. *Acta Psychiatrica Scandinavica* (Suppl. 323) **72**, 1–108.

Weinberg, W. A., Rutman, J., Sullivan, L. *et al.*. (1973). Depression in children referred to an educational diagnostic centre: diagnosis and treatment. Preliminary report. *Journal of Paediatrics*, **83**, 1065–72.

Weissmann, M.,M. (1990). Applying impairment criteria to children's psychiatric diagnosis. *Journal of the American Academy of Child and Adolescent Psychiatry*, **29**, 789–95.

Zeitlin, H. (1986). The natural history of psychiatric disorder in children. Institute of Psychiatry, *Maudsley Monograph No.29.* Oxford University Press, London.

6

The epidemiology of depression in children and adolescents

Adrian Angold and Elizabeth J. Costello

INTRODUCTION

A number of important questions about depression in young people can only be answered from general population studies. In the first instance, given that only a small minority of disturbed children are ever referred for psychiatric treatment (Costello *et al.*, 1993), estimates of the rates of depression in children and adolescents cannot be determined from clinical data. Secondly, though clinical studies have often provided important leads to be followed up in epidemiological studies, the likelihood of referral biases vitiates their use in describing patterns of diagnostic comorbidity with depression and risk factors for depression. In 1987, Angold reviewed the epidemiological literature on this topic (Angold, 1988*a,b*) and concluded that many of the most basic questions were unanswered. The last six years have seen substantial progress, and so we will concentrate here on the more recent literature as it pertains to rates of depression in boys and girls, the effects of age on those rates, comorbidity between depression and other disorders and the identification of risk factors for depression.

The most significant trend over the last decade or so has been the shift toward diagnostic measures of depression based on structured interviews and the DSM-III and DSM-III-R criteria. Although some major studies have continued to use questionnaire measures only, they have often attempted to modify them to better reflect the concepts embodied in the DSM. However, the relationship between such measures and diagnoses based on interviews are not known, and Boyle *et al.*

127

Table 6.1. *Summary of community studies of depression*

Study	Number of subjects interviewed	Age range	% Depressed (weighted back to provide population prevalence where necessary)
New Zealand 9[a]	251	9	4.3
New Zealand 11[b]	786	11	1.8
New Zealand 15[c]	943	15	4.2
Puerto Rico[d]	224	9–16	8.0
New York State 10–13[e]	975	1–10	3.4
New York State 14–16[f]	776	9–18	3.4
New York State 17–20[g]	776	11–20	2.8
Pittsburgh 1[h]	300	7–11	2.0
Pittsburgh 2[i]	278	12–18	3.1
Mid West 7–12[j]	103	7–12	1.9
Mid West 14–16[k]	150	14–16	8.0
Cambridge[l]	368 (girls)	11–16	8.9

[a] Kashani *et al.*, 1983.
[b] Anderson *et al.*, 1987.
[c] McGee *et al.*, 1990.
[d] Bird *et al.*, 1988.
[e] Cohen *et al.*, 1993.
[f] Cohen *et al.*, 1993.

[g] Cohen *et al.*, 1993.
[h] Costello *et al.*, 1988.
[i] Costello *et al.*, 1993.
[j] Kashani & Simonds, 1979.
[k] Kashani *et al.*, 1987.
[l] Cooper & Goodyer, 1993.

(1987*a,b*) found that their DSM-III-like diagnoses agreed poorly with clinician diagnoses of depression. Therefore, studies which report on 'DSM-like' symptom clusters are included in this review. However, this trend towards standardised assessment is offset by the use of highly variable rules for combining information from different informants and different interpretations of the implementation of the DSM (see Fleming & Offord, 1990 for a trenchant review). In particular, some studies combine various depressive categories (such as depression and dysthymia), while others present results for individual disorders (see Table 6.1).

RATES OF DEPRESSION IN CHILDREN AND ADOLESCENTS

Table 6.1 shows the rates of depression found in the major studies in this area. It can be seen that the prevalence estimates vary between 1.8 and 8.9%. (The highest of these values from the Cambridge study refers to 1 year prevalence; the 1 month prevalence was 3.6%. Most studies using the DISC report 6 month prevalence, so the equivalent figure for the Cambridge study must lie somewhere between 3.6% and 8.9%.) Given the small numbers of depressed subjects in each individual study, the confidence intervals around these estimates are sometimes quite wide, even the larger studies, for example, the Dunedin study (Anderson *et al.*, 1987), with a sample size of 786, has a 95% confidence interval of almost ± 1%. It is also worth noting that the reliability and validity of the measures used in these studies are far from perfect. Even when quite narrow confidence intervals result from a particular study, the true rate of disorder may still lie outside those confidence intervals because of inaccurate measurement. Most studies find rates less than 5%, and there is a cluster of studies which found rates of 2–3%, so it seems reasonable to think that the overall rate of depression in children and adolescents is around that figure.

The effects of age on rates of depression

It has often been stated that rates of depression rise between childhood and adolescence and that the female preponderance in depression that has been well substantiated in adulthood does not become apparent until adolescence. The original empirical basis for these propositions was the Isle of Wight studies of Rutter and his colleagues, who found rates of 0.1% in 10-year-olds, but a rate of 1.5% in the same children 5 years later. Also depressed girls only came to outnumber depressed boys at the latter assessment. More recently, several epidemiological studies have generated estimates of the rates of depression in children and adolescents according to DSM-III and DSM-III-R criteria. Rates of depressive disorders by gender and age from reported studies that permit such a breakdown are presented in Table 6.2.

The first question to be decided is how to divide up the age range. Because several studies have reported rates in those over and under the age of 12, we have made the division there. Special thanks are due here to Hector Bird, who provided figures using this age split from the Puerto Rican study for this chapter. A problem with any age split is that pubertal, pubescent and physically mature individuals will be included in both groups, since some girls are already entering puberty by the age of 6, while some boys are still not pubescent by the age of 17. However, a split at age 12 concentrates physically immature individuals in the younger group and more mature individuals in the older group. It would be much preferable to examine this topic with age and maturity

Table 6.2. *Depression rates in boys and girls by age*

Study	No. boys	% Depressed		No. girls	% Depressed
New Zealand 11[b]	414	2.9		376	0.54
New Zealand 15[c]	483	0.8 (MDD)		460	3.0 (MDD)
Puerto Rico 9–11[d]	35	0.8		42	1.4
Puerto Rico 12–16[d]	71	2.2		74	3.4
New York State 10–13[e]	281	1.8		260	2.3
New York State 14–16[f]	246	1.6		262	7.6
New York State 17–20[g]	222	2.7		224	2.7
Pittsburgh 1[h]	130	2.5		148	0.8
Pittsburgh 2i	130	3.4		148	4.9

For references, see Table 6.1. MDD, major depressive disorder.

considered as continuous (or at least ordinal) measures. However, such data are not available from published reports.

Beginning with children under the age of 12, two of the three studies found a higher rate of depression in boys than girls, while the Puerto Rican study found a slight excess of girls. Though it is not possible to calculate the actual rates of depression in boys and girls from the data from Dunedin 9-year-olds presented by Kashani *et al.* they reported that there was no statistically significant difference. Turning to the data on 12 to 17-year-olds, girls have higher rates than boys in all cases except one, though the size of the difference is very variable. The exception here is the Dunedin study, which finds a continuing 5:1 excess of males at age 13. (This study is not included in Table 6.2 because the exact figures could not be calculated from the data presented in the relevant papers). It is worth noting, however, that by the age of 15, this is replaced by a 3:1 excess of depressed girls. Overall, therefore, it does seem that the excess of depressed females that has been repeatedly observed in adults appears only in adolescence. The data also indicate that the rate of depression rises in girls from childhood to adolescence. In every study involving children both above and below the age of 12, the rate of depression is higher in the former. However, the picture in regard to boys is much more confused: In the Puerto-Rican and Pittsburgh studies, the rate in boys rises a little, but in the Dunedin study it falls, while the New York study found essentially similar rates across the range from age 10 to 20. The fact that the Dunedin study used different assessments and data combination procedures at different assessments is a real problem; rates across ages cannot easily be compared, since they refer to different entities. In an attempt to introduce more order into this situation, McGee *et al.* (1990) re-scored the rates for the 11-year-old sample, so that they fell more nearly in line with the procedures used for the 13 and 15-year-old samples. Unfortunately, they also used a hierarchical diagnostic scheme for all ages, so that the diagnosis of depression could be made only in the *absence* of oppositional, conduct or attention deficit/hyperactivity disorder. In the face of high levels of comorbidity, all other workers in the area (and the Dunedin group in its other papers on depression) have chosen to allow the diagnosis of depression regardless of other symptomatology. This seems to be a sensible decision, and it means that the data of McGee *et al.* really do not help with the attempt to trace gender dependent changes in the rates of depression. It would be possible to compare directly the rates for 13 and 15-year-olds in the Dunedin study, but the published data on the former cohort do not give the sample sizes by gender for those actually assessed (these figures are given for the sample interviewed on both occasions, but there is no breakdown by gender for the large number of non-participants). The study by Cohen *et al.*, 1993 allows comparison of 10 to 13-year-olds with 14 to 16-year-olds, but these groups are, in part, made up of the same children assessed at two points in time. While a good justification of this procedure for exploratory data analysis is presented, there must be doubt about its figures being used to provide a formal test of whether the rates of depression change with age in boys and girls.

That leaves just the Puerto Rican and Pittsburgh studies for direct statistical comparison between ages. A logistic regression including gender, age and their interaction as predictors of depression found no significant effect of any of these factors (gender: chi squared = 0.06, P = 0.80; age: chi squared = 2.58, P = 0.11; gender x age: chi squared = 0.01, P = 0.91) in Puerto Rico. A similar analysis of the Pittsburgh data found a 'significant' (no correction for all the other statistical tests done on the Pittsburgh data set) effect of age group, but not of gender or the interaction of gender and age (gender: chi squared = 0.6, P = 0.81; age: chi squared = 4.52, P = 0.03; gender x age: chi squared = 0.61, P = 0.43).

Thus, neither of the two community-based studies in which we can make a straightforward comparison of the rates of depression in childhood and adolescence offer strong evidence for changes associated with gender or age. We are left with rather weak evidence that the rate of depression rises in adolescent girls, but no real idea of what happens in boys, since the data variously point to an increase, a decrease and no change at all. When we turn to the questionnaire-based studies (see

Fleming, Boyle & Offord, 1993 for a helpful review and details of the Ontario study), a similar level of confusion is found, though the evidence probably does point to an overall increase in depression in adolescence. Unfortunately, the only study with assessments on a large enough group of children and adolescents (the Ontario study) used only questionnaire measures and report results for 'emotional disorders' rather than giving figures separately for depressive and anxiety disorders. This very unsatisfactory situation suggests that we really need larger studies of gender and age effects on depression using structured diagnostic interviews with reasonably good levels of reliability before being convinced that there is really any change in the rates of depression between childhood and adolescence.

Before leaving the topic of age, it is worth noting that there are probably changes in the patterns of depressive symptomatology as well as in rates of disorder with age (Angold & Worthman, 1993). The recent epidemiological work of Goodyer and his colleagues (Cooper & Goodyer, 1993; Goodyer & Cooper, 1993) has suggested that this question needs to be followed up in community samples, since they found some changes in individual symptom rates within diagnosis. The problem here is that the small numbers of depressed individuals in each individual study make it difficult to detect real effects unless they are very large but the clinical data also point to the presence of such change (Angold & Costello, 1993).

DEPRESSIVE COMORBIDITY

In contrast to the uncertain situation with regard to the effects of age and gender, the epidemiological data have now demonstrated beyond a doubt that depression is more often associated with other disorders than would be expected from their chance co-occurrence based on the base rates of the individual disorders (Caron & Rutter, 1991; Angold & Cortello, 1993). The Isle of Wight and Inner City studies of Rutter and his colleagues found, more than 20 years ago, that there was a high degree of overlap between emotional and behavioural disorders (Rutter, Tizard & Whitmore, 1970; Rutter et al., 1976) and several studies have quantified this recently in terms of the DSM-III nosology. These recent data are summarised in Figure 6.1 (see Angold & Costello, 1993 for a detailed analysis). The comorbidity rates are so high that one wonders whether there is such a thing as a 'pure' depression before adulthood.

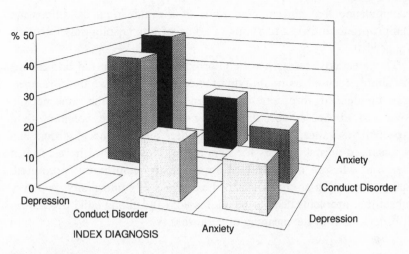

Figure 6.1. Summary of comorbidity rates. Percentage of children with second diagnosis given index diagnosis.

Then again, the adult comorbidity literature suggests that 'pure' depressions are far from being the norm at any time in life (Guze , Woodruff & Clayton, 1971; Shuckit & Winokur, 1972; Robins & Wish, 1977; Wood *et al.*, 1977; Clayton & Lewis, 1981; Boyd *et al.*, 1984; Weissman *et al.*, 1984*d*; Angst & Dobler-Mitkola, 1985; Earls *et al.*, 1988; Helzer, 1988).

It has long been recognised that the simultaneous presence of more than one disorder can complicate both diagnosis and treatment (Feinstein, 1970). The comorbidity issue should cause concern because it has implications for studies of the aetiology, cause, natural history, treatment and nosology of disorders.

Aetiology: We may identify a risk factor (for example, life events) as a potential cause of depression, when in fact it is only related causally to a comorbid condition (e.g. conduct disorder).

Development and course: In the presence of an unmeasured (or measured, but ignored) comorbid condition, observed symptoms that are assumed to be part of the course of depression could in fact be manifestations of the other disorder.

Treatment: Diagnostic homogeneity is critical for treatment trials, since treatment effects on depression may be overwhelmed by differences in outcome related to pre-therapeutic comorbidity, or spuriously inflated because the treatment is actually effective for the comorbid condition rather than depression.

Nosology: Very high levels of comorbidity between two conditions

133

may indicate that current definitions of the individual conditions are inappropriate and that revisions of some of our nosological constructs are needed.

To date, most research on comorbidity in children and adolescents has simply focused on quantifying the coexistence of two or more operationally-defined 'disorders' at the same time and in the same person. As noted above, comorbid conditions are far more common than expected by chance. Thus anxiety disorders and conduct disorders can be regarded as risk factors for depression. However, we have reached the point where a more detailed approach to comorbidity is required. Before presenting an approach to the analysis of comorbidity, two very substantial problems need to be addressed; (a) defining child psychiatric disorders, and (b) the meaning of comorbidity.

The definition of child psychiatric disorders

The statement that two or more conditions are present, implies that we can define and identify each individual condition. However, there are no generally accepted, *empirically-based*, definitions of childhood depression (Rutter, 1986; Angold, 1988*a,b*). We remain uncertain about the necessary and sufficient conditions for identifying a depressive disorder, despite the apparent certainty embodied in the extensive use of DSM-III or DSM-III-R criteria for depression. The same is true of the anxiety disorders, attention deficit/hyperactivity disorders, and conduct and oppositional disorders of childhood (Werry, Reeves & Elkind, 1987). An illustration of the degree to which differences between diagnostic systems can affect the apparent patterns of comorbidity has been provided by Angold & Costello (1991) from a study of parent reports on child psychiatric out-patients obtained by interviewer-based (semi-structured) interview. Diagnoses were generated from the symptom ratings according to both the DSM-III-R and draft ICD-10 criteria. Thirty-one subjects had at least four depressive symptoms (from a list of 25) that were intrusive, occurred in multiple situations, and were not always controllable. Of these 'depressives', 58% had a comorbid conduct disorder, according to the ICD-10 criteria, while only 19% had a comorbid conduct disorder according to the DSM-III-R criteria.

A further problem arises when one considers that the manifestations of individual disorders may change with age. This is most obviously the case for oppositional and conduct disorders, but has also been found for depression, ADHD and autism (Werry, 1986; Marks, 1987; Klein & Mannuzza, 1988; Loeber, 1989; Loeber *et al.*, 1992). If we cannot precisely define each individual morbid state, how can we talk of comorbidity? In fact, a number of approaches are available that will allow us to explore the problem of comorbidity without uncritically adopting any particular diagnostic system. Three of them have been discussed by Angold & Costello (1993).

(1) Examine 'archetypal' cases of the disorders of interest

When diagnostic categories have imprecise borders, the inclusion of mild cases will select, among others, individuals whose 'depression caseness' is in doubt, or in whom depression does not seem to be the most salient feature of the overall clinical picture. If one looks only at severe 'archetypal' cases, then this problem is eliminated. However, diagnostic certainty will only be achieved, in the case of depression, at the cost of rejecting most of the population of interest, and producing findings that apply only to a highly atypical subset of cases. Obviously, this approach is also unhelpful in determining where the lower bounds for a disorder should be.

(2) Examine symptom patterns rather than just diagnoses

Another strategy is to shift the focus from diagnostic categories, and to examine patterns of association amongst symptoms themselves. The most extreme approach is to avoid diagnosis altogether, and concentrate on looking at symptom associations using techniques such as factor analysis, cluster analysis or grade of membership analysis. (See Chapter 5 for a discussion of the use of multivariate analysis in identifying 'depressive constructs', with the broad phenotype of major depression). This has the advantage of eliminating the comorbidity problem, since individuals are usually not considered to be suffering from one or more distinct disorders, but from varying degrees of disturbance or maladaptation (Achenbach & Edelbrock, 1978). In general, such studies regularly identify the distinction between emotional (internalising) and conduct/attention/hyperactivity (externalising) problems (Edelbrock & Achenbach, 1980; Verhulst *et al.*, 1985*a,b*). Within the internalising problem area, there is a substantial degree of agreement over subcategorization into depressive and anxious syndromes. Within the externalising problem area, overactivity and antisocial syndromes usually emerge. These syndromes are similar to, but not identical with, DSM categories (Achenbach *et al.*, 1989). Furthermore, there is considerable overlap between the two main areas of 'internalising' and 'externalising' problems, particularly in severely disturbed, clinically referred children. But it is not clear whether the symptom patterns of children with both internalising and externalising symptoms are different from those whose symptoms lie in one area only. Neither strategy has this been very successful in discriminating between depressive and anxiety disorders in adult studies. A lesser degree of diagnostic agnosticism is also consistent with the use of symptom scales rather than diagnostic categories. For example, it would be quite reasonable to investigate the nature of depressions, defined according to adult criteria, in children. The presence or absence of a particular diagnosis could be used to determine group membership for each subject and then patterns of other symptoms could be examined in the resultant groups. If the depressed children had different conduct symptoms from the non-depressed children, we would have some evidence that Depressive Conduct Disorder is not simply a subcategory of Conduct Disorder. One might then reverse the process to see whether the depressive symptoms of depressed children with a diagnosis of Conduct Disorder differ from those without.

A closer study of symptom patterns could be particularly useful in resolving a major difference between the DSM and ICD nosologies: the use of mixed disorders. ICD-9 (World Health Organization, 1977) and the draft ICD-10 (World Health Organization, 1987) demand that every attempt should be made to allot a single diagnosis to each subject, whereas DSM-III (American Psychiatric Association, 1980), DSM-III-R (American Psychiatric Association, 1987) and DSM-IV (American Psychiatric Association, 1994) permit the more liberal use of multiple diagnostic categories. Thus, where a child manifests a mixture of depressive symptoms and conduct disorder symptoms, the ICD-9 diagnosis would be Mixed Disorder of Conduct and Emotions, and ICD-10 offers the diagnosis of Depressive Conduct Disorder, while separate diagnoses of Conduct Disorder and one of the depressive disorders would be given according to the DSM criteria. The ICD approach arbitrarily solves the problem of comorbidity by doing away with it, at least in part. The patient with mixed symptomatology is assigned to a single diagnostic grouping and is regarded, by definition, as suffering from a single morbid condition.

The availability of data sets that permit both ICD and DSM diagnoses to be made, as well as providing detailed symptoms data for analysis, provides the opportunity to see which diagnostic approach best fits the data – if either does.

(3) Examine mixed and pure disorders as defined by different nosologies in relation to their associations with aetiological factors, biological markers and outcome

This approach offers the best means of enhancing our understanding of the nature of depressive comorbidity. The aim here is to discriminate disorders on the basis of their course, aetiology and pathogenesis. This is a substantial task, requiring the detailed study of multiple disorders simultaneously. Large epidemiological studies and extensive exploratory multivariate analyses will be needed. Examples of this approach can be found in the literature on the course of depression. Harrington *et al.* (1991), in a 15-year clinical follow-up study, found that those with comorbid depression and conduct disorder had adult outcomes similar to the CD group. Using epidemiological data, Fleming, Boyle & Offord (1993) found the opposite for their mixed disorder cases at four-year follow-up. Both studies suffered from having only limited numbers of mixed cases, and from less than optimal assessments of depression in their time 1 observations. Much more work is needed on this topic.

The meaning of comorbidity

It is usually supposed that the presence of two disorders means that two different 'disease processes' are in operation in the same individual. By a 'disease process' we mean the triad of aetiology, pathogenesis and progression that characterises the individual disease (Susser, 1973). However, because of our weak nosological foundations, we must examine a number of other possible meanings. These can be divided into 'methodological interpretations' (possible explanations of patterns of comorbidity as artefacts of the methods of data collection, data aggregation or the nosology itself) and 'substantive interpretations' (possible explanations that suggest that comorbidity is more than an artefact).

Methodological interpretations

We are fortunate that epidemiological studies using structured interview techniques have eliminated three possibilities: that comorbidity results only from referral bias; that it is due to 'illusory correlation' (Chapman & Chapman, 1967; Kellam *et al.*, 1975) generated by unwarranted clinical expectations; or that it is simply due to the detection of a second disorder resulting from an examination that would not have occurred had the first disorder not been present.

However, other method-based interpretations cannot be ruled out at present:

> *(a) Individual conditions share some symptoms in common, so that the presence of one disorder reduces the number of symptoms required for the second disorder to reach the threshold for diagnosis.* For instance, irritability is allowed to be the basic mood state for the DSM-III-R diagnosis of depression. Irritability may be manifested as temper tantrums, arguments, touchiness, anger and resentment or fighting, all of which are included as defining criteria for DSM-III-R Oppositional Defiant Disorder or Conduct Disorder. Thus the presence of one disorder partially fulfils the criteria for the second disorder.
>
> Two further methodological interpretations result from the use of multiple informants to make child and adolescent psychiatric diagnoses. Their effects would, therefore, vary according to the way data from different informants were combined.
>
> *(b) The presence of one disorder makes a parent or teacher more likely to report the presence of a second disorder than would have been the case if the first disorder had not been present.* For instance, a parent who observes that a child seems unhappy might talk to the child about his or her feelings, and include questions about fears and worries that would never have been asked had not the depressive symptoms provided a cue to the fact that something was worrying the child. Then, even if fears and worries were really no more common in depressed children that non-depressed children, the parents of the former could report more anxiety problems because they had explored this area. This problem would not affect patterns of comorbidity in self-report data. A start could be made on addressing this question but checking to see whether patterns of comorbidity are the same in self-reports and reports by others. If they are, then this possible bias is unlikely to be important. If different patterns are observed, then specific studies of how this comes about will be required.
>
> *(c) The use of multiple informants describing the same phenomena in different terms leads to the spurious appearance of multiple disorders.* Most studies have used a decision rule that if either the parent or the child reports the presence of a symptom, then it is regarded as being present. This raises the problem that different individuals may interpret symptoms in different ways. If a child tells a parent that he or she is frightened about

bullying at school and cries every day before going to school, it is possible that the parent may interpret this as a sign of the child's being depressed, and lead to a parental report of depressed mood, while the child's description leads her interviewer to record the presence of anxiety. Thus two symptoms are counted, when only one was present. The fact that comorbidity is found in studies of both children and adults, although the latter rely mainly on self-reports, makes it unlikely that the use of multiple formats is responsible for the phenomenon of comorbidity. However, different approaches to data combination might help to explain the disparities in the rates of comorbidity seen in the epidemiological studies. This topic could be addressed directly in a number of current data sets.

Substantive interpretations

(a) All childhood psychiatric disorders result from the same pathogenic processes. As discussed below, there is little evidence for specific risk factors for depression. Perhaps apparently diverse clinical outcomes are products of a single pathogenic process with variable behavioural manifestations, non-specific responses to a variety of non-specific insults, so that the supposed 'disorders' are nothing more than arbitrary subdivisions unrelated to any useful distinctions between underlying disease processes.

(b) Depressive and anxiety symptoms represent alternative outcomes of the same pathogenetic process, but this process is different from that which results in some other disorders (such as conduct disorder). The broad distinction between the emotional (internalising) disorders and behavioural (externalising) disorders has stood the tests of time and repeated investigation. These two patterns of disturbance may represent different underlying disease processes, while the diagnostic distinctions within each of the higher order groupings may be arbitrary. If so, some of the observed associations would be the spurious products of the nosology itself, while others would result from real differences in underlying disease processes.

(c) Depressive and/or anxiety symptoms result non-specifically from a variety of pathogenetic mechanisms, which are reflected in other symptomatology (such as conduct disorder). This suggestion refers to the possibility that certain supposed disorders represent non-specific accompaniments (epiphenomena) of other underlying disease processes. For instance, perhaps what DSM-III-R labels a Major Depressive Episode is the response of the organism to many types of psychosocial problems (e.g. learning difficulties or conduct disorder).

(d) Depression directly causes disruptive behaviour disorders (or vice versa). This possibility resembles (c), but recognises that separate disease processes are involved in the production of the two conditions, that is one is not simply an epiphenomenon of the other. Thus one disorder (conduct disorder) may have a variety of causes, of which one is the other disorder (depression). To examine this question, comorbid disorders need to be

139

incorporated into risk models for depression that take account of the timing of risk factors.

(e) The presence of some third factor modulates the relationship of depression with other disorders. It is possible that the interplay between the various risk factors may affect the diagnostic outcome; for example, a family history of depression might increase the risk of developing depression in the face of risk factors for some other disorder (e.g. conduct disorder). Here again we need a better understanding of the dynamic interplay amongst risk factors for multiple disorders.

RISK FACTORS FOR DEPRESSION

Models and mechanisms

Several recent epidemiological studies from the UK, America, New Zealand and Canada have reported on associations between a number of putative risk factors for depression and the presence of DSM-III (or similar) diagnoses of depression in children and adolescents. In summary (Costello, 1989), these studies find that low socio-economic status (SES), high life stress, low academic achievement, and various measures of family disruption, disharmony and disorder are associated with the presence of psychiatric disorders in general, with each study finding slightly different patterns of effect. However, no pattern of risk factors has yet appeared that is specifically associated with depression. The non-specificity of risk factors may result, in part, from the crudity of most of our measures of them. For instance, family dysfunction comes in many forms and an overall measure of this potential risk factor may be lumping together apples and oranges. Thus a family with an alcoholic father may have all sorts of problems (Earls *et al.*, 1988; Reich, Earls & Powell, 1988) as may a family with a depressed mother (see below for further discussion), and two such families might score equally highly on a questionnaire about family dysfunction. However, the nature of the difficulties experienced by children in each of these families might be quite different, and associated with substantially different psychiatric outcomes. This suggests that there would be value in looking at risk factors like family dysfunction in a more molecular fashion.

Little attention has been paid to the various possible actions of risk factors, or the important point that in a developing organism, patterns of risk cannot be expected to be static (Costello & Angold, 1993). The task now is to investigate the processes by which risk factors interact to produce the end-point of an identifiable depressive disorder. As Rutter has said:

The research issues (for developmental psychopathology) have been formulated in ways that depart in some respects from those that have been traditional in epidemiology. Most crucially, there is a focus on continuities and discontinuities rather than on rates of disorder as such. The developmental perspective is concerned with continuities and discontinuities over time, and the psychopathologic perspective with continuities and discontinuities over the span of behavioural variation. In both cases the findings are used to examine mechanisms and processes. In other words, the aim is to go beyond the identification of risk factors to the delineation of the chain of operations by which such factors lead to disorder.

Consider the case of depression and conduct disorder. There are four possible combinations of these two diagnoses: (1) neither disorder is present, (2) only depression is present, (3) only conduct disorder is present and (4) both disorders are present. Let A represent a vector of risk factor parameter estimates from, say, a logistic regression of a number of potential risk factors on depression status, in a comparison between non-depressed and purely depressed children. Let B represent a similar vector of risk factor parameters predicting conduct disorder. Let C represent a similar vector of risk factor parameters for depression in those who have conduct disorder, D represent risk factor parameters for conduct disorder in those with depression. If $A \approx B \approx C \approx D$, then we have no evidence that depression and conduct disorder are really different disorders. However, at the other end of the spectrum, if $A \approx C$ and $B \approx D$ and A and B (and C and D) are substantially different, then we have useful evidence that depression and conduct disorder result from different processes. Such a finding would support the nosological distinction between depression and conduct disorder. Cross-checking of results of this sort could involve analysing risk factors for depression, while controlling for comorbid disorders.

Though we have noted that the evidence for changes in the rate of depression in adolescent girls is rather weaker than is usually supposed, it is still the case that the data do point in that direction. There is also some evidence from studies of physical and hormonal development that these changes are differentially associated with a variety of negative outcomes in girls, but much less so in boys (Angold & Costello, 1993). This implies that analyses of risk for depression need to treat boys and girls separately, since here they may have quite different patterns of risk for depression.

Intergenerational non-specificity of risk

Numerous studies have shown that a wide range of psychiatric disorders are more common in the children of psychiatrically disturbed parents than in the children of 'normal' parents (see Rutter & Brown, 1966; Rutter & Quinton, 1984; Quinton & Rutter, 1985). More recently, clear links between parental depression and child psychiatric disturbance have been established (Beardslee *et al.*, 1983; Orvaschel, 1983; Weissman *et al.*, 1984*b,c*, 1986). Having reviewed the literature, Beardslee *et al.* (1983) suggest that the current evidence indicates that about 40% of the children of depressives have a psychiatric disorder of some sort. Recent studies (Winokur *et al.*, 1978; Tsuang *et al.*, 1980; Weissman *et al.*, 1984*a–b*) have found an increase in risk for depressive disorders in the relatives of depressed probands, including their children, according to both parents' and children's own reports. Perhaps the most convincing evidence with respect to childhood and adolescent depression is to be found in the work of Weissman *et al.* (1987), and Orvaschel *et al.* (1988). However, many of these children had other problems as well; in fact, *substance abuse problems in the children showed a stronger relationship with parental depression than did childhood depression itself* in Weissman's study, while Orvaschel also found *an increased risk of attention deficit disorder* .

There is overwhelming evidence that disordered family functioning is involved in the aetiology of a wide range of child psychiatric problems (Rutter, 1981) but the issue requires detailed exploration specifically in relation to childhood depression. There are also strong suggestions that depressed adults often exhibit poor parenting skills (Raskin *et al.*, 1971; Weissman *et al.*, 1972; Weissman *et al.*, 1974; Parker, 1979*a,b*, 1981, 1982; Cytryn *et al.*, 1984; Davenport *et al.*, 1984; Gaensbauer *et al.*, 1984; Ainsworth & Wittig, 1992) as well as other defects of social functioning (John & Weissman, 1991). However, we are far from identifying specific links between each adult disorder and its childhood equivalent. Rutter & Quinton (1984) have argued that the degree of disturbance of the parent's psychosocial dysfunction is more important than the clinical diagnosis as a predictor of childhood disorder. Even in their work, an independent effect of parental depression as a predictor of childhood disorder was found. However, there is little to support the idea that these factors are specific precipitants of depressive syndromes as opposed to other emotional and behavioural syndromes, such as conduct disorder. Thus comorbidity appears as an issue both in individuals over time, and across generations.

CONCLUSIONS

This review of epidemiologic studies published in the last six years supports earlier evidence of a 2 to 4% prevalence rate in children, rising after puberty. The question of whether, and when, rates in boys and girls diverge is still not resolved, but most evidence points to increasing rates in adolescent girls.

Recent epidemiological data have confirmed that depressive comorbidity occurs much more commonly than would be expected on the basis of chance co-occurrence, and have ruled out some obvious possible explanations for it. It seems that comorbidity is thus a real problem for developmental psychopathology. Developmental epidemiology offers a number of strategies for addressing the problem.

While generic risk factors for depression have been described, these overlap substantially with risk for other disorders. We need to identify specific causal pathways to depression and epidemiological approaches have the great advantage that they avoid the problems of referral bias. Developmental epidemiology has a large and difficult agenda to face in relation to depression, but the tools are available, and we should expect substantial progress in the near future.

REFERENCES

Achenbach, T. M., Conners, C. K., Quay, H. C. *et al.* (1989). Replication of empirically derived syndromes as a basis for taxonomy of child/adolescent psychopathology. *Journal of Abnormal Child Psychology*, **17**, 299–323.

Achenbach, T. M. & Edelbrock, C. S. (1978). The classification of child psychopathology: A review and analysis of empirical efforts. *Psychological Reviews*, **85**, 1275–301.

Ainsworth, M. D. S. & Wittig, B. A. (1992). Attachment and exploratory behaviour of one-year olds in a Strange Situation. In: *Determinants of infant behaviour IV*, pp. 111–36, Methuen & Co., London.

American Psychiatric Association (1980). *Diagnostic and statistical manual of mental disorders – DSM-III.* 3rd edn.,Washington, DC.

American Psychiatric Association (1987). *Diagnostic and statistical manual of mental disorders – revised – DSM-III-R*, 3rd edn., American Psychiatric Association, Washington, DC.

American Psychiatric Association (1994). *Diagnostic and statistical manual of mental disorders – DSM-IV*, 4th edn. American Psychiatric Association, Washington DC.

Anderson, J. C., Williams, S., McGee, R. & Silva, P. A. (1987). DSM-III disorders in preadolescent children: Prevalence in a large sample from the general population. *Archives of General Psychiatry*, **44**, 69–77.

Angold, A. (1988a). Childhood and adolescent depression I: Epidemiological and aetiological aspects. *British Journal of Psychiatry*, **152**, 601–17.

Angold, A. (1988*b*). Childhood and adolescent depression II: Research in clinical populations. *British Journal of Psychiatry*, 153, 476–92.

Angold, A. & Costello, E. J. (1991). Developing a developmental epidemiology. In *Rochester Symposium on Developmental Psychology*, *3* (ed. D. Cicchetti & S. Toth), pp.75–96. Laurence Earlbaum Associates, Hillsdale, NJ.

Angold, A. & Costello, E. J. (1993). Depressive comorbidity in children and adolescents: Empirical, theoretical, and methodological issues. *American Journal of Psychiatry* 150, 1779–91.

Angold, A. & Worthman, C. M. (1993). Puberty onset of gender differences in rates of depression: A developmental, epidemiologic and neuroendocrine perspective. *Journal of Affective Disorders*, 29, 145–58.

Angst, J. & Dobler-Mikola, A. (1985). The Zurich study VI: A continuum from depression to anxiety disorders? *European Archives of Psychiatry and Neurological Sciences*, 235, 179–86.

Beardslee, W. R., Bemporad, J. R., Keller, M. B. & Klerman, G. L. (1983). Children of parents with major affective disorder: A review. *American Journal of Psychiatry*, 140, 825–31.

Bird, H. R., Canino, G., Rubio-Stipec, M. *et al.* (1988). Estimates of the prevalence of childhood maladjustment in a community survey in Puerto Rico: The use of combined measures. *Archives of General Psychiatry*, 45, 1120–6.

Boyd, J. H., Burke, J. D., Gruenberg, E. *et al* (1984). Exclusion criteria of DSM-III: A study of co-occurrence of hierarchy-free syndromes. *Archives of General Psychiatry*, 41, 983–9.

Boyle, M. H., Offord, D. R., Hofmann, H. G. *et al.* (1987*a*). Ontario Child Health Study: I. Methodology. *Archives of General Psychiatry*, 44, 826–31.

Boyle, M. H., Offord, D. R., Hofmann, H. G. *et al.* (1987*b*). Ontario child health study. I. Methodology. *Archives of General Psychiatry*, 44, 826–31.

Caron, C. & Rutter, M. (1991). Comorbidity in child psychopathology: Concepts, issues and research strategies. *Journal of Child Psychology and Psychiatry*, 32, 1063–80.

Chapman, L. J. & Chapman, J. P. (1967). Genesis of popular but erroneous psycho-diagnostic observations. *Journal of Abnormal Psychology*, 74, 271–80.

Clayton, P.J. & Lewis, C.E. (1981). The significance of secondary depression. *Journal of Affective Disorders*, 3, 25–35.

Cohen, P., Cohen, J., Kasen, S. *et al.* (1993). An epidemiological study of disorders in late childhood and adolescence: 1. Age and gender specific prevalence. *Journal of Child Psychology and Psychiatry*, 34, 851–67.

Cooper, P. J. & Goodyer, I. (1993). A community study of depression in adolescent girls: I. Estimates of symptom and syndrome prevalence. *British Journal of Psychiatry* 163, 369–74.

Costello, E. J. (1989). Developments in child psychiatric epidemiology. *Journal of the American Academy of Child and Adolescent Psychiatry*, 28, 836–41.

Costello, E. J. & Angold, A. (1993). Developmental epidemiology. In *Manual of Developmental Psychopathology* (ed. D. Cicchetti & D. Cohen), pp. 25–30. Wiley, New York

Costello, E. J., Burns, B. J., Angold, A. & Leaf, P. J. (1993). How can epidemiology improve mental health services for children and adolescents? *Journal of the American Academy of Child and Adolescent Psychiatry*, 32, 1106–13.

Costello, E. J., Costello, A. J., Edelbrock, C. *et al.* (1988). Psychiatric disorders in pediatric primary care: Prevalence and risk factors. *Archives of General Psychiatry*, 45, 1107–16.

Cytryn, L., McKnew, D. H., Zahn-Waxler, C. *et al* . (1984). A developmental view of affective disturbances in the children of affectively ill parents. *American Journal of Psychiatry*, **141**, 219–22.

Davenport, Y. B., Zahn-Waxler, C., Adland, M. L., & Mayfield, A. (1984). Early child-rearing practices in families with a manic-depressive parent. *American Journal of Psychiatry*, **141**, 230–5.

Earls, F., Reich, W., Jung, K. G. & Cloninger, C.R. (1988). Psychopathology in children of alcoholic and antisocial parents. *Alcoholism: Clinical and Experimental Research*, **12**, 481–7.

Edelbrock, C. & Achenbach, T. M. (1980). A typology of child behavior profile patterns: Distribution and correlates for disturbed children aged 6–16. *Journal of Abnormal Child Psychology*, **8**, 441–70.

Feinstein, A. R. (1970). The pre-therapeutic classification of co-morbidity in chronic disease. *Journal of Chronic Diseases*, **23**, 455–68.

Fleming, J. E., Boyle, M. H. & Offord, D. R. (1993). The outcome of adolescent depression in the Ontario child health study follow-up. *Journal of the American Academy of Child and Adolescent Psychiatry*, **32**, 28–33.

Fleming, J. E. & Offord, D. R. (1990). Epidemiology of childhood depressive disorders: A critical review. *Journal of the American Academy of Child and Adolescent Psychiatry*, **29**, 571–80.

Gaensbauer, T. J., Harmon, R. J., Cytryn, L. & McKnew, D. H. (1984). Social and affective development in infants with a manic-depressive parent. *American Journal of Psychiatry*, **141**, 223–9.

Goodyer, I. M., & Cooper P. J. (1993). A community study of depression in adolescent girls: II. The clinical features of identified disorder. *British Journal of Psychiatry*, **163**, 374–80.

Guze, S. B., Woodruff, R. A. & Clayton, P. J. (1971). Secondary affective disorder: A study of 95 cases. *Psychological Medicine*, **1**, 426–8.

Harrington, R., Fudge, H., Rutter, M. *et al.* (1991). Adult outcomes of childhood and adolescent depression: II. Links with antisocial disorders. *Journal of the American Academy of Child and Adolescent Psychiatry*, **30**, 434–9.

Helzer, J. (1988). *National Institute on Drug Abuse Research Monograph Series* 81. *Problems of Drug Dependence*. NIDA, Office of Science,Washington, DC.

John, K. & Weissman, M. M. (1991). Familial and psychosocial measurement. In *The measurement of depression: Clinical, biological, psychological, and psychosocial perspectives*. (ed. A. J. Marsella, R. M. A. Hirschfeld & M. Katz), pp. 1–71. Guilford Press, New York.

Kashani, J. H., Beck, N. C., Hoeper, E. W. *et al.* (1987). Psychiatric disorders in a community sample of adolescents. *American Journal of Psychiatry*, **144**, 584–9.

Kashani, J. H., McGee, R. O., Clarkson, S. E. *et al.* (1983). Depression in a sample of 9-year-old children. *Archives of General Psychiatry*, **40**, 1217–23.

Kashani, J. H. & Simonds, J. F. (1979). The incidence of depression in children. *American Journal of Psychiatry*, **136**, 1203–5.

Kellam, S. G., Branch, J. D., Agrawal, K. C. & Ensminger, M. D. (1975). *Mental health and going to school: The woodlawn program of assessment, early intervention, and evaluation*. University of Chicago Press, Chicago, IL.

Klein, R. G. & Mannuzza, S. (1988). The long-term outcome of the attention deficit disorder/hyperactivity syndrome. In *Attention deficit disorder and hyperkinetic syndrome* (ed. T. Sagvolden, J. M. Borchgrevink & R. Archers), pp. 71–9. Erlbaum, Hillsdale, NJ.

Loeber, R. (1989). Development and risk factors of juvenile antisocial behavior and delinquency. *Clinical Psychology Review*, **9**, 1–41.

Loeber, R., Green, S. M., Lahey, B. B *et al.* (1992). Developmental sequences in the age of onset of disruptive child behaviors. *Journal of Child and Family Studies*, **1**, 21–41.

Marks, I. (1987). The development of normal fear: a review. *Journal of Child Psychology and Psychiatry*, **28**, 667–97.

McGee, R., Feehan, M., Williams, S. *et al.* (1990). DSM-III disorders in a large sample of adolescents. *Journal of the American Academy of Child and Adolescent Psychiatry*, **29**, 611–9.

Orvaschel, H. (1983). Parental depression and child psychopathology. In *Childhood psychopathology and development* (ed. S.B. Guze, F.J. Earls & J.E. Barrett), pp. 53–63. Raven Press, New York.

Orvaschel, H., Walsh-Allis, G., Ye, W. & Walsh, G.T (1988). Psychopathology in children of parents with recurrent depression. *Journal of Abnormal Child Psychology*, **16**, 17–28.

Parker, G. (1979a). Parental characteristics in relation to depressive disorders. *British Journal of Psychiatry*, **134**, 138–47.

Parker, G. (1979b). Reported parental characteristics in relation to trait depression and anxiety levels in a non-clinical group. *Australian and New Zealand Journal of Psychiatry*, **13**, 260–4.

Parker, G. (1981). Parental reports of depressives: An investigation of several explanations. *Journal of Affective Disorders*, **3**, 131–40.

Parker, G. (1982). Parental representations and affective symptoms: Examination for an hereditary link. *British Journal of Medical Psychology*, **55**, 57–61.

Quinton, D. & Rutter, M. (1985). Family pathology and child psychiatric disorder: A four year perspective study. In *Longitudinal studies of child psychology and psychiatry* (ed. A. R. Nicol), pp. 157–201. Wiley, Chichester.

Raskin, A., Boothe, H. H., Reatig, N. A. *et al.* (1971). Factor analyses of normal and depressed patients' memories of parental behavior. *Psychological Reports*, **29**, 871–9.

Reich, W., Earls, F. & Powell, J. (1988). A comparison of the home and social environments of children of alcoholic parents. *British Journal of Addiction*, **83**, 831–9.

Robins, L. N. & Wish, E. (1977). Childhood deviance as a developmental process: A study of 223 urban black men from birth to 18. *Social Forces*, **56**, 448–73.

Rutter, M. & Brown, G. W. (1966). The reliability and validity of measures of family life and relationships in families containing a psychiatric patient. *Social Psychiatry*, **1**, 38–53.

Rutter, M. (1981). Epidemiological/longitudinal strategies and causal research in child psychiatry. *Journal of the American Academy of Child Psychiatry*, **20**, 513–44.

Rutter, M. (1986). The developmental psychopathology of depression: Issues and perspectives. In *Depression in young people: Issues and perspectives.* (ed. M. Rutter, C. Izard & P. Read), pp. 3–30. Guilford Press, New York.

Rutter, M., Graham, P., Chadwick, O. F. D. & Yule, W. (1976). Adolescent turmoil: Fact or fiction? *Journal of Child Psychology and Psychiatry*, **17**, 35–56.

Rutter, M. & Quinton, D. (1984). Parental psychiatric disorder: Effects on children. *Psychological Medicine*, **14**, 853–80.

Rutter, M., Tizard, J. & Whitmore, K. (1970). In *Education, health, and behaviour.* Longman, London.

Shuckit, M. A. & Winokur, G. (1972). A short term follow up of women alcoholics. *Diseases of the Nervous System*, **33**, 672–8.

Susser, M. (1973). *Causal thinking in the health sciences: concepts and strategies in epidemiology.* Oxford University Press, New York.

Tsuang, M.T., Winokur, G. & Crowe, R.R. (1980). Morbidity risks of schizophrenia and affective disorders among first degree relatives of patients with schizophrenia, mania, depression and surgical conditions. *British Journal of Psychiatry*, **137**, 497–504.

Verhulst, F. C., Akkerhuis, G. W. & Althaus, M. (1985*a*). Mental health in Dutch children: (I) a cross-cultural comparison. *Acta Psychiatrica Scandinavica*, **72**, 1–108.

Verhulst, F. C., Berden, G. F. M. G. & Sanders-Woudstra, J. A. R. (1985*b*). Mental health in Dutch children: (II) the prevalence of psychiatric disorder and relationship between measures. *Acta Psychiatrica Scandinavica*, **72**, 1–45.

Weissman, M. M., Gammon, G. D., John, K. *et al.* (1987). Children of depressed parents: Increased psychopathology and early onset of major depression. *Archives of General Psychiatry*, **44**, 847–53.

Weissman, M. M., Gershon, E. S., Kidd, K. K. *et al.* (1984*a*). Psychiatric disorders in the relatives of probands with affective disorders: The Yale University-National Institute of Mental Health collaborative study. *Archives of General Psychiatry*, **41**, 13–21.

Weissman, M. M., John, K., Merikangas, K. R. *et al.* (1986). Depressed children and their parents: General health and psychiatric problems. *American Journal of Diseases of Children*, **140**, 801–5.

Weissman, M. M., Klerman, G. G., Paykel, E. S. *et al.* (1974). Treatment effects on the social adjustment of depressed patients. *Archives of General Psychiatry*, **30**, 771–8.

Weissman, M. M., Leckman, J. F., Merikangas, K. R., Gammon, G. D. & Prusoff, A. (1984*b*). Depression and anxiety disorders in parents and children: Results from the Yale family study. *Archives of General Psychiatry*, **41**, 845–852.

Weissman, M. M., Paykel, E. S. & Klerman, G. L. (1972). The depressed woman as a mother. *Social Psychiatry*, **7**, 98–108.

Weissman, M. M., Prusoff, B. A., Gammon, G. D. *et al.* (1984*c*). Psychopathology in the children (ages 6–18) of depressed and normal parents. *Journal of the American Academy of Child Psychiatry*, **23**, 78–84.

Weissman, M. M., Wickramaratne, P., Merikangas, K. R. *et al.* (1984*d*). Onset of major depression in early adulthood: Increased familial loading and specificity. *Archives of General Psychiatry*, **41**, 1136–43.

Werry, J. S. (1986). Diagnosis and assessment. In *Anxiety disorders of childhood* (ed. R. Gittelman), pp. 73–99.Wiley, Chichester.

Werry, J. S., Reeves, J. C. & Elkind, G. S. (1987). Attention deficit, conduct, oppositional, and anxiety disorders in children: I. A review of research on differentiating characteristics. *Journal of the American Academy of Child and Adolescent Psychiatry*, **26**, 133–143.

Winokur, G., Behar, D., Vanvalkenburg, C. & Lowry, M. (1978). Is a familial definition of depression both feasible and valid? *Journal of Nervous and Mental Disease*, **166**, 764–768.

Wood, D., Othmer, S., Reich, T. *et al.* (1977). Primary and secondary affective disorder. I. Past social history and current episodes in 92 depressed inpatients. *Comprehensive Psychiatry*, **18**, 201–210.

World Health Organization, (1977). *Manual of the international classification of diseases, injuries, and causes of death*, 9th edn, pp. 157. World Health Organization: Geneva, Switzerland.

World Health Organization, (1987). ICD-10: 1987 draft of Chapter V. In *Mental, behavioural and developmental disorders*. World Health Organization, Geneva.

7

Family-genetic aspects of juvenile affective disorders

Michael Strober

INTRODUCTION

Recent epidemiologic and family studies show that affective disorders are becoming increasingly prevalent in the juvenile population (Klerman & Weissman, 1989). The factors underlying these temporal changes in rates of illness are little understood, although both genetic and environmental effects can be assumed. The validity of these conditions as diagnostic entities in young people remains an important area for further research.

Disturbances of mood in young people encompass a wide range of clinical phenomena and associated risk factors. That there is overlap in the syndromic expression of depression in juveniles and adults is well documented (Ryan et al., 1987); but clinical heterogeneity does not mean there is a single common disorder across all age groups. For example, there clearly are cases of prepubertal (major) depression that breed true over time and recur through adolescence (Kovacs et al., 1984; Hammen et al., 1990); indeed, one recent follow-up study examining the adult psychiatric status of children and adolescents meeting operational criteria for depression showed that prospective continuity with adult major depression was much stronger among postpubertal subjects (Harrington et al., 1990). A subsequent analysis of data from this cohort illustrates, as well, how immensely important it is to take into account the non-depressive comorbid states in mapping developmental linkages to establish evidence for nosologic validity. Specifically, when the cohort was stratified by the presence versus absence of coexist-

149

ing conduct disorder, only the purely depressed subjects were strongly predisposed to adult depressions, whereas comorbidity of depression and conduct disorder during childhood was strongly predictive of adult alcoholism and criminality. These differential patterns of continuity are in line with clinical studies (Nurcombe *et al.*, 1989; Seifer *et al.*, 1989) which suggest an increasing incidence of adult-like depressive states with onset of puberty.

An important empirical question, then, is how research methodologies may be usefully applied in child psychiatry in investigations of nosologic validity and the search for specific susceptibility factors and mediators of symptom expression and course of illness. This chapter focuses on the relevance of family-genetic studies to these issues. Substantive findings will be highlighted, along with methodological and conceptual problems that arise when applying this perspective to the study of causal influences. Since critical appraisals of this literature have appeared elsewhere (Beardslee *et al.*, 1983; Orvaschel, 1983; Weissman, 1988, 1990; Downey & Coyne, 1990; Hammen, 1991), the present chapter will be more selective in its focus on recent controlled studies, and on studies that shed light on possible mediators of juvenile age-of-onset.

FAMILY DATA IN JUVENILE DEPRESSION: PROSPECTS AND CAVEATS

Evidence that unipolar and bipolar affective disorders are transmitted across generations is impressive (see Tsuang & Faraone, 1990). This fact makes the family study a highly informative complement to other conventional methods in testing the diagnostic validity of juvenile affective conditions. The intuitive appeal and straightforward simplicity of the family study are important virtues. If depression in juveniles is a valid entity then lifetime risk of affective disorders in their adult relatives will be significantly greater than in the general population. Likewise, psychiatric assessment of the school-age offspring of affectively ill parents, when combined with longitudinal, prospective follow-up designs, should not only demonstrate concordance between parent and child diagnostic status, but illuminate risk and protective factors, as well as developmental effects on phenotypic expression of underlying vulnerabilities. The informativeness of family study data concerning juvenile affective disorder is, however, offset by significant challenges to their interpretation. As noted by others (Downey & Coyne, 1990; Coyne, Downey &

Boergers, 1992), research on children of depressed parents has paid surprisingly little attention to the unrepresentativeness of these samples, methodological complexities, and the potential impact of contextual factors on measures of psychopathological adjustment in such a group. For example, with rare exception, studies of this type have recruited ill parents through treatment centres; but since the majority of affectively disturbed adults do not seek treatment these families may not be truly representative of the larger population. Only scant data are available on the psychiatric status of offspring of depressed adults in the community (Beardslee *et al.*, 1988) to allow some gauge of the generality of findings from treated samples. Equally problematical is the assumption, usually inferred if not made explicit in these studies, that parent–child concordance for diagnostic status is accounted for by simple intergenerational transmission of risk. Yet conventional approaches to matching and statistical control may be inadequate to the task of separating spurious from causal influences in the multifactorial pathways of psychiatric risk linking parent to child (Coyne *et al.*, 1992). Moreover, given that genetic and environmental effects are perfectly confounded in studies of intact families, and that diagnostic criteria for major depression are likely to encompass multiple disorders with distinct heritable and developmental antecedents, it becomes apparent how daunting is the challenge of dissecting transmissible risk into genetic, psychological, and situational components. It is likely the case that 'depressed' offspring of affectively ill adults are a mixed lot, including true forms of inherited illness along with phenocopies arising from a combination of sources: chronic strains and adversities that accompany parental psychiatric impairment; lowered self-concept and peer rejection; deviant parenting behaviours resulting from depression; the effects of psychopathology in co-parents; and marital conflict, to cite but a few. Empirical data attesting to the power of these variables in mediating associations between parent and child maladjustment are substantial (Downey & Coyne, 1990; Hammen, 1991; Coyne *et al.*, 1992). Since these dysphorogenic stresses often cluster in families but are not particular to any one psychiatric disorder, they may spuriously inflate estimates from family data of the magnitude and specificity of affective risk transmitted from parent to child. Such cautions do not imply that the family study is too confounded to have practical or heuristic value in child psychiatry. On the contrary; as descriptive data on juvenile depression rapidly accumulates and methods in psychiatric genetics become more refined, the study of genetic and environmental risk factors in juvenile-onset affec-

151

tive disorders becomes an even more promising and clinically important endeavour. At this juncture, however, any review of the family-genetic literature must give proper acknowledgement to these complexities.

THE OFFSPRING OF AFFECTIVELY ILL PARENTS

At least 11 studies have utilised modern case-control methods and principles in assessing parent–child resemblance for affective disorder. Klein, Depue & Slater (1985) examined 37 offspring, 15 to 21 years of age, of 24 patients with bipolar illness and 22 offspring of adults with non affective psychiatric disorders. Index and control parents were recruited through in-patient and out-patient treatment programmes of several large urban hospitals. Diagnoses were based on a review of medical records and personal interviews using the Schedule for Affective Disorders and Schizophrenia (SADS; Endicott & Spitzer, 1978) and Research Diagnostic Criteria (RDC; Spitzer, Endicott & Robins, 1978). Diagnoses in offspring, based on RDC and DSM-III criteria, were established through personal interviews using the lifetime version of the SADS conducted by assessors who were blind to parental diagnostic status. Final diagnoses were determined independently by two experienced clinicians.

Gershon *et al.* (1985) reported diagnoses by DSM-III criteria in 29 children, 6 to 17 years of age, of bipolar parents recruited through the affective disorders programme at the National Institute of Mental Health, and 37 children of normal control families. History of psychopathology in the offspring was obtained from separate parent and child interviews using the Kiddie-SADS (K-SADS; Orvaschel *et al.*, 1981). Although interviews with offspring were often conducted with knowledge of the parent's diagnostic status, final diagnoses were decided by two child psychiatrists who blindly evaluated parent and child interview forms. Beardslee, Schultz & Selman (1987) evaluated 108 offspring, 11 to 19 years of age, of adults with affective disorder (mainly unipolar major depression), and 64 offspring from a randomly selected sample of community control families free of psychiatric illness. Index families were recruited, in part, from subjects at the Boston site of the National Institute of Mental Health (NIMH) Collaborative Study of the Psychobiology of Depression (Katz & Klerman, 1979). Lifetime psychopathology in the offspring was assessed using the Diagnostic Interview for Children and Adolescents (DICA; Herjanic & Reich,

1982), administered separately to parent and child by independent assessors who were blind to parental diagnostic status. DSM-III diagnoses were made by combining parent and child data using predetermined consensus rating procedures. Breslau, Davis & Prabuclzi (1987) reported rates of major depression and anxiety disorders in 331 mother–child dyads obtained from a geographically based probability sample. Psychiatric history information on mother and child was obtained by personal interview using adult and child versions of the Diagnostic Interview Schedule (Robins *et al.*, 1981; Costello *et al.*, 1984). With rare exception, the same interviewer examined mother and child; however, final DSM-III diagnoses were derived by computer algorithms. Rates of disorder are reported separately for children 8 to 17 years of age, and 18 to 23 years of age. Mothers' diagnostic status was trichotomised into (a) generalised anxiety only, (b) major depression, of whom 80% had concurrent generalised anxiety, and (c) neither major depression nor generalised anxiety.

The study by Weissman *et al.* (1987) compared rates of disorder in 125 children, 6 to 23 years of age, of 56 unipolar depressed adults and 95 children of 35 controls without any history of psychiatric illness. Depressed adults were probands involved in the Yale Family Study of affective disorders, recruited through treatment clinics at the Yale University Depression Research Unit. History of psychiatric disorder in the offspring was determined by independent K-SADS interviews of parent and child conducted blind to parental diagnosis. DSM-III diagnoses were determined by consensus using a best estimate procedure in which two clinicians independently and blindly examined all available sources of information.

The study by Hammen *et al.* (1987) included 19 offspring of 13 mothers with recurrent unipolar depression, 12 offspring of 9 mothers with bipolar illness, 18 offspring of 14 mothers with chronic physical disease, and 35 offspring of 22 mothers free of psychiatric disorder. Offspring ranged in age from 8 to 16. Affectively ill mothers were recruited through both private and public treatment facilities. Medical controls were obtained through advertisement in newsletters of the American Diabetes Association and Arthritis Foundation, and through specialty medical practices. Normals were recruited from schools matched demographically to socioeconomic profiles of the affective probands and medically ill controls. Information on the child's psychiatric history was obtained from separate K-SADS interviews with mother and child by different interviewers. In spite of efforts to keep child interviewers blind to maternal diagnosis, violations of the blind occurred in an unspecified proportion of cases. Diagnoses were based on DSM-III criteria, although procedures used in assigning diagnoses are not described. Orvaschel, Walsh-Allis & Ye (1988) studied 61 children of 34 parents with recurrent unipolar major depression recruited from a larger pool of subjects enrolled in clinical trials at the University of Pittsburgh Western Psychiatric Institute, and 45 children from a random community sample matched on income level and education in which neither parent met any lifetime criteria for major psychiatric illness. School-age subjects ranged in age from 6 to 16. DSM-III diagnoses were based on separate K-SADS interviews of mother and child by a single interviewer. It is not stated whether interviewers were blind to parental diagnosis, nor are procedures for reaching diagnostic consensus described. To avoid the possible confound of treatment-seeking bias on reported rates of psychiatric illness in young offspring of depressed parents, Beardslee *et al.* (1988) reported on a sample of families randomly selected without knowledge of psychiatric history from a large pool of enrolees in a health maintenance organisation. Potential subjects were told they would be participating in a study of psychosocial adjustment, and since results of the research interviews were not volunteered to parents, selection bias was minimised. Diagnoses in adults were established by SADS-L interviews and RDC. Subjects consisted of 89 school-age children from 49 families in which one or both parents had affective illness, 19 children from 11 families in which one or both parents had non affective psychiatric illness, and 45 children from 21 families in which neither parent had a history of psychiatric disorder. The majority of affectively ill parents suffered from primary unipolar major depression. Consensus DSM-III diagnoses in children were based on separate and independent DICA interviews of parent and child by assessors who were blind to parental diagnostic status.

In a study by Welner & Rice (1988), rates of psychiatric disorders were compared in 60 school-age children of parents with affective disorder, mainly unipolar type, 43 children from unscreened community control families, and 15 children from unscreened medically ill control families. Ill parents were recruited from subjects at the St Louis site of the NIMH Collaborative Study of the Psychobiology of Depression. Controls were selected from a pool of names who were acquaintances of first-degree relatives of these subjects, and from patients treated in the dialysis unit of the Washington University Medical Center. DSM-III diagnoses were based on DICA interviews of parent and child conducted by different assessors, each of whom was blind to parent diagnosis. Best estimate diagnoses were determined by consensus judgement of the two clinicians.

Klein *et al.* (1988) studied 47 offspring, 14 to 22 years of age, of 24 primary unipolar depressives recruited through in-patient services of a large university medical center. Two control groups were employed: 33 offspring of 19 adults with chronic rheumatoid arthritis or orthopaedic disease, and 38 offspring of adults without any personal or family history of psychiatric illness. Normal controls were drawn from random sampling of adults living in the same community as the index depressed families. Offspring were personally and blindly interviewed with a modification of the lifetime SADS. Final diagnoses were made blindly by a single interviewer using DSM-III, DSM-III-R, and RDC.

Sylvester, Hyde & Reichler (1988) examined rates of major depression and anxiety disorders in 125 children, 7 to 17 years of age, from 72 families. Twenty-seven were offspring of a parent with major depression, 50 were offspring of a parent with panic disorder, and 48 were from families without psychiatric disorder. Separate and independent interviews were conducted blind to parental diagnosis using the DICA. Procedures used in reaching final diagnoses are not described.

Rates of affective diagnoses among offspring examined in these studies are given in Table 7.1. A wide variation in rates is evident, especially for major depression. This is not unanticipated given inter-study differences in diagnostic instruments, training and skill of interviewers. procedures for rendering study diagnoses, ascertainment of adult probands; and the inevitable differences among clinicians in thresholds applied for determining 'caseness'. Even so, in the nine studies that include unipolar, or mainly unipolar, disorder in the index adult proband, a clear association between parent and offspring affective disorder is found. The risk of major depression in these offspring ranges from 9 to 47%, the average being 25%. For offspring of normal controls, the range is 0 to 24%, the average being 7%. Moreover, in 4 of the 11 studies, major depression was non-existent among offspring of normal controls.

Only three studies employed medically ill controls (Hammen *et al.*, 1987; Klein *et al.*, 1988; Welner & Rice, 1988); nonetheless, rates of major depression in their offspring are low (17, 0, and 5%, respectively), and they are low, as well, in offspring of mixed psychiatric controls (Klein *et al.*, 1985; Beardslee *et al.*, 1988). On the other hand, two studies indicate widely divergent rates of major depression in offspring of adults with anxiety disorders – 12% from Breslau *et al.* (1987) compared

Table 7.1. *Affective disorder among school-age offspring of affectively ill adults and controls by DSM-III criteria*

| Study | Parent diagnosis | Rates/100 in offspring | | |
		Major depression	Dysthymia	Bipolar[a]
Gershon et al., 1985	BP	10	–	3
	NC	14	–	0
Klein et al., 1985	BP	3	3	27
	PC	5	0	0
Breslau et al., 1987	MD	16	–	–
	AN[b]	12	–	–
	NC	8	–	–
Beardslee et al., 1987	AD	18	12	–
	NC	0	0	–
Hammen et al., 1987	UP	47	32	–
	BP	25	8	–
	MC	17	6	–
	NC	9	3	–
Weissman et al., 1987	UP	38	–	–
	NC	24	–	–
Beardslee et al., 1988	AD	20	17	–
	PC	0	0	–
	NC	0	2	–
Klein et al., 1988	UP	9	15	6
	MC	0	3	0
	NC	0	0	0
Orvaschel et al., 1988	UP	15	15	2
	NC	0	2	0
Sylvester et al., 1988[c]	MD	37	–	–
	AN[d]	48	–	–
	NC	21	–	–
Welner et al., 1988	AD	23	–	–
	MC	5	–	–
	NC	5	–	–

BP, bipolar illness; MD, major depression, polarity unspecified; UP, unipolar major depression; AD, affective disorder mainly unipolar type; AN, anxiety disorder; MC, medically ill control; NC, no psychiatric illness control.
[a] Bipolar I, hypomania; Bipolar II, cyclothymia combined.
[b] Generalised anxiety.
[c] Rates reported based on psychiatric interview of child.
[d] Majority of adult probands diagnosed panic disorder.

to 48% from Sylvester et al. (1988). However, this latter figure is not entirely unexpected given evidence of similar genetic liabilities influencing risk to major depression and anxiety disorders (Merikangas, 1990; Kendler et al., 1992).

Taken together, these data suggest that major depression is roughly 3- to 4-fold more likely in juvenile offspring of adults with unipolar affective disorder in comparison to offspring of normal, medically ill, and non affective, but psychiatrically ill adults. By contrast, two of the three studies (Gershon *et al.*, 1985; Klein *et al.*, 1985) that included adult probands with bipolar illness found no association with major depression in offspring. An exception is the study by Hammen *et al.* (1987), in which major depression was nearly 3-fold more prevalent in offspring of bipolars compared to offspring of normal controls, but roughly one-half the rate observed in offspring of unipolar depressed adults.

In the six studies that give rates of dysthymia, an association between parent and offspring affective status is supported. The risk among offspring of unipolar adults ranges from 8 to 32%, compared to 0 to 6% among offspring of controls. In two studies (Klein *et al.*, 1985; Hammen *et al.*, 1987), dysthymia is reported in 8% of offspring with bipolar illness. Pooling these results, dysthymia is roughly 7-fold more prevalent in offspring of affectively ill adults compared to offspring of controls.

Only four studies give rates of bipolar conditions among offspring. In two studies (Gershon *et al.*, 1985; Klein *et al.*, 1985) the index parental diagnosis is bipolar illness, and unipolar depression in the others (Klein *et al.*, 1988; Orvaschel *et al.*, 1988). Most noteworthy is the fact that all cases of bipolar illness occur in offspring of affectively ill parents, the majority of these receiving diagnoses of cyclothymia or hypomania.

Non affective conditions among offspring

Although not consistent across studies, rates of non affective psychiatric disorders are higher among offspring of affectively ill parents compared to offspring of controls. In seven studies (Gershon *et al.*, 1985; Beardslee *et al.*, 1987; Hammen *et al.*, 1987; Weissman *et al.*, 1987; Beardslee *et al.*, 1988; Klein *et al.*, 1988; Welner & Rice, 1988) rates of conduct disorder range from 11 to 47%, compared to 0 to 17% among offspring of controls – an average 4-fold greater risk. Five studies (Gershon *et al.*, 1985; Weissman *et al.*, 1987; Beardslee *et al.*, 1988; Orvaschel *et al.*, 1988; Welner & Rice, 1988) report rates of attention deficit disorder; the rates range from 5 to 20% in offspring of affectively ill parents compared to 5 to 8% in offspring of controls – an average 2-fold increased risk. Substance abuse is reported in five studies (Beardslee *et al.*, 1987; Hammen *et al.*, 1987; Weissman *et al.*, 1987; Beardslee *et al.*, 1988; Klein *et al.*, 1988) to occur in 10 to 26% of offspring of affectively ill parents, compared to 3 to 8% in offspring of control – an average 2.7-fold increased risk. And in seven studies (Hammen *et al.*, 1987; Weissman *et al.*, 1987; Beardslee *et al.*, 1988; Klein *et al.*, 1988; Orvaschel *et al.*, 1988; Sylvester *et al.*, 1988; Welner & Rice, 1988), rates of anxiety disorders in offspring of affectively parents ranged from 5 to 47%, compared to 9 to 27% in offspring of controls – a nearly 2-fold increased risk.

Unfortunately, these studies do not make clear to what extent these rates reflect comorbidity of affective and non affective diagnoses within individual offspring as opposed to clustering of non affective diagnoses among the larger group of offspring at risk. The importance of this distinction has been discussed by Merikangas (1990) and by Cloninger *et al.* (1988, 1990), who showed how spurious conclusions about the clinical boundaries of familialy transmitted disorders can be reached in genetic epidemiologic studies by failing to pay close attention to patterns of diagnostic covariation within individuals and between individuals within families. Thus, the association of affective and non affective diagnoses in these offspring studies is open to multiple interpretations: (a) affective illness and certain non affective psychiatric disorders in children may reflect variable expressions of a common transmitted liability, (b) one disorder predisposes to another, (c) certain conditions are non-specific effects of environmental disruption arising from parental depressive illness, (d) they are aetiologically distinct conditions that aggregate in families because of parental assortative mating for particular diagnostic syndromes.

Considering these possibilities, it is reasonable to assume that fundamentally different mechanisms are operating to a greater or lesser degree in the transmission of risk between parent and child. Thus, in some families a child's depression might signify a true homotypic pattern of genetic inheritance, in others a non-specific demoralisation reaction to parental disease and its sequelae, or to the functional impairment resulting from antecedent non affective psychopathology present in the child. In a similar vein, the co-occurrence of depression and substance abuse might be independent of genetic factors, but explained by the frequent use of alcohol and other drugs by depressed adolescents to self-medicate negative affect states. To the extent that conduct disorders and substance abuse often co-aggregate in families (West & Prinz, 1987), the clustering together of all three diagnoses is not unexpected.

However, a common genetic propensity seems unlikely given evidence of independent familial transmission of alcoholism and affective disorders (Merikangas *et al.*, 1985).

By contrast, the co-occurrence of anxiety and depression amongst offspring of depressed parents may well reflect the operation of common, or overlapping, familial-genetic determinants, as previously noted. Along the same lines, longitudinal follow-up data from the Zurich cohort study (Angst *et al.*, 1990) shows that upwards of one-half of subjects who present initially with pure anxiety develop prominent depressive illness over time. In short, certain anxiety and depressive conditions may lie on a common genetic continuum of clinical phenotypes transmitted by affectively ill parents to their children.

Identification of specific risk factors

Several studies provide information about specific familial and parental variables possibly associated with elevated risk for general psychiatric impairment, and depressive disorder in particular. Keller *et al.* (1986) reported on the power of measures of the severity and chronicity of parental depression, family discord, and demographic variables in predicting impairment in a cohort of 72 children with at least one biological parent with a history of depressive disorder. Marital discord and a more severe and chronic course of depression in parents were associated with greater overall functional impairment in their offspring and an increased risk of a DSM-III diagnosis of some sort. However, these effects varied by sex of the affected parent; children from families where mother was depressed exhibited greater functional impairment than did children from families with paternal depression.

With regard to predictors of specific diagnostic outcomes, Orvaschel *et al.* (1988) found no association between sex of the affected parent and specific diagnosis in the child, nor were number of lifetime episodes of depression in the affected parent or symptom severity at the time of intake into the study related to specific diagnosis in the children. However, positive findings are reported in two studies. In the study by Welner & Rice (1988), maternal depression and paternal alcoholism were associated with elevated risk for depression in offspring of depressed parents, whereas divorce was a significant predictor of conduct disorder. Klein *et al.* (1988) showed that the odds of a diagnosis of dysthymia in offspring of unipolar depressed adults were increased significantly if the family contained major affective disorder in the coparent or in a first-degree relative of the affected parent or unaffected coparent, chronicity of parental depression, or early-onset of parental illness.

Further evidence of the potential importance of parental and familial variables in predicting diagnostic status in the children of unipolar adults is found in an important study by Warner *et al.* (1992). These investigators examined the rate of new incident cases of depression, time to recovery, and risk of recurrence during a 2-year period in offspring of unipolar depressed adults and offspring of normal controls. All of the new incident cases developed in offspring of depressed adults, and were predicted by previous subclinical depressive symptoms and an antecedent diagnosis of conduct disorder. Within this subset, recurrence was associated with a pre-existing diagnosis of dysthymia, whereas time to recovery was more protracted in offspring with prepupertal-onset of depression, the majority of whom had parents with multiple episodes of depression.

In critically evaluating possible reasons for the highly variable expression of psychopathology among offspring of parents with affective illness, Merikangas and colleagues (1988*a,b*) have called attention to powerful effects of parental concordance for psychiatric disorder on the transmission of specific vulnerabilities. They found that comorbidity and parental assortative mating for alcoholism significantly increased the risk of substance abuse and antisocial conduct in offspring, whereas comorbidity and assortative mating for anxiety disorder in the parent or parental dyad sharply increased the risk for anxiety and depressive disorders among offspring. These findings make it evident that one cannot ignore the nature of parental mating types when attempting to unravel familial mechanisms through which risk of specific pychopathologies are transmitted between generations.

In short, the studies highlighted in this section suggest that general measures of parental illness and quality of marital interaction may predict a broad range of outcomes in overall psychosocial adaptation in children while having little association with nosologically discrete diagnoses. At the same time, certain indices of parent illness and familial liability, whether genetically or environmentally mediated, may be informative predictors of symptom development in high-risk individuals.

PSYCHIATRIC ILLNESS IN ADULT RELATIVES OF AFFECTIVELY ILL JUVENILES

Five case-control family studies begin with children or adolescents as probands and give rates of affective disorder in adult biological relatives. An important advantage of this so-called 'bottom-up' approach is that the validating index – the form and distribution of illness in pedigrees – is better defined clinically and nosologically.

Livingston *et al.* (1985) determined rates of psychiatric disorder in 58 first- and second-degree relates of 11 children with major depression, and 69 relatives of 12 controls with anxiety disorder. The probands ranged in age from 6 to 12 and were diagnosed by DSM-III criteria following structured clinical interviews using the DICA. Although polarity of illness in depressed probands is not defined, it can be assumed that the majority are non-bipolar. Diagnoses of relatives were derived from FH-RDC interviews evaluated independently and blindly by two psychiatrists.

A study by Strober *et al.* (1988) examined lifetime rates of psychiatric illness in 523 first- and second-degree relatives of adolescent-age probands with bipolar illness, and 321 first and second-degree relatives of 31 carefully matched schizophrenic controls. Proband diagnoses based on RDC criteria were established through SADS interviews and a review of all hospital records. Over 80% of first-degree relatives were interviewed personally using the SADS; family history interviews (FH-RDC; Andreasen *et al.*, 1977) were used to establish diagnoses for second-degree relatives. Interviewers were fully blind to proband diagnosis and the narrative summaries were separately coded to avoid bias from knowledge of familial illness. All diagnoses were determined by a single clinician who assigned best-estimate diagnoses according to RDC.

Mitchell *et al.* (1989) studied 169 parents of 94 probands with major depression and 65 parents of 38 non-depressed psychiatric controls. Probands ranged in age from 7 to 17. Diagnoses were based on K-SADS interviews using RDC, however polarity of illness in depressed probands is not specified. Diagnoses of controls included anxiety disorder, 9; conduct disorder, 6; parent–child conflict, 5; attention deficit disorder, 4; gender identity disorder, 1; and adjustment disorder, 13. Virtually all mothers, and slightly more than half the fathers, were directly interviewed using the SADS and RDC; FH-RDC interviews were used to obtain diagnostic information on unavailable relatives. All interviews of relatives were conducted blind to proband status.

Puig-Antich and colleagues (1989) studied 503 first- and second-degree relatives of 48 prepubertal probands with major depression, 165 relatives of 20 non-depressed psychiatric controls, and 302 relatives of 27 never-ill controls. Of the 48 depressed probands, five had histories of manic or hypomanic episodes. All probands were assessed using the K-SADS. The diagnosis of major depression was based on RDC whereas DSM-III criteria were used to diagnose controls. Of the 20 non-depressed controls, 19 had some form of anxiety disorder. Never-ill controls were obtained through random sampling in an urban school whose sociodemographic characteristics resembled those of the depressed probands. Mothers were assessed directly using the SADS and provided FH-RDC information to diagnose fathers and second-degree relatives. Although attempts were made to keep interviewers blind to proband status, this condition was broken in roughly one-third of patient proband families.

Kutcher & Marton (1991) studied 81 first-degree relatives of 23 adolescent probands with bipolar illness, 95 relatives of 26 unipolar depressives, and 83 relatives of 24 normal controls. Patients were assessed using the K-SADS and diagnosed according to DSM-III criteria. Controls were solicited from local church groups and through advertisement. Relatives' diagnoses were based exclusively on the FH-RDC method with mothers serving as the informant in the majority of cases; it is unclear whether or not these interviews were blind to diagnosis of the proband.

Results of these studies appear in Table 7.2, which gives lifetime rates of unipolar and bipolar illness among relatives of probands. Several methodological points must be taken into account in considering the implications of these data, and in comparing results across studies. First, only two studies (Puig-Antich *et al.*, 1989; Kutcher & Marton, 1991) include a control group of never-ill probands and their relatives. Second, with one exception (Strober *et al.*, 1988), these studies rely primarily on the family history method for determining illness in relatives, a procedure more prone to imprecision. Third, in three of the studies (Livingston *et al.*, 1985; Puig-Antich *et al.*, 1989; Kutcher & Marton, 1991) interviewers were not blind to diagnosis of the proband, or the blind was broken in a substantial minority of cases.

In spite of these shortcomings, the results indicate that relatives of juvenile probands with major depression or bipolar illness are several times more likely to develop affective disorders than individuals in the general population, where the average lifetime expected morbidity has

Table 7.2. *Lifetime rates of unipolar and bipolar affective disorder among adult first-degree relatives of adolescent probands*

Study	Proband diagnosis	Rate per 100 Unipolar	Bipolar
Livingston *et al.*, 1985	MD	24	0
	AN	30	13
Strober *et al.*, 1988	BP	15	15
	SZ	4	0
Mitchell *et al.*, 1989	MD	46	1
	PC	37	3
Puig-Antich *et al.*, 1989	AD	34	4
	PC	20	2
	NC	16	0
Kutcher & Marton, 1991	BP	19	15
	UP	20	5
	NC	4	1

MD, major depression, polarity unspecified; AD, affective disorder, mainly unipolar type; BP, bipolar illness, UP, unipolar depression; AN, anxiety disorder; SZ, schizophrenia; PC, non-affectively ill psychiatric controls; NC, normal controls.

been estimated at roughly 7% (Tsuang & Faraone, 1990). However, at first glance the results seem to offer only partial support for distinct familial transmission. Two studies (Livingston *et al.*, 1985; Mitchell *et al.*, 1989) failed to find a higher lifetime risk of affective disorder among relatives of index probands compared to relatives of controls. There is, however, a related confound in both: the selection of anxiety disorder as a comparison group in the study by Livingston *et al.*, and the presence of anxiety disorder in one-quarter of the control probands studied by Mitchell *et al.* This is problematic since, as previously noted, longitudinal and family studies support at least some association between affective and anxiety disorders in aetiologic factors. As such, the negative findings are not unanticipated; nor is the lack of differentiation between relatives of depressed probands and relatives of psychiatric controls in rates of affective disorder reported by Puig-Antich *et al.* (1989) unexpected given the predominance of anxiety disorder diagnoses in control probands. In short, if 'true' cases of affective disorder are nested within anxiety disorder controls then implications of these data with regard to the specificity of familial transmission are greatly limited.

These caveats aside, evidence of familial transmission is strong in the studies by Strober *et al.* (1988) and Kutcher & Marton (1991), both showing a several-fold increase in rates of affective disorders in relatives of unipolar and bipolar probands compared to controls. The study by Strober *et al.* is noteworthy in that it shows a clear familial separation of bipolar illness and schizophrenia in adolescence. And while a lower relative risk is reflected in the comparison between relatives of depressed and normal control probands in the study by Puig-Antich *et al.* (1989), the rate of affectation among relatives of depressed probands is still twice that of relatives of normals. Moreover, this relative risk increases to 2.5 if the analysis is restricted to depressed probands without concurrent conduct disorder. By contrast, the risk of affective disorders among relatives of depressed probands with conduct disorder is no different from that in relatives of normal controls. These findings lend added support for the nosologic separation of depressive syndromes with and without antisocial behaviour.

EARLY AGE-OF-ONSET AND FAMILIAL AGGREGATION

Disorders with non-Mendelian inheritance and variable age-of-onset are generally believed to have complex and heterogeneous familial aetiologies. For this reason, there is increasing interest in identifying more discrete subforms of affective illness in order to improve the precision and replicability of genetic analyses.

A considerable literature exists on the relationship between age-of-onset and density of familial loading in both unipolar and bipolar illness (see Tsuang & Faraone, 1990; Moldin, Reich & Rice, 1991). In most studies, age 40 is the cut-off used to stratify probands into early- and late-onset subgroups. With some exceptions, they indicate that the lifetime risk of affective disorder is significantly greater among relatives of probands with early-onset disease.

However, recent evidence suggests that this particular stratification results in considerable loss of information in estimating the magnitude of the age effect on familial aggregation. Three recent family studies of unipolar depression show that as the age cut-off is extended downward, familial morbid risk increases in almost linear fashion. In studies by Weissman *et al.* (1984) and Kupfer *et al.* (1989), relatives of probands with onset of illness before age 20 had a two-fold increased risk for affective illness compared to relatives of probands with later onset. A similar trend has also been detected in the juvenile offspring of depressed parents examined by Weissman *et al.* (1988) as part of the Yale Family Study. In this study, children aged 6 to 23, of parents with an onset of major depression before age 20, had 1.5 to 1.7 times the risk of major depression compared to offspring of parents with later age-of-onset, and had a 14-fold increased risk of pre-pubertal onset of depressive disorder.

Concerning bipolar illness, Rice *et al.* (1987) applied a segregation analysis to family data from 187 bipolar I probands stratified by age-of-onset into separate liability classes. Transmissible liability was assumed to be related inversely to age-of-onset and was derived by taking the log age-of-onset, subtracting the mean for the proband's birth cohort and dividing by the standard deviation. When a mixed multifactorial-autosomal major locus model was examined ignoring age-of-onset, major locus transmission was rejected. However, relatives of probands whose age-of-onset was one standard deviation or more below their cohort-specific mean had twice the morbid risk of bipolar illness compared with relatives of probands in the adjacent liability class. When age-of-onset in probands was modelled as a covariate in the segregation analysis, single major locus transmission provided a better fit to the data than multifactorial-polygenic inheritance. These authors suggest that age-of-onset be treated as an important parameter in efforts to reduce aetiologic heterogeneity in quantitative and molecular genetic analyses.

In their family study of bipolar adolescent probands, Strober *et al.* (1988) modelled an age-of-onset effect by subdividing probands on the presence or absence of pre-pubertal onset of psychiatric abnormality. Two findings of note emerged: there was a very high ratio of bipolar to unipolar cases among affected relatives of probands with prepubertal-onset of psychopathology; and relatives of this subgroup had 3.5 times the risk for bipolar illness compared to relatives of probands who had no major signs of psychiatric disorder prior to the onset of their affective illness (29.4% vs. 8.6%). These risk estimates are especially compelling in that they greatly exceed those reported in family-genetic studies of adult bipolar probands (see Gershon, 1990; Tsuang & Faraone, 1990).

More recently, an analysis of family morbid risk data from the Amish study of bipolar illness (Pauls, Morton & Egeland, 1992) lends yet additional support to the idea that juvenile onset delimits a more severe or familial subform of disease. In this study, relatives of probands with onset of illness before age 20 had a 3-fold increase in risk of bipolar I illness compared to relatives of probands with later age-of-onset, and a 1.6-fold increase in the combined risk of bipolar and unipolar conditions.

Finally, work by Baron *et al.* (1990) raises the interesting possibility of an association between early-onset bipolar illness and X-linked inheritance. Reanalysing previously published data on five large multiplex pedigrees, the authors compared several clinical parameters of illness in these X-linked pedigrees to general samples of familial bipolar probands reported in the literature. Affected cases from X-linked pedigrees were found to develop their illness at an earlier age and had a higher ratio of bipolar to unipolar type illness. The authors postulate that an X-linked variant of bipolar illness may be over-represented among individuals with early-onset of disease.

CONCLUSIONS

Several different lines of inquiry point to the validity of depressive disorder in children and adolescents. In spite of this, some qualifications to our current knowledge are in order.

Depression clearly is among the most prominent types of psychopathology in offspring of parents with affective disorder, unipolar major depression in particular; however, psychopathology in general is widespread in these samples thus raising questions about the mechanisms underlying parent–child resemblance for depression and the coaggregation of affective and non affective conditions. Heritability of depressive vulnerability is doubtless one important causal factor; but it may be too rigid a conclusion that depression in children of depressed parents is determined solely by genetic factors when other pathogenic influences are displayed in these families in varying degrees. A more parsimonious view holds that the cumulative impact of these adverse family circumstances may well be sufficient in intensity and chronicity to mediate the development of affect disturbance of some type in certain offspring of depressed parents. But what clinical features, if any, differentiate these environmental phenocopies from genetically transmitted depressive states remains unclear at present. In addition to specific transmissible effects of parental affective disorder, psychiatric outcome in offspring is also influenced heavily by patterns of parental concordance for psychopathology. Parental matings involving depression and anxiety appear to significantly increase liability for both conditions in offspring, whereas parental alcoholism elevates risk to offspring of conduct problems and substance abuse. Hence, available evidence indicates the significance of multifactorial processes underlying the varying forms of psychopathology in high-risk children. Exactly how the effects of these different transmitted liabilities are mediated and then potentiated by environmental risk factors with which they inevitably correlate emerge as questions of enormous complexity for future research.

One reasonably solid conclusion we can draw from family studies of early-onset probands is that this variable is a robust marker of aetiologic heterogeneity. In both unipolar and bipolar illness, the association between juvenile age-of-onset and increased familial loading of affective disorder is remarkably consistent across studies. Whether specific genes are, in fact, critical determinants of early-onset subforms of disease remains unknown; however, the speculation is an intriguing one. Alternatively, age-of-onset may be independent of genetic liability but rather mediated by exposure to various environmental risk and protective factors at early and sensitive periods of development.

Clearly, the in-depth study of juvenile populations will be a necessary part of future efforts at elucidating genetic mechanisms and gaining a better understanding of the unfolding biological and environmental processes linked to onset of disease. In this endeavour, the study of multiply affected pedigrees identified through cases of juvenile-onset depression and bipolar illness may provide a new, relevant source of data in the search for disease susceptibility genes. Ultimately, the developmental perspective to emerge from these bridging efforts will add new strands of knowledge on the causes, sequelae and treatment of affective disorders across the life span.

REFERENCES

Andreasen, N. C., Endicott, J., Spitzer, R. L. & Winokur, G. (1977). The family history method using diagnostic criteria. *Archives of General Psychiatry*, **34**, 1229–35.

Angst, J., Vollrath, M., Merikangas, K. & Ernst, C. (1990). Comorbidity of anxiety and depression in the Zurich Cohort, Study of Young Adults. In *Comorbidity of mood and anxiety disorders* (ed. J. D. Maser & C. R. Cloninger), pp. 123–38. American Psychiatric Press. Washington, DC.

Baron, M., Hamburger, R., Sandkuyl, L. A. *et al* . (1990). The impact of phenotypic variation on genetic analysis: application to X-linkage in manic-depressive illness. *Acta Psychiatrica Scandanavica*, **82**, 196–203.

Beardslee, W. R., Bemporad, J., Keller, M. B. & Klerman, G. L. (1983). Children of parents with affective disorders. *American Journal of Psychiatry*, **140**, 825–32.

Beardslee, W. R., Keller, M. B., Lavori, P. W. *et al.* (1988). Psychiatric disorder in adolescent offspring of parents with affective disorder in a non-referred sample. *Journal of Affective Disorders*, **15**, 313–22.

Beardslee, W. R., Schultz, L. H. & Selman, R. L. (1987). Level of social-cognitive development, adaptive functioning, and DSM III diagnoses in adolescent offspring of parents with affective disorders: implications of the development of the capacity for mutuality. *Developmental Psychology*, **23**, 807–15.

Breslau, N., Davis, G. C. & Prabuclzi, K. (1987). Searching for evidence on the validity of generalised anxiety disorder: psychopathology in children of anxious mothers. *Psychiatry Research*, **20**, 285–97.

Cloninger, C. R., Martin, R. L., Guze, S. B. & Clayton, P. J. (1990). The empirical structure of psychiatric comorbidity and its theoretical significance. In *Comorbidity of mood and anxiety disorders* (ed. J. D. Maser & C. R. Cloninger), pp. 439–62. American Psychiatric Press, Washington, DC.

Cloninger, C. R., von Knorring, A. L., Sigvardsson, S. & Bohman, M. (1988). Clinical predictors of familial psychopathology: principles, methods, and findings. In *Relatives at risk for mental disorders* (ed. D. L. Dunner, E. S. Gershon & J. E. Barrett), pp. 9–30. Raven Press, New York.

Costello, A. J., Edelbrock, C., Dulcan, M. K. *et al.* (1984). Development and testing of the NIMH Diagnostic Interview Schedule for Children in a clinic population. Center for Epidemiologic Studies, National Institute of Mental Health, Rockville.

Coyne, J. C., Downey G. & Boergers, J. (1992). Depression in families: a systems perspective. In *Developmental perspectives on depression* (ed. D. Cicchetti & S. L. Toth), pp. 251–82. University of Rochester Press, Rochester.

Downey G. & Coyne, J. C. (1990). Children of depressed parents: an integrative review. *Psychological Bulletin*, **108**, 50–76.

Endicott, J. & Spitzer, R. L. (1978). A diagnostic interview: the Schedule for Affective Disorders and Schizophrenia. *Archives of General Psychiatry*, **35**, 837–44.

Gershon, E. S. (1990). Genetics. In *Manic-depressive illness* (ed. F. K. Goodwin & K. R. Jamison), pp. 373–401. Oxford University Press, Oxford .

Gershon, E., McKnew, D., Cytryn, L. *et al.* (1985). Diagnosis in school-age children of bipolar affective disorder parents and normal controls. *Journal of Affective Disorders*, **8**, 283–91.

Hammen, C. (1991). *Depression runs in families.* Springer-Verlag, New York .

Hammen, C., Burge, D., Burney, E. & Adrian, C. (1990). Longitudinal study of diagnoses in children of women with unipolar and bipolar affective disorder. *Archives of General Psychiatry*, **47**, 1112–7.

Hammen, C., Gordon, D., Burge, D. *et al.* (1987). Maternal affective disorders, illness, and stress: risk for children's psychopathology. *American Journal of Psychiatry*, **144**, 736–41.

Harrington, R., Fudge, H., Rutter, M. *et al.* (1990). Adult outcomes of childhood and adolescent depression. *Archives of General Psychiatry*, **47**, 465–73.

Herjanic, B. & Reich, W. (1982). Development of a structured psychiatric interview for children: agreement between child and parent on individual symptoms. *Journal of Abnormal Child Psychology*, **10**, 307–24.

Katz, M. M. & Klerman, G. L. (1979). Introduction: over-view of the clinical studies program. *American Journal of Psychiatry*, **136**, 49–51.

Keller, M., Beardslee, W., Dorer, D. *et al.* (1986). Impact of severity and chronicity of parental affective illness on adaptive functioning and psychopathology in children. *Archives of General Psychiatry*, **43**, 930–7.

Kendler, K. S., Neale, M. C., Kessler, R. C. *et al.* (1992). Major depression and generalised anxiety disorder: same genes, (partly) different environments? *Archives of General Psychiatry*, **49**, 716–22.

Klein, D., Clark, D., Dansky, L. & Margolis, E. T. (1988). Dysthymia in the offspring of parents with primary unipolar affective disorder. *Journal of Abnormal Psychology*, **97**, 265–76.

Klein, D., Depue, R. A. & Slater, J. F. (1985). Cyclothymia in the adolescent offspring of parents with bipolar affective disorder. *Journal of Abnormal Psychology*, **94**, 115–27.

Klerman, G. L. & Weissman, M. M. (1989). Increasing rates of depression. *Journal of the American Medical Association*, **261**, 2229–35.

Kovacs, M., Feinberg, T. L., Crouse-Novak, M. *et al.* (1984). Depressive disorders in childhood. II. A longitudinal study of the risk for a subsequent major depression. *Archives of General Psychiatry*, **41**, 643–9.

Kupfer, D. J., Frank, E., Carpenter, L. L. & Neiswanger, K. (1989). Family history in recurrent depression. *Journal of Affective Disorders*, **17**, 113–19.

Kutcher, S. & Marton, P. (1991). Affective disorders in first degree relatives of adolescent onset bipolars, unipolars, and normal controls. *Journal of the American Academy of Child and Adolescent Psychiatry*, **30**, 75–8.

Livingston, R., Nugent, H., Rader, L. & Smith, R. C. (1985). Family histories of depressed and severely anxious children. *American Journal of Psychiatry*, **142**, 1497–9.

Merikangas, K. R. (1990). Comorbidity for anxiety and depression: review of family and genetic studies. In *Comorbidity of mood and anxiety disorders* (ed. J. D. Maser & C. R. Cloninger), pp. 331–48. American Psychiatric Press, Washington, DC.

Merikangas, K. R., Leckman, J. F., Prusoff, B. A. *et al.* (1985). Familial transmission of depression and alcoholism. *Archives of General Psychiatry*, **42**, 367–72.

Merikangas, K. R., Prusoff, B. A. & Weissman, M. M. (1988a). Parental concordance for affective disorders: psychopathology in offspring. *Journal of Affective Disorders*, **15**, 279–90.

Merikangas, K. R., Weissman, M. M., Prusoff, B. A. & John, K. (1988b). Assortative mating and affective disorders: psychopathology in offspring. *Psychiatry*, **51**, 48–57.

Mitchell, J., McCauley, E., Burke, P. *et al.* (1989). Psychopathology in parents of depressed children and adolescents. *Journal of the American Academy of Child and Adolescent Psychiatry*, **28**, 352–7.

Moldin, S. O., Reich, T. & Rice, J. (1991). Current perspectives on the genetics of unipolar depression. *Behaviour Genetics*, **21**, 211–42.

Nurcombe, B., Seifer, R., Scioli, A. *et al.* (1989). Is major depressive disorder in adolescence a distinct diagnostic entity? *Journal of the American Academy of Child and Adolescent Psychiatry*, **28**, 333–42.

Orvaschel, H. (1983). Parental depression and child psychopathology. In *Childhood psychopathology and development* (ed. S. B. Guze, F. J. Earls & J. E. Barrett), pp. 53–66. Raven Press, New York.

Orvaschel, H., Walsh-Allis, G. & Ye, W. (1988). Psychopathology in children of parents with recurrent depression. *Journal of Abnormal Child Psychology*, **16**, 17–28.

Orvaschel, H., Weissman, M. M., Padian, N. & Lowe, T. L. (1981). Assessing psychopathology in children of psychiatrically disturbed parents: a pilot study. *Journal of the American of Child Psychiatry*, **20**, 112–22.

Pauls, D. L., Morton, L. A & Egeland, J. (1992). Risks of affective illness among first-degree relatives of bipolar I Older-Order Amish probands. *Archives of General Psychiatry*, **49**, 703–8.

Puig-Antich, J., Goetz, D., Davies, M. *et al.* (1989). A controlled family history study of prepubertal major depressive disorder. *Archives of General Psychiatry*, **46**, 406–20.

Rice, J., Reich, T., Andreasen, N. C., Endicott, J. *et al.* (1987). The familial transmission of bipolar illness. *Archives of General Psychiatry*, **44**, 441–50.

Robins, L. N., Helzer, J. E., Croughan, J. & Ratcliff, K. S. (1981). The National Institute of Mental Health Diagnostic Interview Schedule. *Archives of General Psychiatry*, **38**, 381–7.

Ryan, N. D., Puig-Antich, J., Ambrosini, P. *et al.* (1987). The clinical picture of major depression in children and adolescents. *Archives of General Psychiatry*, **44**, 854–61.

Seifer, R., Nurcombe, B., Scioli, A & Grapentine W. L. (1989). Is major depressive disorder in childhood a distinct diagnostic entity? *Journal of the American Academy of Children and Adolescent Psychiatry*, **28**, 935–41.

Spitzer, R. L., Endicott, J. & Robins, E. (1978). Research Diagnostic Criteria: rational and reliability. *Archives of General Psychiatry*, **35**, 773–82.

Strober, M., Morrell, W., Burroughs, J. *et al.* (1988). A family study of bipolar I illness in adolescence: early onset of symptoms linked to increased family loading and lithium resistance. *Journal of Affective Disorders*, **15**, 255–68.

Sylvester, C. E., Hyde, T. S. & Reichler, R. J. (1988). Clinical psychopathology among children of adults with panic disorder. In *Relatives at risk for mental disorders* (ed. D. L. Dunner, E. S. Gershon & J. E. Barrett), pp. 87–102. Raven Press, New York.

Tsuang, M T. & Faraone, S. V. (1990). *The genetics of mood disorders*. Johns Hopkins University Press, Baltimore.

Warner, V., Weissman, M. M., Fendrich, M. *et al.* (1992). The course of major depression in the offspring of depressed parents: incidence, recurrence, and recovery. *Archives of General Psychiatry*, **49**, 795–801.

Weissman, M. M. (1988). Psychopathology in the children of depressed parents: direct interview studies. In *Relatives at risk for mental disorders* (ed. D. L. Dunner, E. S. Gershon & J. E. Barrett), pp. 143–59. Raven Press, New York.

Weissman, M. M. (1990). Evidence for comorbidity of anxiety and depression: family and genetic studies of children. In *Comorbidity of mood and anxiety disorders* (ed. J. D. Maser & C. R. Cloninger), pp. 349–66. American Psychiatric Press, Washington, DC.

Weissman, M. M., Gammon, G. D., John, K. *et al.* (1987). Children of depressed parents: increased psychopathology and early onset of major depression. *Archives of General Psychiatry*, **44**, 847–53.

Weissman, M. M., Warner, V., Wickramaratne, P. & Prusoff, B. A. (1988). Early-onset major depression in parents and their children. *Journal of Affective Disorders*, **15**, 269–78.

Weissman, M. M., Wickramaratne, P., Merikangas, K. R. *et al.* (1984). Onset of major depression in early adulthood: increased familial loading and specificity. *Archives of General Psychiatry*, **41**, 1136–43.

Welner, Z. & Rice, J. (1988). School-aged children of depressed parents: a blind and controlled study. *Journal of Affective Disorders*, **15**, 291–302.

West, M. O. & Prinz, R. J. (1987). Parental alcoholism and childhood psychopathology. *Psychological Bulletin*, **102**, 204–218.

8

Life events and difficulties: Their nature and effects

Ian M. Goodyer

INTRODUCTION

A life event is an environmental circumstance that has an identifiable onset and ending and may carry a potential for altering an individual's present state of mental or physical well-being. Such circumscribed happenings should be discriminated from other forms of longer-term social experience which may carry the same or similar effects but do not have readily identifiable onsets or endings. When the latter are considered undesirable they are generally referred to as long-term difficulties. Life events and difficulties have been the subject of much investigation as potential causes of major depression in adults and more recently in children and adolescents (Brown & Harris, 1978; Goodyer, 1991; Berney et al., 1991).

The psychiatrist Adolf Meyer was the first modern practitioner to suggest that life events need not be catastrophic or particularly unusual to be pathogenic (Meyer, 1951). He developed the use of life charts to systematically determine the temporal relationships between life experiences of many kinds and subsequent onsets of psychiatric disorder. This clinical method was further developed in the 1960s by Holmes & Rahe (1967), who devised a questionnaire to provide a summation of the quantity of environmental change in a person's life. Life change was hypothesised as the process which altered the chances of well-being. The life change score was used as a non-specific risk indicator for physical and mental illnesses. The 1970s and 1980s saw major advances in the investigation of life experiences as causal factors in the onset of psychi-

171

atric disorders. Firstly, Paykel noted the importance of discriminating between desirable and undesirable life changes (Paykel, 1974). Paykel also demonstrated that major undesirable events such as bereavements and divorce (collectively termed exit events) did not always result in clinical depression in adults and many episodes of depression were not preceded by major undesirable life events (Paykel, 1978). Secondly, Lazarus & Folkman (1984) emphasised that intrinsic psychological processes, notably cognitive appraisal, mediate or modulate the effects of life experiences on individual behaviour. Thirdly, Brown & Harris (1978) emphasised the importance of recording the specific nature and context of each recent life experience. Brown & Harris demonstrated that it was possible to reliably record the qualitative differences in the content of life experiences between individuals. These researchers also demonstrated that qualitative life event information could be rated reliably thereby comparing the latent psychological effects of socially differing events between individuals with and without depression. Such a procedure captures the coherence of individual experience whilst at the same time making it possible to draw general inferences about underlying psychopathological mechanisms from disparate happenings. Goodyer and colleagues adapted the advances of Paykel and Brown & Harris to investigate the impact of recent life experiences on school-age children but emphasised that, in addition to recording the nature and context of each experience, the child's developmental status must be taken into account when recording and rating the potential impact of recent life experiences (Goodyer, Kolvin & Gatzanis, 1985; Goodyer, 1991). Goodyer and colleagues also introduced the notion of measuring major life events over a childs lifetime by interview with a parent (Goodyer & Altham, 1991a). Sandberg and colleagues have incorporated the measurement of chronic experiences and major happenings over a child's lifetime into a systematic assessment of environmental experiences (Sandberg et al., 1993).

THE NATURE AND CHARACTERISTICS OF LIFE EXPERIENCES

Phenomenology

Events and experiences occur throughout a person's life and may be classified according to a number of criteria. Firstly, by their time of occurrence, i.e. they may be recent (days, weeks or months) or more distant in time; secondly, by their social characteristics, such as being family or school focused; thirdly, by their hedonic qualities, that is to say the degree to which an event, regardless of its social characteristics may be viewed as desirable; fourthly, by whether or not it is in the individual's best interests (regardless of its degree of desirability – not everything one likes or wants is good for you!); fifthly, by the social consequences, such as permanently altering the status quo in a child's life following bereavement or divorce or birth of a sibling (often referred to as exit and entry events) and sixthly, by the latent psychological characteristics that may be postulated as carried by an event. These potential latent effects include a diverse range of constructs, the most frequently used being loss (either real, such as bereavement, or perceived such as loss of a cherished idea or belief), physical danger to the self or disappointment (indicating unfulfilled expectations).

Events and experiences may also be classified according to their dependence on an individual's own behaviour. Thus events may be brought about by individuals influencing their environments or they may be independent of the individuals' own actions. Finally, it is important to determine the precedence of experiences to an individual's behaviour. For example, a causal question such as: do recent undesirable life events contribute to the onset of psychiatric disorder? requires an evaluation of the impact of events that *precede* the onset of an episode of disorder and are *independent* of illness-related behaviour. By contrast, a question which asks: do greater levels of undesirable life experiences occur to individuals with previous psychiatric disorder? requires an evaluation of events that *follow* after an episode of disorder but should include experiences *dependent* (i.e. occurring as a consequence of previous psychopathology) on previous illness as well as those independent of such illness. This is because in some individuals subsequent undesirable life experiences may arise as a consequence of previous illness or illness-related behaviour. The relative contribution of both dependent and independent life experiences to subsequent social adjustment and/or episodes of psychopathology can then be determined.

Measuring events – some issues for childhood

In adult studies the patient is invariably the person interviewed about recent stressful life events. But can we expect children reliably and validly to report recent adversities in their lives? We cannot be sure that adults' concepts and perceptions of threat, undesirability and other dimensions of events are necessarily the same as those of young people themselves (Monck & Dobbs, 1985; Yamamoto *et al.*, 1987).

Recent findings have shown, for example, that children's and adults' perceptions of the impact of recent life events are not entirely comparable (Rende & Plomin 1991). Parents may overestimate the general level of undesirability of recent events and children and their parents may vary on the degree of upsettingness of individual events. This study was small but together with previous findings (Brown & Cohen, 1988) indicates that children are indeed capable of reporting recent life events and rating their degree of upsettingness.

The correspondence between children's and adult's ratings may be a function of age. Thus the older the child the greater the correspondence with adults for the number of events reported and their degree of undesirability, suggesting that with maturity variation in the perception of events, as undesirable or not, becomes more stable (Brown & Cohen, 1988). The correspondence between adolescents' (who are free of current depression) and adults' ratings of the degree of undesirability of recent life events is high, indicating that subjective ratings of the impact of life events is as potentially valid as those of adults rating the adolescents' account of the events (Goodyer, Secher & Altham, 1994).

With these methodological features in mind, the rest of this chapter will consider the role of recent and past life events and ongoing life difficulties as social factors in the onset and outcome of individuals with major depression. Reference to research on adults is made where the findings are relevant to understanding the role of life experiences in the onset, course and outcome of depression in children and adolescents.

LIFE EVENTS AND THE ONSET OF DEPRESSION

In studies of adults it is only events that carry a moderate to severe degree of threat or undesirable negative impact that are significantly associated with the onset of an episode of major depression (Brown & Harris, 1978; Paykel, Myers & Dienelt, 1969). In recent years a number of refinements to event measurement have occurred in order to improve our understanding of the nature of undesirability. Classifying events according to some form of permanent and personal loss has received most study (Paykel *et al.*, 1980). Such exit events (i.e. events that result in the permanent removal of an individual from a person's social field) have been reported as significantly more common in depressives than in controls (Paykel *et al.*, 1969). A number of other studies in adults confirm that separations and losses are significantly more common in depressives than controls (Paykel *et al.*, 1980; Finlay-Jones & Brown, 1981). The converse entrance events (the permanent entry into a person's social field) are not associated with depression (Paykel *et al.*, 1969). There is also a suggestion that exits, undesirable and uncontrollable interpersonal disruptions, are reported more by depressed than anxious adults (Barrett, 1979). The latter findings suggest that some specificity may exist between the nature of undesirable events and depression. However, separations have been shown to precede other non-depressive disorders indicating that the relationship between depression and loss events is not entirely specific (Paykel & Cooper, 1992).

In recent years there has been increasing evidence to support the clinical observation that children and adolescents exposed to undesirable events and difficulties in the recent past are at a significantly increased risk for major depression and other types of psychopathology (Goodyer, 1991; Berden, Althaus & Verhulst, 1990). As with findings in adults it is only *moderate to severely* undesirable life events which are significantly associated with depressive disorders in school-age children (Goodyer *et al.*, 1985, 1988). Depressed children are also more likely to experience multiple losses over their own lifetime than controls (Goodyer & Altham 1991*a*). There is also the suggestion that bereavement events during the school age years, but not in the pre-school years, provoke the onsets of depressive disorder (Berney *et al.*, 1991).

These findings are not however specific to major depression and are found in other disorders including obsessive-compulsive disorder and anxiety states. The possible exception is that of bereavement during the school age years, which appears to result in greater risk for depression than other forms of psychiatric disorder (Berney *et al.*, 1991).

Some 50% of depressive episodes in young people are preceded by either an undesirable event or difficulty or a combination of both (Goodyer *et al.*, 1988; Goodyer, Wright & Altham, 1989; Goodyer, 1991). Undesirable events are therefore neither necessary nor sufficient to explain the onset of an episode of depression. Clearly, many other factors besides recent events and difficulties are important in the onset of depression.

Dimensions of life events

Refining the event measure can improve the specificity of the association between recent events and depression. This appears to be true mainly for refinements that relate to the underlying or latent psychological constructs that an event has, rather than a reclassification on descriptive social characteristics. For example, Miller and colleagues (1987) categorised events on six psychological dimensions (loss, threat, social action, hopeless situation, uncertain outcome, choice of action) and found that the number and pattern of these characteristics within a single event provided a better estimate for predicting adult depression than any one single dimension alone. These improvements in event measurement can be important in improving the magnitude of the association between events and depression.

Brown and colleagues refined their original concept of threat and investigated specific qualities of events (Brown, Bifulco & Harris, 1987). Firstly, long-term threat was dichotomised into upper and lower, indicating whether a threat was imminent or had already occurred. Secondly, six types of loss were considered: (i) death, (ii) separation, (iii) unemployment, (iv) physical illness, (v) disappointment, (vi) loss of a cherished idea. The first four of these classes of loss are identifiable in terms of social experience, i.e. they have an identifiable frame of reference. The last two classes are latent psychological constructs. The first of these is closely connected to social experience and therefore may be recognised by others The second is more abstract and less likely to be immediately apparent from a description of the event.

The last two concepts were not easy to discriminate, and careful definitions were used to assist in maintaining independence of the ratings. Thus, disappointment was defined as an event which resulted in an undesirable revision of a previous life experience. By contrast, loss of a cherished idea is a disruption of an expectation of trust, faithfulness or commitment, which may lead the individual to question these qualities in herself (these measures have so far only been reported in women). A rating of loss of a cherished idea therefore excludes a rating of previous experiences and is made on the basis of undesirable changes to ideas. This rating is therefore an attempt to measure the symbolic appraisal of loss. The concept of danger to the self is further divided into present danger and anticipated danger, which might occur in the future as a consequence of an event in the present. The results confirmed that these more sophisticated multidimensional ratings of events improves the specificity of the association between recent events and the onset of depression. The findings also suggested that depression is more likely when recent events match a woman's past undesirable experience. It appears possible that recent disappointments and/or loss of a cherished idea are components of a psychological mechanism that provokes onsets of major depression in women. It is apparent, however, that such a mechanism is dependent on having a previous similar experience. This suggests the negative reconsideration of the recent event is more likely when there has been a 'double exposure' of the experience.

Dimensional ratings of recent life events reported by adolescents in the community suggest that a single loss event is relatively common and less of a risk for depression than a recent disappointment (Goodyer *et al.*, 1994). Children exposed, however, to two or more losses over their lifetime (i.e. a double exposure) do appear to be at increased risk for depression or anxiety – this important issue is discussed detail in a later section of this chapter.

Disappointments represent the failure of a previously held expectation suggesting that the difference between expectation and real outcome of an event is the process determining the degree of impact on a child. The mechanisms of action of disappointments may be due to an unrealistic cognitive set of expectations about the outcome of an event which increases the likelihood of an 'event outcome' being considered as disappointing.

Childhood loss and adolescent depression

The substantive literature on loss and separation in childhood has clearly shown that brief separations from parents or other caregivers does not carry long-term risk for psychiatric disorder in middle childhood or adolescence (Wolkind & Rutter, 1985). When separations are permanent, such as removal into care or loss of parent by death, the long-term consequences are determined by the quality of the child's relationship prior to separation and the subsequent care arrangements for the child (Rutter, 1985). Thus the long-term effects are determined by the antecedent *and* consequential effects of the separation rather than the immediate reaction of the child to the separation per se. Longitudinal studies on children raised in care have confirmed that such early separation experiences exert adverse effects on the quality of subsequent interpersonal relationships (Quinton & Rutter, 1988; Rutter, 1990).

Bowlby proposed that early loss of a parent predisposes to depression in adult life through the development of cognitive-affective schemas that lowered self-image and self-efficacy when confronted with subsequent undesirable life events (Bowlby, 1980). The possibility that such a model may be relevant for depression in adolescence is suggested from some recent findings on early loss events.

Firstly, there is a surprising dearth of longitudinal studies on the long-term impact of permanent loss and separation. Little is known, for example, of the outcome of bereaved children beyond the first year following the loss (Van Eerdewegh et al., 1982). What evidence there is suggests, however, that such children do not demonstrate florid bereavement reactions beyond a few weeks. They do, however, continue to report higher levels of emotional symptoms than controls at 14 months. It is not known whether children with such 'sub-clinical' levels of emotional symptoms are at greater long-term risk for depression than children without such symptoms. It may be that such children are indeed at risk when faced with subsequent undesirable life events, but as yet this question has not been systematically investigated (see Berney et al., 1991, for an account of cross-sectional findings on the impact of bereavement).

Investigating the potentially causal effect of early loss, such as bereavement, for later depression in young persons is indeed difficult and complex because it requires extremely long-term follow-up of a large cohort of children, systematically and repeatedly assessed for life events and difficulties. In order to determine the appropriate period for follow-up a knowledge of the expected rate of such losses per unit time in the population at large would also be required. In practical terms, such a study is very unlikely to occur. A first step, however, would be to conduct retrospective studies determining if there is, in fact, a significant increase of loss events in the lives of children with current psychiatric disorder compared with those without such a disorder. A few such studies have been reported. For example, adolescents with psychotic illnesses and anorexia nervosa are significantly more likely to have experienced death of a first degree relative in childhood than community controls (Hellgren, Gillberg & Enerskog 1986; Råstam & Gillberg 1992). Less than a quarter of these cases experienced such a loss indicating that such 'exit events' are neither necessary nor sufficient for the subsequent onset of disorder in most cases. It remains unclear, however, how such loss exerts undesirable effects for subsequent disorder in the small but significant minority of such cases.

178

A study using in-depth interview procedures has recently been reported, in which permanent loss and separation events were recorded retrospectively from mothers. Such a life history procedure allows for a long-term view of early experiences on current functioning (Goodyer & Altham, 1991a).

The method of collecting 'long-term exit events' in an interview procedure is reliable and not subject to distortions of recall, even for exit events being recalled 5 years or more distant. The findings showed a significant association between current depression and multiple (two or more) losses or separations in a child's life but not for a single such experience. Currently there is some evidence to support the notion that loss in childhood increases the risk for depression in adolescence. The specificity of the association is unclear but appears to depend on being at least 'doubly exposed' to events with the same psychological connotation. A longitudinal 'catch up' study comparing rates of depression and other disorders in adolescents bereaved, divorced or separated as children would considerably illuminate the question of specificity.

It is important to note that many children who were exposed to multiple losses (including bereavements) remain well (Goodyer & Altham, 1991b). As noted with the studies on undesirable events, early loss events appear neither necessary nor sufficient to account for depression in adolescence.

Confiding relations and friendships

There has been a rapidly growing literature on the role of social support as influencing the risk for subsequent depression in adults (Paykel & Cooper, 1992). In the majority of studies social support is taken to mean the availability and adequacy of a confiding relationship (see e.g. Brown & Harris, 1978). There is some evidence that a confiding relationship decreases the risk of depression in adults who are exposed to recent undesirable life events (Brown & Harris, 1978). Perhaps more apparent is that the lack of a confiding relationship is a substantial risk for onsets of depression (Paykel & Cooper, 1992). The relationship between social supports and recent life events is complex and methods of measurement and statistical analysis have varied across studies. Overall the view is that the absence of social support is an independent causal factor in the onset of depression and poor social support at the time of depression is related to a longer course.

179

In children and adolescents, confiding relationships with a parent have also been noted to decrease the risk of psychopathology in general (Rutter, 1985). The role of a confiding relationship as a specific protective feature against depression has not been investigated. There is good evidence that depressed children have impaired relationships with parents and siblings during depression and to some extent following recovery (Puig-Antich *et al.*, 1993). There is also some evidence that poor friendships act as a risk factor for subsequent depression (Goodyer *et al.*, 1989). However, the finding is non-specific in that poor friendships predisposes to anxiety and probably some behavioural disorders as well. What little evidence there currently is suggests that impaired friendships are independent risks from undesirable life events for both anxious and depressive conditions (Goodyer, 1991). The potential mechanisms and processes that exist when a child is exposed to two or more risks such as undesirable life events and deficits in friendships are discussed later in this chapter.

There are complex issues surrounding the origins of friendship development and many factors that may influence a child's popularity and quality of relationship with peers, including family relationships in the pre-school years, temperament and personal achievements (Goodyer, 1991; Dunn & Maguire 1992). The possibility that impairments in friendships is itself a consequence of other earlier risk factors has yet to be determined.

EVENTS, ONSETS AND OUTCOME OF DEPRESSION – PROSPECTIVE STUDIES

The majority of the findings discussed above come from case-control studies conducted on community and clinical populations. Ideally, the causal link between life events and psychiatric disorder would be strengthened by studying events as they occur in the community, following up the population at risk as a consequence of the event, and noting the rate of illness in the days, weeks and months after event occurrence. The incidence of depression occurring within days and weeks of an event would give the best estimation of the causal association of events to disorder, as it reflects the proportion of new-onset cases. This would be entirely true if all known causal factors of depression were measured concurrently and prospectively. Under such circumstances the relative contribution of events could be accurately established. Major depression is, however, a heterogeneous condition with a range of causal mechanisms and processes some of which may be heavily dependent on preceding life events and others not at all. It is not surprising, therefore, that given the current state of knowledge about the syndrome, even longitudinal studies are unlikely to provide more that improved estimates of the mechanisms and magnitude of association between events and disorder. The specificity of the associations between environmental events and disorder is clearly dependent upon a valid classification of depression as much as it is upon events.

Studies on adults

Andrews (1981) reported a community-based prospective study of events occurring in 407 adults initially free from symptoms and found that the incidence of neurotic symptoms was significantly associated with life events that had occurred in the 4 months prior to symptom onset. The size of the association was similar to that of other retrospective studies. Andrews examined the path analysis of events to symptoms and found that 8 months later the association between events and symptoms was negligible and that previous symptoms were a better prediction of present symptoms than previous life events. A possible interaction between persistent symptoms and life events was noted.

A different longitudinal strategy was used with community samples by Tennant and colleagues (Tennant, Bebbington & Hurry, 1981). They examined the relationship between life events and the remission of neurotic disorders in adults . In this study, the authors concluded that 30% of all remissions were due to a 'neutralising' life event, defined as an event which specifically neutralised the impact of an earlier threatening life event. This appeared to be true for anxious and depressive conditions.

Miller and colleagues (Miller *et al.*, 1987) suggested that the duration, course and nature of depression was related to the form and timing of the life event. Events rated as likely to be of uncertain outcome were associated with illnesses of relatively longer duration, whereas events involving impaired interpersonal relations were associated with continuing illnesses. Events containing neither of these factors were associated with transient disorders of a few weeks' duration only.

Brown and colleagues (Brown, Adler & Bifulco, 1988; Brown, Lemyre & Bifulco, 1992) suggested that some events may exert a positive influence on the outcome of disorder because they intrinsically alter the person's appraisal of their life circumstances for the better, through the instillation of hope for the future. Such events have been referred to as 'fresh start' events. The hedonic qualities of fresh start events do not indicate their effects. Thus such events may often possess undesirable qualities in themselves, such as a serious personal accident, sudden unemployment or divorce. In such circumstances some individuals appear to use this negative experience for the better. There is no evidence, as yet, that children and adolescents are able to do this.

The onsets of depression in adults appear to be most strongly associated with undesirable events whose disappointing qualities are perceived as their own personal failure in relationships rather than the failures of a partner (Brown et al., 1988). By contrast, children and adolescents appear equally at risk from undesirable events whether or not they perceive them as resulting from their own personal failures (Goodyer et al., 1990b). Friendship failures perceived as the fault of another may indeed be an important and psychopathological form of disappointment.

In adults, events that result in a failure to meet expectations are associated with longer episodes of illness. By contrast, events which instill hope for the future appear to improve the opportunity of recovery. A reappraisal of one's own life may occur through private experiences of illnesses and personal failures. To date there is no evidence that such a set of processes are important for children or adolescents.

It is also apparent, however, that in many depressed cases in adults, events that precede or follow onsets of depression do not markedly influence outcome (Paykel & Cooper, 1992). A host of other factors may modify individual differences in response to events and outcome of disorder. These include both genetic and other environmental factors, ranging from biochemical through to family and other social experiences, temperament and coping strategies.

Studies in childhood and adolescence

There is currently only one published prospective longitudinal study on the influence of life events and difficulties on the outcome of childhood psychopathology (Goodyer et al.,1991). This small preliminary study investigated the role of life events and friendships in the recovery of 8 to 16-year-olds with a clinical diagnosis of anxiety or depression who had attended a child psychiatry clinic. The findings suggested that in the 14 to 28 months between onset of disorder, referral to the clinic and follow-up from discharge, the subjects were exposed to less undesirable events and significant improvements occurred in the confiding relations for their mothers. These findings were the same for both anxious and depressed subjects. Interestingly, neither the reduction in exposure to undesirable life events nor the improvement in maternal confiding predicted the child's recovery (defined as the absence of any mental state abnormalities). Failure to recover was predicted, however, by friendship difficulties occurring *after* onset of disorder, particularly for those with a diagnosis of depression. The possibility that an episode of depression increases the risk for *subsequent* friendship difficulties is suggested by these findings. In other words, psychopathology appears to increase the likelihood of children promoting, through their own maladaptation, long-term difficulties in their peer group environment.

MECHANISMS AND PROCESSES

The evidence that recent undesirable life events are of some non-specific importance in the onset of major depression in childhood and adolescence is reasonably strong. Far less clear is how these events exert their effects. Why is it that some children appear more sensitive than others when exposed to the same or similar circumstances? There is a need for life events research to move beyond a description of events as factors and determine the *mechanisms* by which they act and the *processes* which result in effects (Rutter, 1990). To date there has been no such specific research in major depression. The rest of this chapter discusses potential mechanisms and processes of life events and family and social difficulties on the basis of the few results available from cross-sectional studies that are currently reported.

Associations between recent undesirable events

Timing

If exposure to undesirable events provokes onset of depression then the prevalence of such events should be greater closer to onset. In the one case-control study to date that has measured the timing of events over a 12-month period, events occurred throughout the 12 months prior to the onset of disorder, but clustered in the 16 weeks closest to the onset of symptoms, supporting the inference that events cause disorder (Goodyer *et al.*, 1987).

Number of events

The onset of depression may be dependent in some circumstances on the number of events that an individual is exposed to. Currently there is some evidence that multiple event exposure does indeed increase the likelihood of psychiatric disorder in some cases (Goodyer et al., 1985, 1987). The mechanisms for this effect remain unclear; some individuals may be exposed to two or more recent events that are socially unconnected to each other increasing the general burden of social adversities in the child's life, for others a psychosocial connection may exist in which previous events increase the likelihood of further similar event occurrence.

The argument for multiple unconnected recent undesirable events as a causal aspect of depression in young people does not seem strong at present. Rather the current evidence suggests that such a 'dose–response' model is more appropriate for explaining some behaviour and adjustment disorders.

The co-occurrence of recent undesirable life events with other recent adversities

Few depressed school-age children are in fact exposed only to undesirable life events prior to the onset of their disorder. Over half of these patients are likely to be exposed to undesirable events and another type of recent difficulty, either within their family or within their friendships, in the year before the current episode of disorder (approximately 10% are exposed to no such adversities, Goodyer et al., 1990a, Goodyer & Altham, 1991b). The co-occurrence of different types of environmental adversities raises two rather different but related questions. Firstly, do recent undesirable life events exert negative effects in the presence of other more persistent difficulties? Secondly, do undesirable life events occur as a consequence of such difficulties?

Additivity

Additivity is defined as an increase in the magnitude of risk for disorder due to the presence of two or more social circumstances each with a known degree of risk. The magnitude of risk in additive circumstances is obtained by multiplying the known risks carried by each undesirable experience. As can be seen from Figure 8.1, this does not result in a simple summation of the quantity of risk.

The figure shows that each of these three risk circumstances occurring alone carries odds of between 3- and 5-fold (i.e. lonely mothers = 3.5, maternal distress = 5.5, life events = 5), rising to between 15 and nearly 20 fold increased risk for two circumstances occurring together and almost 100 fold for all three (as a consequence of multiplying the known odds, i.e. 3.5 x 5.5 x 5 = 96.25 fold an increase in risk). This additive model suggests that, even in the presence of many social adversities, the prevention or amelioration of a single risk circumstance may substantially decrease the likelihood of anxiety or depression in some secondary school-age children.

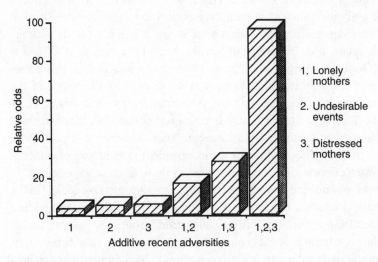

Figure 8.1. Cumulative effects of recent family adversities in anxious and depressed 8- to 16-year-olds.

Connectivity

Two undesirable experiences may be causally connected even when they exert additive effects. For example, one adversity may facilitate the onset of another. Mothers with a lifetime history of episodes of psychiatric disorder, notably depression, report a significantly increased rate of recent undesirable life events that exert a negative impact on their offspring (Goodyer et al., 1993). These findings indicate that some families are 'life event prone' and that children and adolescents in such families are more likely to be exposed to undesirable life events. The clinical implication is that ameliorating episodes of psychiatric disorder in parents may diminish the occurrence of undesirable life events focused on the child, thereby reducing the risk of psychiatric disorder in the child. (NB. There may also be a common origin in a third factor not measured which may account for the occurrence of both the measured factors; such a possibility has yet to be investigated in childhood emotional disorders.)

Independent Cumulation

Some concurrent environmental risks, whilst additive in their effects, may be truly independent in their origins. For example, about a third of anxious or depressed school-age children are exposed to both undesirable life events and friendship difficulties prior to the onset of their disorder (Goodyer, Wright & Altham, 1990a). The analyses of this cross-sectional data indicated that there was no significant difference in the co-occurrence of adverse events and poor friendships for either cases or controls. This suggests that there is no causal connection between these two different undesirable circumstances. These children were therefore exposed to both risks, indicating an independent cumulation of undesirable life experiences. The co-occurrence of these adverse experiences, in fact, gives an additive risk of 4.9 (friends) x 5.5 (events) or 26.95 fold, a substantive increase. The implications here are that school-age children with friendship difficulties are an important group for mental health surveillance whether or not such children or adolescents come from disharmonious families. In addition, it cannot be assumed by clinicians that, in such cases, treatment focused on the family will result in cessation of concurrent difficulties in the child's friendships.

Multiplicativity

There are some undesirable events or difficulties which, when they occur, carry no significant risk for subsequent psychiatric disorder on their own. In the presence of other risk circumstances, however, they potentiate the liability for an episode of disorder. The resultant interaction is termed a multiplicative effect to illustrate the importance of the potentiating effects of an apparently neutral circumstance on a known active one. Two rather different multiplicative processes, vulnerability and enhancement, have been described which, although similar in effect, differ in the precedence of the potentiating and active risk circumstances to each other.

Vulnerability

Women with three or more children and/or lacking a confiding relationship are much more likely to become depressed following exposure to threatening (provoking) life events than women exposed to similar life events but with fewer children and/or a confiding relationship (Brown & Harris, 1978) . In such circumstances, three or more children or lacking a confiding relationship are termed vulnerability factors because alone they carry no appreciable increase in risk but potentiate the effects of the provoking agent, recent life events. In this 'vulnerability factor-provoking agent model', the vulnerability circumstance *precedes* the provoking circumstance.

This vulnerability-provoking agent model has yet to be comprehensively tested in depressed children and adolescents. The current sparse evidence suggests, however, that recent undesirable life events and difficulties involving family or peer relationships all act as provoking agents rather than vulnerability factors, even when some undesirable circumstances are shown to precede others by months or even years (Goodyer 1991; Goodyer *et al.*, 1988, 1990*a*; Goodyer & Altham 1991*a*).

Enhancement

A second form of multiplicative risk process occurs when a potentiating risk factor occurs *following* that of an existing provoking agent. Under these conditions, the action of the second circumstance is enhancing the already existing risk.

For example, about 50% of school age children with anxious or depressive disorders experience desirable life events in the 12 months prior to the onset of their disorder, the same proportion as controls (Goodyer *et al.*, 1990*a*). These findings indicate that, alone, events which constitute recent desirable achievements appear to exert no effects (good or bad) on the risk for anxiety and depression. The importance of

187

the *absence of achievements* becomes clear, however, when considered in association with the quality of recent friendships.

The findings shown in Figure 8.2 indicate that, in the *presence* of friendship difficulties and an *absence* of recent desirable achievements, there is a marked increase in the likelihood of anxiety and depression beyond that already known for friendship difficulties alone. No achievements is concurrent with, or follows, friendship difficulties but *does not precede it*. Having no social achievements therefore enhances the already known risks carried by existing friendship difficulty.

When these analyses were repeated for the absence of social achievements and the presence of recent undesirable life events (most of which are family focused), no such negative enhancement was found. These findings suggest some differences in mechanisms of risk between predominantly peer related and predominantly family related adverse experiences.

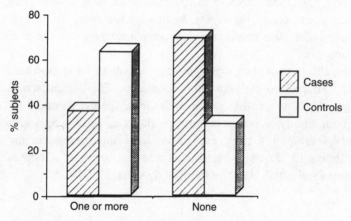

Figure 8.2. The negative enhancing effect of no desirable events in the presence of poor friendships.

Lifetime exits and current adversities

When the relative contribution of multiple exit events together with other events and difficulties preceding the onset of emotional disorders (family life events and maternal difficulties and distress; friendship difficulties/no desirable achievements) are analysed, the findings point to an effect for early exits that is independent of, and not accounted for, by either set of recent social adverse experiences (Goodyer & Altham,

1991*a*). The mechanisms by which multiple lifetime losses and/or separations exert their effects remain unclear. The findings suggest that such experiences may influence the child's mental representation of social relationships and his or her subsequent interpersonal behaviour. Other mechanisms are equally possible, however. For example, multiple loss and/or separation may initiate a chaining of undesirable ongoing experiences (i.e. a form of connectivity), such as chronically impaired family relations which are responsible for subsequent disorder in the child. The issue requires further research and may provide much needed insights into the influence of loss experiences on social-cognitive development in middle childhood, an area to date somewhat neglected by developmental science.

RESILIENCE TO ADVERSE EVENTS AND DIFFICULTIES

A persistent finding in the studies discussed are the proportion of subjects (perhaps as many as one in five) who, despite exposure to undesirable events and difficulties, are not cases of anxiety or depression – even when the increased risk for depression or anxiety is increased between 13- and 100-fold. A substantial proportion of school-age children and adolescents are resilient in the face of multiple adversities. There is, as yet, little research that has addressed the specific question, why are some children resilient in the face of such marked social difficulties (Rolfe *et al.*, 1990)? Rutter has indicated some of the current issues and controversies surrounding the concept of resilience in young persons (Rutter, 1990). The little that we currently know indicates that intrinsic psychological processes, such as affective-cognitive appraisal, are important in determining an individual's response to adverse life experiences (Lazarus & Folkman, 1984). Such a mediating mechanism seems particularly attractive to explain the sensitising effect of childhood losses for subsequent adolescent depression. Less clear, but of potential importance in determining both risk and resilience to environmental adversity, are physiological processes such as cortisol response to novel and arousing circumstances and individual differences in levels of sex hormones as organising influences on mood and behaviour (Goodyer *et al.*, 1991*b*; Buchanan, Eccles & Becker, 1992).

CONCLUSIONS

Specificity of life events and depression

A further striking feature of the findings discussed in this chapter is the lack of any clear specific associations between any one pattern of social adversities and the subsequent onset of major depression. To date the findings indicate that an onset of major depression *or* anxiety may occur as a consequence of a range of recent life events and difficulties from either the familial or peer group domain. The social mechanisms and processes elucidated so far fail to predict the form and type of disorder. Furthermore the 'vulnerability-provoking agent', model described by Brown & Harris (1978) for depression in adults (particularly women) appears less applicable to children and adolescents. The research so far suggests a 'provoking-amplification' model in which recent life events and difficulties in the main exert direct effects on the likelihood of disorder and the undesirable effects may be enhanced by further adversities, particularly those related to social achievement. Indeed there is compelling evidence to consider the quality of peer group experiences and the child's perception of their own social worth as particularly important in onset and outcome of depression. Some depressed young people are at risk for recurrent major depression because of a person–environment interaction increasing peer group (but not family) difficulties and perhaps impairing the capacity for evolving confiding relationships in adolescence and young adult life. The role of chronic social difficulties, such as persistent marital discord, family violence and unemployment appear more relevant to conduct disorders than major depression. It has to be said, however, that the concurrent measurement of chronic difficulties and recent life events and difficulties has yet to be systematically carried out in depressed children and adolescents (Sandberg *et al.*, 1993). Furthermore the interpersonal aspects of life events such as impaired family communication and level of critical comment between family members have only recently begun to be investigated (Asarnow *et al.*, 1993; Puig-Antich *et al.*, 1993). The relationship of these process measures of interpersonal behaviour to previous levels of life events and difficulties and subsequent onsets of depression remain unclear. Finally the notion of diagnosis itself needs careful scrutiny. It is possible that the specificity of events to diagnosis is dependent on delineating subgroups of depression based on patterns of depressive and non-depressive symptoms. This issue together with that of comorbidity of diagnoses is discussed in detail in Chapters 6 and 5 respectively. An example of such an association is suggested by the finding that early childhood loss appears to be more frequent in depressed adolescents with a clinical picture dominated by depressive cognitions rather than somatic or physiological symptoms (Berney *et al.*, 1991).

Future research clearly requires a combined approach both in terms of the design of studies and collaboration between behavioural and neuroscientists. Epidemiological studies of children and adolescents at high risk for depression combined with studies of a clinical population of already depressed children will be required so that sufficient numbers of subjects can be followed longitudinally. Such studies will be able to elucidate the social, psychological and physiological components that contribute to the onset, course and outcome of depression in young people.

REFERENCES

Andrews, G. (1981). A prospective study of life events and psychological symptoms. *Psychological Medicine*, **11**, 795–801.

Asarnow, J. R., Goldstein, M. J., Tompson, M., Guthrie, D. (1993). One year outcomes of depressive disorders in child psychiatric in-patients: the evaluation of the prognostic power of a brief measure of expressed emotion. *Journal of Child Psychology and Psychiatry*, **34**, 129–38.

Barrett, J. E. (1979). The relationship of life events to onset of neurotic disorders. In *Stress and mental disorder* (ed. J.E. Barrat), pp. 87–109. Raven Press, New York.

Berden, G. F. M. G., Althaus, M. & Verhulst F. C. (1990). Major life events and changes in the behavioural functioning of children. *Journal of Child Psychology and Psychiatry*, **31**, 949–60.

Berney, T. P., Bhate, S. R., Kolvin, I. *et al.* (1991). The context of childhood depression: the Newcastle childhood depression project. *British Journal of Psychiatry*, **159**, (suppl. 11), 28–35.

Bowlby, J. (1980). *Attachment and loss. Vol 3: Loss, sadness and depression.* Basic Books, New York.

Brown, G. W., Adler, Z. & Bifulco, A. (1988). Life events, difficulties and recovery from chronic depression. *British Journal of Psychiatry*, **152**, 487–98.

Brown, G. W., Bifulco, A. & Harris, T. O. (1987). Life events vulnerability and onset of depression; some refinements. *British Journal of Psychiatry*, **150**, 30–42.

Brown, G. W. & Harris,T. (1978). *The social origins of depression.* Tavistock Press, London.

Brown, G. W., Lemyre, L. & Bifulco, A. (1992). Social factors and recovery from anxiety and depressive disorders: a test of specificity. *British Journal of Psychiatry*, **152**, 44–54.

Brown, L. P. & Cohen, E. L. (1988). Children's judgements of event upsettingness and personal experience of stressful events. *American Journal of Community Psychology*, **16**, 123–35.

Buchanan, C. N., Eccles, J. S, Becker, J. B. (1992). Are adolescents the victims of raging hormones: evidence for activational effects of hormones on moods and behaviour at adolescence. *Psychological Bulletin* **111**, 62–107.

Dunn, J. & McGuire, S. (1992). Sibling and peer relationships in childhood. *Journal of Child Psychology and Psychiatry*, **33**, 67–106.

Finlay Jones, R. & Brown, G. W. (1981). Types of stressful life event and the onset of anxiety and depressive disorders. *Psychological Medicine*, **11**, 803–15.

Goodyer, I. M. (1991). *Life experiences, development and psychopathology*. John Wiley, Chichester.

Goodyer, I. M. & Altham, P. M. E. (1991*a*). Lifetime exit events in anxiety and depression in school-age children – I. *Journal of Affective Disorders*, **21**, 219–28.

Goodyer, I. M. & Altham, P. M. E. (1991*b*). Lifetime exit events in anxiety and depression in school-age children – II. *Journal of Affective Disorders*, **2**, 229–38.

Goodyer, I. M., Cooper, P. J., Vize, C & Ashby, L. (1993). Depression in 11 to 16 year old girls: the role of past parental psychopathology and exposure to recent life events. *Journal of Child Psychology and Psychiatry*, **34**, 1103–17.

Goodyer, I. M., Germany, E., Gowrusankur, J. & Altham, P. M. E. (1991*a*). Social influences on the course of anxious and depressive disorders in school-age children. *British Journal of Psychiatry*, **158**, 676–84.

Goodyer, I. M., Herbert, J., Moor, S. & Altham, P. M. E. (1991*b*). Cortisol hypersecretion in depressed school aged children and adolescents. *Psychiatry Research* **37**, 237–44.

Goodyer, I. M., Kolvin, I. & Gatzanis, S. (1985). Recent undesirable life events and psychiatric disorders of childhood and adolescence. *British Journal of Psychiatry*, **47**, 512–23.

Goodyer, M., Kolvin, I. & Gatzanis, S. (1987) The impact of recent life events in psychiatric disorders of childhood and adolescence. *British Journal of Psychiatry*, **151**, 179–85.

Goodyer, I. M., Secher, S. & Altham P. M. E. (1994) T*he perception of recent life events by adolescents in the community*, Developmental Psychiatry Section, research report no. 3, University of Cambridge

Goodyer, I. M., Wright, C. & Altham, P. M. E. (1988). Maternal adversity and recent stressful life events in anxious and depressed children. *Journal of Child Psychology and Psychiatry*, **29**, 651–67.

Goodyer, I. M., Wright, C. & Altham, P. M. E (1989). Recent friendships in anxious and depressed school age children. *Psychological Medicine*, **19**, 165–74.

Goodyer, I. M., Wright C. & Altham P. M. E. (1990*a*). Friendships and recent life events in anxious and depressed school-age children. *British Journal of Psychiatry*, **156**, 689–98.

Goodyer, I. M, Wright, C. & Altham, P. M. E. (1990*b*). Recent achievements and adversities in anxious and depressed school-age children. *Journal of Child Psychology and Psychiatry*, **31**, 1063–77.

Hellgren, L., Gillberg, C., & Enerskog, I. (1986). Antecedents of adolescent psychosis: a population-based study of school health problems in children who develop psychosis in adolescence. *Journal of the American Academy of Child and Adolescent Psychiatry*, **26**, 351–55.

Holmes, T. & Rahe, R (1967). The social readjustment rating scale. *Journal of Psychosomatic Research*, **11**, 213–18.

Lazarus, R.S. & Folkman, S. (1984) *Stress, appraisal and coping*. Springer, New York.

Meyer, A. (1951). The life chart and the obligation of specifying positive data in psychopathological diagnosis. In *The collected papers of Adolf Meyer Vol III* (ed. E. E. Winters), pp. 21–6. Johns Hopkins Press, Baltimore.

Miller, P. McC., Ingham, J. G., Kreitman, N. B. *et al.* (1987). Life events and other factors implicated in onset and in remission of psychiatric illness in women. *Journal of Affective Disorders*, **10**, 203–6.

Monck, E, Dobbs, R. (1985). Measuring life events in an adolescent population: methodological issues and related findings. *Psychological Medicine*, **15**, 841–50.

Paykel, E. (1974). Life stress and psychiatric disorder. Chapter in: *Stressful life events: their nature and effects*, pp. 42–51. John Wiley, New York.

Paykel, E. S. (1978). The contribution of life events to causation of psychiatric illness. *Psychological Medicine*, **8**, 245–53.

Paykel, E. & Cooper, Z. (1992). Life events and social stress. In *Handbook of Affective Disorders* (ed. E. Paykel), pp. 149–71. Churchill Livingstone, Edinburgh.

Paykel, E. S., Emms, E. M., Fletcher, J. & Rassaby, E. S. (1980). Life events and social support in puerperal depression. *British Journal of Psychiatry*, **139**, 339–46.

Paykel, E., Myers, J, K. & Dienelt, M. N. (1969). Life events and depression: a controlled study. *Archives of General Psychiatry*, **32**, 327–33.

Puig-Antich, J., Kauffman, J., Ryan, N. D. *et al.* (1993). The psychosocial functioning and family environment of depressed children. *Journal of the American Academy of Child and Adolescent Psychiatry*, **32**, 244–54.

Quinton, D. & Rutter, M. (1988). *Parenting breakdown: the making and breaking of intergenerational links*. Avebury, Aldershot.

Råstam, M. & Gillberg, C. (1992). Background factors in anorexia nervosa. *European Child and Adolescent Psychiatry*, **1**, 54–65.

Rende, D. & Plomin, R. (1991). Child and parent perceptions of the upsettingness of major life events. *Journal of Child Psychology and Psychiatry*, **32**, 627–33.

Rolfe, J., Masten A.S., Cicchetti, D. *et al.* eds. (1990) *Risk and protective factors in the development of psychopathology*. Cambridge University Press, Cambridge.

Rutter, M. (1985). Family and school influences on behavioural development. *Journal of Child Psychology and Psychiatry*, **3**, 349–68.

Rutter, M. (1990). Psychosocial resilience and protective mechanisms. In *Risk and protective factors in the development of psychopathology* (ed. J. Rolfe, A. S. Masten, D. Cicchetti *et al.*), pp. 181–214, Cambridge University Press, Cambridge.

Sandberg, S., Rutter, M., Giles, S. *et al.* (1993). Assessment of psychosocial experiences in childhood: methodological issues and some illustrative findings. *Journal of Child Psychology and Psychiatry*, **34**, 879–99.

Tennant, C., Bebbington, P. & Hurry, J. (1981). The role of life events in depressive illness. Is there a substantive causal relation? *Psychological Medicine*, **11**, 379–89.

Wolkind, S. & Rutter, M. (1985). Separation, loss and other family relationships. In *Child psychiatry: Modern approaches* (ed. M. Rutter, & L. Herzov), pp. 34–58. Blackwells, Oxford.

Van Eerdewegh, M.. Bieri, M., Parilla, R. & Clayton, P. (1982). The bereaved child. *British Journal of Psychiatry*, **140**, 23–9.

Yamamoto, K., Soliman, A., Parsons, J. & Davis, O. C., Jr. (1987). Voices in unison: stressful events in the lives of children in 6 countries, *Journal of Child Psychology and Psychiatry*, **6**, 855–64.

9

Adolescent depression: Neuroendocrine aspects

Stan Kutcher and Stephen Sokolov

INTRODUCTION

The development of criterion-based diagnostic systems has been an impetus for the investigation of the neurobiological underpinnings of psychiatric disturbance in children and adolescents. Although, to date, insufficient knowledge exists to specifically identify the aetiologies of various disorders, studies of clinical and normative populations have led to a veritable explosion of knowledge about the neuroendocrine aspects of psychiatric disorders. As a result of these investigations, the specificity of current diagnostic systems has been questioned, the pathophysiology of various psychiatric disorders has been explored and simplistic models which previously has been invoked to explain both normal and pathological behaviour (for example: adolescent turmoil is due to hormones) are no longer tenable.

Neuroendocrine studies in adolescent depression have arisen from the influence of similar research in adult populations, and some of the earliest work in this field was an attempt to determine if the neurobiological features found in adult depressives would also be present in children and adolescents. Similar findings, it was argued, would provide further evidence for the presence of depressive disorders in younger populations and thus lend credibility to the diagnostic classification of child and adolescent depression. This work of pioneering investigators has been further developed by the realisation of the different central nervous system and neurohormonal aspects of adolescents compared to adults. Furthermore, the complexities of adolescent neuroendocrinology with its developmentally determined differences that occur rapidly during a few years of the life cycle have added a dimension of complexity that is not usually addressed in studies of adult populations. Thus, the study of the neuroendocrinology of adolescent mood disorders has become an important area of investigation in its own right.

This importance is further substantiated by the recent realisation that depressive disorders are, by and large, adolescent onset disorders (Christie *et al.*, 1989; Weissman & Klerman, 1992). The prevalence rate of major depression changes from about 1% pre-pubertally to the adult levels of about 8% by age 19. That the onset of this disorder occurs during a phase of a major central nervous system reorganisation concurrently with the onset of puberty suggests that an understanding of these issues may advance our knowledge of the aetiology of depression, an idea that receives further support from the well-known relationship between organic disorders of the central nervous and endocrine systems and depression. Some authors have even suggested that neuroendocrine studies of depression should occur primarily in the adolescent population, free from the confounds of antidepressant treatments and previous episodes.

Neuroendocrine studies in adolescent depression have two complementary but different purposes. First, they are an attempt to determine the biological aetiology of depression. According to this model, depression is the symptomatic expression of a final common pathway of central nervous system (CNS) dysfunctions that may involve a number of neurotransmitter systems (Siever & Davis, 1985). The systems most commonly postulated to be involved include the noradrenergic, serotonergic and cholinergic systems, with disturbances possibly occurring at the level of deficiencies or excesses of specific neurotransmitters, functioning of various receptors, or in second messenger systems (Coppen, 1967; Heninger & Charney, 1987; Charney *et al.*, 1990). Neuroendocrine strategies provide a 'window on the brain' model (a method of indirectly assessing CNS functioning) useful in the study of putative CNS disturbances by assessing differences in neuroendocrine functioning between depressed adolescents and normal controls. Significant differences in peripheral measures of neuroendocrine variables between depressed teenagers and normal controls are postulated to reflect differences in CNS functioning between groups. These presumed CNS differences are then further proposed to reflect CNS dysregulation associated with the depressed state or trait.

As such, neuroendocrine strategies have inherent limitations. Measurements of monoamine metabolities in peripheral fluids are not exact reflections of monoamine metabolism in the central nervous system. For example, only about 50% of dopamine metabolites measured in the urine and up to 30% of noradrenaline metabolites measured in plasma originate in the CNS (Kopin, Gordon & Jimmerson, 1983; Riddle, Anderson & McIntosh, 1986). Even further removed from presumed CNS pathology are baseline and challenge paradigm evaluations of thyroid and growth hormone, cortisol, prolactin, and other hormones. These studies are even more problematic as, in addition to the developmental changes in hormone secretions, the effect of diet, physical activity, baseline levels of arousal, difficulties in laboratory measurement and the generalised stress response may all influence the findings or interpretation (Johnson *et al.*, 1992). However, given these limitations, such studies still advance our understanding of the neurobiology of depression in the adolescent population. These studies may also provide clues as to pharmacological treatments or physiological parameters that may aid in diagnosis, predicting treatment outcome or relapse.

This chapter will review the current literature on various neuroendocrine studies in adolescent depression. Wherever possible, it will also briefly summarise relevant physiological information about various endocrine systems and also, succinctly review selected adult findings in similar areas of investigation, to highlight similarities and differences to adolescent studies in findings where they occur.

GROWTH HORMONE

The hypothalamic pituitary growth hormone axis (HPGH) provides a good model for evaluating central nervous system (CNS) functioning. The HPGH axis is under serotonin, histamine, acetylcholine, norepinephrine and dopamine control at the level of the hypothalamus (Checkley, 1980; Dieguez, Page & Scanlon, 1987). Growth hormone (GH) release from the pituitary is regulated by the interplay of the above neurotransmitters, either by direct hypothalamic action or through their effect on intermediate compounds such as growth hormone releasing hormone (GHRH) or somatostatin (GHRF). Thus, disturbances in various paramaters (basal secretion and stimulated secretion) of the HPGH axis, if found in adolescents with major depression, could be understood as reflecting disordered CNS neurotransmission, and would be best viewed as a 'downstream' marker of CNS dysfunction.

Growth hormone secretion from the anterior pituitary is controlled

197

by an intricate balance of central nervous system peptides including somatatostatin and GHRH. While somatostatin is widely distributed in the CNS, GHRH is localised primarily in the arcuate and ventromedial nuclei of the hypothalamus. GH is released from the pituitary in a pulsatile pattern, primarily in response to the interaction between somatostatin and GHRH, with somatostatin acting as to decrease the GHRH stimulated GH release by signalling the offset of each secretory phase. Additionally, adrenocortical hormones and corticotropic releasing hormone (CRH) also play a modulating role on somatotropin functioning.

Neuropeptide control of GH is exceedingly complex with noradrenergic, cholinergic and serotonergic systems all involved. Furthermore, nocturnal GH secretion may be under different neuropeptide control (primarily serotonergic) than daytime GH secretion (primarily noradrenergic). Thus, clinical evaluation of the GH axis may involve time-of-day effects, with studies conducted during the day to evaluate CNS control mechanisms that differ from those active nocturnally.

Developmentally, basal GH secretion declines significantly with age. The daily pattern of GH secretion also changes, with significantly fewer GH peaks and a lower night to day secretory ratio occurring with increased age (Finkelstein et al., 1972; Zadik et al., 1985). Furthermore, recent studies have shown similar age effects in growth hormone binding protein (GHBP) with progressive increases in GHBP during the first two decades of life (Daughaday & Trivedi, 1991) and decreases in GHBP beginning sometime in the third decade of life (Hattori et al., 1991). The response of GH to GHRH, however, is relatively consistent throughout life, therefore suggesting that the developmental change in GH basal secretion is due to changes in the secretory patterns of GHRH or somatostatin occurring at the hypothalamic level (Gelato & Merriam, 1986).

Basal growth hormone secretion

Basal GH secretory studies in depressed adults do not show consistent findings, with reports of nocturnal hypersecretion (Schilkrut, Chandra & Oswald, 1975), hypersecretion over a 24-hour period (Mendlewicz et al., 1985) and hypersecretion prior to sleep onset (Linkowski et al., 1987a,b). However, Jarrett, Miewald & Kupfer (1990) reported a reduction in GH secretion occurring during the initial 3 hours following sleep onset and Rubin, Poland & Lesser (1990) were not able to determine any differences in 24-hour secretory profiles between adult depressives and controls. In Rubin's study, however, both male and female depressives had much higher GH secretory peaks during the 24:00 to 02:00 hour period compared to controls. The lack of significance in this report may be due to the large standard deviation of serum GH values in the sample.

Studies of basal GH secretion in adolescent samples have also been contradictory. Kutcher *et al.* (1989, 1991) have reported that adolescents with major depressive disorder hypersecrete GH at night with the period between 24:00 and 02:00 hours showing the greatest difference compared to normal controls. This difference occurred independently of sleep disturbances and the amount of slow wave sleep prior to the first REM (rapid eye movement) period. These findings parallel those reported by Puig-Antich *et al.* (1984*a,c*) in depressed children. However, Dahl *et al.* (1992) did not find significant differences in nocturnal GH secretion between depressed teenagers and controls. The reasons for the discrepant findings are not clear but may reflect different patient populations, different comorbid conditions or different study techniques.

Stimulated growth hormone secretion

Studies of GH stimulation in depressed adults have shown a variety of results, usually with blunting of GH reported to a variety of stimuli including: insulin induced hypoglycaemia; clonidine, dextroamphetamine and desmethylimipramine (Sachar, Finkelstein & Hellman, 1971; Gregoire *et al.*, 1977; Checkley, 1981; Charney, Heninger & Ternberg, 1982; Siever *et al.*, 1982; Amsterdam *et al.*, 1987*a,b*). However, not all investigators have found this pattern in either insulin-induced hypoglycaemia (Koslow *et al.*, 1982; Amsterdam & Maislin, 1991) or dextroamphetamine stimulation (Halbreich *et al.*, 1982). Finally, a number of studies have demonstrated GH blunting to GHRH (Lesch *et al.*, 1987; Risch, Ehlers & Janowsky, 1988), although not all investigators have demonstrated this (Eriksson *et al.*, 1988; Thomas *et al.*, 1989).

Studies of GH stimulation in depressed children have demonstrated GH blunting to both insulin induced hypoglycaemia (Puig-Antich *et al.*, 1984*b*) and clonidine challenge (Jensen & Garfinkel, 1990). In depressed adolescents, Jensen & Garfinkel (1990) demonstrated a similar blunted GH response to clonidine stimulation. Ryan, Puig-Antich & Rabinovich (1988) showed GH blunting in response to intramuscular desipramine challenge in teens with major depression, with maximal blunting found in the most suicidal of the depressives. Waterman *et al.* (1991) did not find any significant differences between depressed adolescents and normal controls in the GH response to dextroamphetamine. There are no reports to our knowledge of GH responses to GHRH in depressed teenagers.

Somatostatin and growth h:ormone

Somatostatin has been reported to be decreased in adult depressives but has not been evaluated in depressed adolescents (Rubinow, Gold & Post, 1983; Agren & Lundqvist, 1984). However, low somatostatin levels fit the paradigm of high nocturnal GH secretion reported by Kutcher *et al.* (1989, 1991) and blunted GH responses to a variety of stimulation tests including GHRH on the basis of reduced daytime pituitary reserve secondary to nocturnal hypersecretion. In any case, although the studies are not conclusive, the available evidence suggests that depressed adolescents exhibit a disturbance of the GH axis that is probably reflective of CNS dysregulation, possibly primarily in the serotonin system (Kutcher *et al.*, 1991).

THYROID HORMONE

The hypothalamic–pituitary–thyroid axis has been studied in response to historical observations of mood alteration in the presence of thyroid disease and as a putative window on CNS processes in depression (Bauer & Whybrow, 1988; Joffe, 1990; Joffe & Sokolov, 1994). While there is a voluminous literature on the thyroid and adult mood disorders, the adolescent literature is more limited.

Neuronal regulation of the thyroid axis at the hypothalamic and pituitary level is not well understood in humans. On the basis of animal studies, it is known that the hypothalamus receives neuronal input via dopaminergic, noradrenergic, and serotonergic pathways originating in the mid-brain. In animals, dopamine seems to play a stimulatory role in TRH secretion mediated through D_2 receptors.

In the pituitary, noradrenergic fibres stimulate TSH release through activation of the adenylate cyclase system. Dopamine, somatostatin and glucocorticoids inhibit TSH release by decreasing pituitary response to TRH stimulation (Scanlon, 1991; Larsen & Ingbar, 1992). The role of the central serotonergic system has been reviewed elsewhere with reports of both an inhibitory and stimulatory effect on TSH secretion (Krulich, 1982; Scanlon, 1991). This may reflect the plethora of serotonin receptor subtypes and the observation that different serotonin subsystems may have opposite physiological effects.

At the level of the thyroid gland, noradrenergic, cholinergic and peptidergic nerves innervate and terminate along the follicles and the blood vessels supplying them. Adrenergic fibres activate the adenylate cyclase system promoting colloid droplet formation and thyroid hormone release. Noradrenaline stimulates thyroid hormone secretion under basal conditions and inhibits thyroid hormone release under conditions of TSH stimulation. Acetylcholine inhibits TSH induced thyroid hormone secretion while vasoactive intestinal peptide (VIP), a peptidergic neurotransmitter, stimulates basal thyroid hormone secretion and potentiates thyroid hormone secretion in response to TSH. To complicate matters further, VIP and acetylcholine may coexist in nerves in the thyroid and the two may be released together when these nerves are stimulated. However, at this time, the exact role of neural mechanisms of thyroid regulation in depression remains unclear (Ahren, 1986; Larsen & Ingbar, 1992).

Developmental considerations may apply when assessing thyroid function in the paediatric or adolescent age group and this reinforces the necessity for utilising age and sex matched controls. In a recent study by Garcia et al. (1991), TSH response to TRH stimulation increased linearly with age in prepubertal children. Although present in both sexes, the increase by age was most marked in girls.

Basal thyroid secretion

Numerous reports of basal thyroid hormone levels in adult depression exist in the literature with the most consistent findings being elevated (but within the euthyroid range) levels of T4 in depressives relative to controls with or without an elevation of some measure of free T4 thought to be secondary to increased T4 production. Additionally, studies that have followed thyroid indices through the course of the depressive episode demonstrate a decrease in T4 and/or free T4 with antidepressant or electroconvulsive therapy and it has been reported that the magnitude of the decrease in T4 has been correlated with the magnitude of the treatment response to these modalities (Dewhurst et al., 1968; Whybrow et al., 1972; Hatotami et al., 1974; Kirkegaard et *al.*, 1975, 1977; Linnoila *et al.*, 1979; Gold, Pottash & Extein, 1981; Kirkegaard, 1981; Kirkegaard & Faber, 1981; Baumgartner *et al.*, 1988; Joffe & Singer, 1990*b*; Kirkegaard, Korner & Faber, 1990; Kirkegaard & Faber, 1991; Styra, Joffe & Singer, 1991).

Thus, findings with respect to basal thyroid function in the adult literature suggest that major depression in this age group is associated with relative thyroid over-activity and that this resolves with recovery.

Reports of basal thyroid function in adolescent depression have been few. Carstens, Taljaard & Van Zyl (1990) reported that basal values of free T4 in patients and controls were within the normal laboratory range but were significantly elevated in depressed subjects compared to normal controls (Carstens *et al.*, 1990). Sokolov, Kutcher & Joffe (1994) assessed baseline thyroid function in a group of adolescents with DSM III-R major depressive disorder and bipolar disorder, manic phase at the time of their first psychiatric hospitalisation. Depressed and bipolar subjects were found to have a significantly elevated total T4 when compared to normal controls. All thyroid indices, however, were within the normal range. Kutcher *et al.* (1991) described no significant group differences between depressed adolescents and normal controls in nocturnal secretions of T4 or free T4. Nocturnal TSH, however, was significantly elevated in about one-third of the depressed group suggesting that a suprapituitary mechanism may be implicated in the findings of thyroid axis dysregulation. Therefore, despite a more limited adolescent literature, findings within this age group also seem to support an association between over-activity of the thyroid axis and depression.

Stimulated TSH secretion

The TRH Stimulation Test has been used extensively in numerous studies of depressed adult patients and has been reviewed elsewhere (Kirkegaard, 1981; Loosen, 1986; Bauer & Whybrow, 1988; Joffe 1990; Joffe & Sokolov, 1994). Despite some inconsistencies in methodology, a blunted TSH response to TRH stimulation has been generally noted in 25–30% of depressed adults. However, certain exogenous and endogenous factors are known to influence the TSH response to TRH. These factors include age, sex and caloric intake (Larsen & Ingbar, 1992). What is more, a blunted TSH response to TRH stimulation is not specific to major depression and may be found in individuals without psychiatric illness or in persons with anorexia nervosa (Gold *et al.*, 1980), alcoholism (Loosen, 1986), borderline personality disorder (Garbutt *et al.*, 1983), and schizophrenia (Baumgartner, 1986).

Although the pathophysiology is unclear, a blunted TSH response in depression may represent overactivity of the thyroid axis. This may be understood as follows. First, the TSH response to TRH is sensitive to feedback inhibition by elevated levels of thyroid hormone. A blunted TSH response may then result from the higher levels of T4 in patients with depression (Joffe & Sokolov, 1994). Second, elevated TRH in the cerebrospinal fluid has been observed in patients with endogenous depression (Kirkegaard *et al.*, 1979; Banki *et al.*, 1988). Since repeated injections of TRH result in a progressively more blunted TSH response to TRH stimulation (Linnoila *et al.*, 1979; Winokur *et al.*, 1984) a blunted TSH response in depression may in fact arise from chronic exposure of the pituitary to excessive TRH secretion. This would presumably result in either receptor down-regulation at the pituitary level, depletion of pituitary stores of TSH, or both. Therefore, it can be taken that studies of stimulated TSH secretion in depressed adults, along with studies of basal thyroid function, provide further evidence of an association of relative thyroid over-activity with depressive illness.

Investigations of the TSH response to TRH in adolescent depression are few. Chabrol, Claverie & Moron (1983) noted that only 2 out of 20 adolescent outpatients referred for suicidal ideation exhibited a blunted TSH response to TRH (Chabrol *et al.*, 1983). However, none of these patients met DSM III criteria for major depressive disorder. Kahn (1987) reported that 33% of adolescents with major depression showed TSH blunting compared to 43% of substance abusers and 17% of psychiatric controls (Kahn, 1987). In another study, Kahn (1988) reported that 37% of adolescents with MDD showed a blunted TSH response to TRH. However, high rates of TSH blunting were again present in adolescents with substance abuse, conduct disorders and adjustment disorders. No significant differences were found between diagnostic groups. Brambilla *et al.* (1989) studied a small group of medication-free dysthymic children and adolescents. Compared to controls, dysthymics did not differ with respect to TSH responses to TRH stimulations. Carstens *et al.* (1990) reported that 17% of his study population showed a blunted TSH response to TRH, an insignificant difference from controls. Taken together, these findings suggest that up to one-third of adolescent depressions may show TSH blunting to TRH, a frequency comparable to findings in adults. The specificity and significance of these findings, however, remain unclear.

As in the adult literature, patterns of basal thyroid dysfunction in the absence of thyroid illness have been found in some adolescents with depression as well as other psychiatric disorders. With respect to TSH response to TRH stimulation, findings are inconsistent in children and adolescents. This may be due in part to variations in the dose of TRH employed as well as due to age and sex effects (Garcia et al., 1991). Furthermore, the evidence to date suggests that the TRH stimulation test is of little diagnostic utility in this age group. Of interest, however, is that in both basal secretion and in response to TRH stimulation, about one-third of adolescent depressives may show deranged TSH parameters. Whether this constitutes a specific subgroup or other particular features of adolescent depression remains a question for further study.

CORTISOL

Corticotropin-releasing hormone (CRH) originating mainly in the paraventricular nucleus of the hypothalamus causes an immediate and dose-dependent release of adrenocorticotropic hormone (ACTH) from the anterior lobe of the pituitary, and is considered to be the major regulator of pituitary secretory ACTH activity (Rivier & Plotsky, 1986). Glucocorticoids, secreted from the adrenals under the influence of ACTH, and ACTH itself, exert a complicated pattern of inhibition on CRH-induced ACTH release through a variety of feedback mechanisms that exhibit both immediate and long-term effects (Axelrod & Reisine, 1984; Aguilera et al., 1987). Both acute and chronic stress intimately affect the hypothalamic–pituitary–adrenal (HPA) axis, with direct effects on the amount and patterns of circulating glucocorticoids (Hauger et al., 1989; Johnson et al., 1992). Additionally, studies of primates and other species have suggested that significant stresses occurring during the neonatal period may alter HPA responses to stress occurring later in life and that these responses may reflect developmentally induced susceptibility to depression (Thomas, Levine & Arnold, 1968; Gold, Goodwin & Chrousos, 1988; Kalin & Takahashi, 1988). These features of the HPA axis, particularly its role in the stress response, make evaluation of its function in depression somewhat problematic as a variety of stressors that may be non-specific to depression can affect the functioning of this system. However, given these caveats, the evaluation of the HPA axis in depression may have some utility.

Neurotransmitter regulation of CRH is exceedingly complex and involves the input of the cholinergic, catecolaminergic, indolaminergic systems and other substances such as GABA, histamine, and angiotensin ll (Pepper & Kreiger, 1984; Johnson *et al.*, 1992). Plasma ACTH and cortisol levels exhibit a diurnal variation with highest amounts found during the early morning (just prior to awakening) and the nadir located in the late afternoon or early evening. Episodic secretory spikes are superimposed on this daily rhythm (Kreiger *et al.*, 1971). This circadian rhythm of HPA activity is thought to be driven by an endogenous central nervous system pacemaker located in the suprachiasmatic nucleus of the hypothalamus (Moore & Eichler, 1972; Stokes & Sikes, 1987) and this pattern apparently persists throughout the life cycle.

Basal cortisol secretion

Studies assessing cortisol activity in both urine and serum have described 24-hour hypersecretion of cortisol, with increased numbers of secretory episodes and a loss of the afternoon/early evening nadir with a resulting flattening of the circadian curve in many but not all adult depressives. Additionally, a phase advance of one to three hours in the early morning cortisol rise has been described (Doig *et al.*, 1966; Sachar *et al.*, 1973; Stokes *et al.*, 1984; Linkowski *et al.*, 1987*a,b*). Although some studies report contradictory results, this increase in cortisol secretion may be secondary to an increased incidence of daily ACTH pulses (Holaday, Martinez & Natelson, 1977; Kirkegaard & Carroll, 1980; Nasr *et al.*, 1983; Follenius *et al.*, 1987; Mortola *et al.*, 1987; Krishnan *et al.*, 1990). Cortisol and CRH levels in the cerebral spinal fluid have been reported as elevated in some adult depressives (Traskman *et al.*, 1980; Stokes *et al.*, 1984; Nemeroff *et al.*, 1984) and while all investigators have not demonstrated this phenomenon (Jimmerson *et al.*, 1980), it can be generally concluded that many depressed adults show perturbations in the basal tone of the HPA axis during the depressive episode.

Studies of basal cortisol secretion in adolescent depressives are few but generally do not parallel the adult findings. Dahl *et al.* (1989) failed to find any significant differences in the 24-hour cortisol secretory profiles of teenage depressives compared to normal controls. In another report using a similar study methodology, Dahl *et al.* (1991) found that some depressed adolescents showed significantly elevated cortisol levels compared to normal controls but only near the time of sleep onset. Of interest, is that most of these differences were accounted for by a sub-group of suicidal in-patient adolescents. Kutcher *et al.* (1991) were not able to demonstrate any significant differences in nocturnal cortisol secretion between adolescent depressives and normal controls. Similarly, Kutcher & Marton (1989), using a neuroendocrine day study paradigm reported that elevated afternoon cortisol secretion occurred in less than one-third of depressed adolescents.

Finally, Kutcher *et al.* (1991) reported that less than 10% of depressed adolescents showed any individual abnormalities in their nocturnal cortisol secretion profiles. Those who demonstrated nocturnal hypersecretion showed elevated serum cortisol levels beginning early in the morning, suggesting a phase advance in the cortisol secretory rise. Of interest is that these patients were characterised by severe guilty ruminations, suggesting a differential HPA effect in those depressed teenagers who exhibited quasi-delusional symptomatology. Goodyer *et al.* (1991), using sophisticated mathematical modelling, demonstrated in a small number of subjects that 24-hour cortisol rhythms may change following recovery from depression. Although no control groups were available for comparison, these findings taken together suggest that sub-tle alterations in baseline cortisol secretion may occur in adolescent depressives, particularly in subgroups, but further detailed investigations are needed.

HPA axis stimulation tests

Dexamethasone suppression test

Non-suppression of serum cortisol by dexamethasone has been fre-quently reported in depressed adults (Carroll, Curtis & Mendels, 1976; Brown & Shuey, 1980; Carroll *et al.*, 1981; Brown, 1984; Rubin *et al.*, 1987), but the specificity of this test has not been demonstrated and recent investigations have raised questions about the exact mechanism of dexamethasone suppression itself (Miller *et al.*, 1992). Current con-sensus, however, is that the DST has little diagnostic validity (Holsboer *et al.*, 1986) in this population. Its current application, however, may be in its use as a state marker which has utility in assessing treatment response. For example, adult depressives who show initial DST non-suppression tend to show DST normalisation on clinical recovery. Persistent DST non-suppression despite symptomatic improvement may be associated with impending relapse (Greden *et al.*, 1983; Holsboer, Steiger & Maier, 1983; Kutcher & Shulman, 1985; Grunhaus *et al.*, 1987; Charles *et al.*, 1989; Coryell, 1990).

Studies of DST in adolescent depressives have been the most frequently reported of the neuroendocrine evaluations in this population, partly perhaps because of the ease in administration of this procedure. Unfortunately, most reports do not provide an assessment of basal cortisol dynamics so the relationship of the DST to basal cortisol secretion cannot be evaluated. Taken as a whole, DST non-suppression in depressed adolescents has been reported in 14 to 80% (Extein *et al.*, 1982; Robbins *et al.*, 1982, 1983; Targum & Capodanno, 1983; Ha, Kaplan & Foley, 1984; Klee & Garfinkel, 1984; Freeman *et al.*, 1985; Emslie *et al.*, 1987; Evans *et al.*, 1987; Kahn, 1987; Woodside, Brownstone & Fisman, 1987; Appleboom-Fondu, Kerkhofs & Mendlewicz, 1988; Casat & Powell, 1988; Birmaher *et al.*, 1992; Dahl *et al.*, 1992) of the populations studied. Taken together, the findings from these studies suggest that the sensitivity of the DST for adolescent depression is about 40%. Specificity estimates are difficult to determine because of a lack of studies utilising non-depressed psychiatric control groups. Thus, the DST in adolescent depression has little diagnostic utility.

However, there are suggestions that the DST may identify specific subgroups of adolescent depressives. Chabrol *et al.*, (1983); Robbins & Alessi, (1985) and Kutcher *et al.*, (1991) have reported that DST non-suppression in depressed teenagers is associated with suicidal behaviours. These findings are similar to those reported by Pfeffer, Stokes & Shindledecker (1991) in a sample of pre-pubertal patients in whom suicidality, regardless of a depressive diagnosis, was associated with DST non-suppression. Whether this test indeed defines a depressive subtype with a distinct HPA axis difference or is merely a reflection of the increased arousal or physiological stresses associated with a suicide attempt, however, is not clear.

Furthermore, Dahl *et al.* (1992) in a carefully controlled study of 27 adolescents with MDD and 34 normal controls were not able to demonstrate any relationship between DST non-suppression and suicidality, thus, this issue awaits further study. The same is true for other potential DST non-suppression and specific MDD characteristics such as clinical status, endogenous MDD subtype and premorbid state (Robbins *et al.*, 1983; Klee & Garfinkel, 1984; Freeman *et al.*, 1985; Dahl *et al.*, 1992).

Finally, at this time, there has been insufficient evaluation of the potential utility of the DST in the assessment of the state aspects of adolescent depression. Specifically, it is not clear whether persistence of DST non-suppression concurrently with symptomatic recovery is predictive of early relapse, if DST non-suppression predicts response to antidepressant treatment, or if DST non-suppression may be a marker of a specific subtype of depressive disorder in teenagers.

Corticotropin releasing hormone (CRH) stimulation test

CRH is a synthetic analogue which stimulates ACTH release from the anterior pituitary. Studies of adult depressives have shown blunted ACTH responses to CRH regardless of serum cortisol levels (Gold *et al.*, 1984; Amsterdam *et al.*, 1987*a,b*; Holsboer, Gerken & Stalla, 1987). These findings taken together with elevated serum cortisol level and elevated cerebrospinal fluid CRH levels, suggest that a suprapituitary abnormality is responsible for the derangements of the HPA axis found in adult depressives.

CRH stimulation studies have been reported in childhood but not in adolescent depressives. Thus, the HPA axis has been insufficiently studied in terms of the CNS control factors of HPA axis functioning in depressed teens. However, it would be expected that similar to findings in the basal cortisol secretions and DST non-suppression studies, CRH stimulation of ACTH may not show the same blunting of ACTH reported in adult studies.

Certainly, CNS developmental factors or repeated depressive episode effects may be at issue in comparing adolescent to adult HPA findings. Accumulated stress effects associated with increasing age may impair HPA axis responses to new stressors, thus older patients may show DST non-suppression when younger patients do not. Furthermore, some evidence exists to suggest that even when age effects are controlled for, patients with repeated episodes of depression show increased basal cortisol secretion (Halbreich *et al.*, 1984) and abnormal cortisol responses to the combined DST-CRH stimulation tests (von Bardeleben & Holsboer, 1991) compared to same age normal controls. This suggests that multiple depressive episodes may themselves impact on the functioning of the HPA axis.

Thus, the reported lack of findings of HPA axis abnormalities in studies of adolescent depressives may reflect either an age-dependent CNS maturational issue or the lack of previous depressive episodes. In this scenario, the HPA axis abnormalities found in studies of adult depressives may not reflect primary abnormalities of CNS function, but may instead be the result of the CNS effects of repeated episodes of the illness – a type of neuroendocrine scar.

MELATONIN

Interest in the retino–hypothalamic–pineal axis in depression has stemmed from clinical observations that depressed patients exhibit sleep disruptions and the hypothesis that these may reflect disturbances of sleep regulation that are associated with pineal gland light/dark cycle rhythmicity. Further interest stems from the observation that melatonin secretion may be negatively correlated with cortisol secretion and is under noradrenergic control. Melatonin has then been investigated as a potential indicator of both noradrenergic disturbance in depression and of circadian rhythm disturbance.

The pineal gland is a small CNS structure embryologically derived from cells of the roof of the third ventricle and located posterior to the posterior commisure. In mammals the pineal receives light input originating from the retina. The retina transmits information pertaining to light and dark via the retinohypothalamic tract to the superchiasmatic nucleus (SCN) which is located in the hypothalamus and acts as a pacemaker for a number of hormonal rhythms. Fibres from the SCN descend to regulate preganglionic neurons in the lateral cell columns of the spinal cord. From there, postganglionic nerves from the superior cervical ganglia (SCG) convey impulses to the pineal gland (Reiter, 1989; Reichlin, 1992). Without light input, pineal rhythms will persist as driven by the SCG pacemaker. However, these rhythms are no longer synchronised to the light-dark cycle. There is evidence that in some vertebrates, the pineal also receives input from thalamic, hypothalamic, epithalamic, and mesencephalic areas (Reiter, 1989).

Melatonin is the principle hormonal product of pineal gland metabolism (Lerner et al., 1958). Melatonin secretion follows a diurnal profile with most being synthesised and secreted at night. The principal rate-limiting step is the conversion of serotonin to melatonin by serotonin-N-acetyl transferase (NAT). Concentrations of NAT may vary 100-fold within a few minutes and parallel the rise and fall in plasma melatonin content. Melatonin synthesis and secretion is activated within minutes of exposure to darkness and is stopped by exposure to light. The route by which melatonin reaches the pituitary and hypothalamus is not entirely clear (Reiter, 1989; Reichlin, 1992) but at least in primates, it is secreted into the blood.

At the site of the pituitary and hypothalamus, melatonin appears to have anti-gonadotropic effects but the precise end-organ effects of this hormone are still not completely known. Administration of melatonin is known to inhibit luteinising hormone (LH) and GH secretion. Behavioural effects of melatonin include sleepiness, increased REM sleep, increased number of alpha waves on EEG (Reichlin, 1992), and possibly an exacerbation of dysphoric symptoms in patients with existing depression (Carman et al., 1976).

Neurotransmitter regulation of melatonin secretion is complicated and not fully understood. The nocturnal rise in melatonin is mediated by noradrenaline (NE) via sympathetic innervation from the superior cervical ganglia. Adrenergic receptors of alpha 1 and beta 1 subtypes are found on pinealocyte membranes. In rats and probably humans, the number of pineal beta 1-adrenoreceptors increase at night. This is most likely to allow maximal stimulation of melatonin production by NE. In humans, the role of pineal alpha-adrenergic receptors is unclear but may serve to potentiate beta-adrenergic mediated melatonin production.

Other factors that may affect pineal melatonin production include extremely low frequency electrical fields, age, sex, calcification of the pineal, stress, and ingestion of alcohol (Wilson, 1988; Reiter, 1989; Reichlin, 1992). Developmentally, melatonin secretion decreases with advanced age (Reiter, 1989). Animal studies suggest that night-time, more reliably than daytime, melatonin secretion is blunted by stress and that this mechanism appears to be mediated by cortisol (Joshi et al., 1986; Troiani et al., 1987, 1988).

Basal melatonin secretion

In the investigation of the role of melatonin in adult depression, plasma melatonin, urinary melatonin, and urinary 6-sulphatoxy melatonin (its principal metabolite) have been studied. However, studies have generally included patients taking a variety of medications, used different assay techniques, and did not use closely matched controls, which makes generalisation from them problematic.

Some cross-sectional data suggests a 'low melatonin syndrome' in depressive illness characterised by low nocturnal melatonin secretion inversely related to serum cortisol levels. Claustrat, *et al.* (1984) reported that depressed adults showed a significantly lower amplitude of nocturnal melatonin secretion than controls. Nair, Hariharasubramanian & Pilapil (1984) found that depressed patients had a nocturnal melatonin secretion that was lower in magnitude when compared to normal controls. Beck-Friis *et al.* (1985) reported significant correlations between a low maximal nocturnal melatonin secretion and retardation symptoms, parental loss before the age of 17, and absence of suicidal behaviour in depressed adults. Thompson *et al.* (1985) and McIntyre *et al.* (1986) described lower nocturnal melatonin secretion in depressives than controls. Wetterberg *et al.* (1979, 1982, 1984) reported that adult depression was characterised by an elevation of nocturnal cortisol secretion and a decrease in melatonin secretion. Taken together, these studies suggested that disturbances in the hypothalamic–pituitary adrenal axis and the retino–hypothalamic–pineal axis in depression might be of diagnostic utility and may provide evidence of noradrenergic disturbance associated with depression.

However, recently, contradictory studies have been reported. Thompson *et al.* (1988) and Rubin *et al.* (1992) were not able to demonstrate lower nocturnal or 24-hour melatonin secretion in depressed adults compared to rigorously matched normal controls. Their studies suggest that the previous findings of decreased secretion of melatonin in depression may be related to factors that influence melatonin secretion independent of the presence of depressive illness. Studies of melatonin secretion using a within-subjects design and comparing basal melatonin secretion during the depressed state to the recovery state have been contradictory. Mendlewicz *et al.* (1980) and Wetterberg *et al.* (1984) found no differences while Halbreich *et al.* (1981) reported that depressives improving with desipramine (DMI) treatment showed lower daytime melatonin levels than non-responders. Thompson *et al.* (1985) and Kennedy & Brown (1992), however, reported elevated serum melatonin and urinary 6-sulphatoxy melatonin in DMI treated depressives, suggesting a direct noradrenergic stimulation of melatonin secretion secondary to DMI effect. Thus, at this time the understanding of basal melatonin secretion in adult depression is not yet clear.

Melatonin: longitudinal studies

Several investigators have studied melatonin secretion in patients in the acutely ill and later in the recovered phase. Mendlewicz *et al.* (1980) reported results on four depressed women whose 24-hour pattern of melatonin secretion was measured first in the depressed phase and then after treatment with amitriptyline (Mendlewicz *et al.*, 1980). Nocturnal melatonin secretion was not elevated from daytime secretion in three of the depressed women in either the depressed or well state. Halbreich *et al.* (1981) studied 32 patients with an RDC diagnosis of endogenous depression treated with desipramine. After treatment, responders had significantly lower levels of daytime melatonin compared to non-responders. In both responders and non-responders, serum melatonin levels correlated negatively with plasma levels of desipramine. Responders showed a stronger negative correlation than non-responders. This inverse relationship was thought to be related to pineal beta-adrenergic receptor down-regulation in response to desipramine. Patients studied by Wetterberg (Wetterberg *et al.*, 1984) on remission showed no difference in nocturnal melatonin secretion compared to the acutely ill phase. Souetre *et al.* (1989) investigated melatonin secretion in 16 endogenously depressed patients and 15 of them in the recovered (antidepressant-treated) state. In the recovered state, nocturnal peaks of TSH and melatonin were significantly lower in depressed patients versus normals.

Investigations of basal melatonin secretion in the child and adolescent literature are few. Cavallo *et al.* (1987) studied a group of five early/mid pubertal and four pre-pubertal depressed boys who were medication-free for at least 3 months and 10 male controls (Cavallo *et al.*, 1987). Mean-24 hour and mean overnight plasma melatonin were significantly lower in depressed patients versus normal. However, Waterman *et al.* (1992) studied nocturnal 6-hydroxymelatonin sulphate levels in 31 prepubertal depressed subjects and showed no significant difference in this melatonin metabolite compared to normal controls. Differences in methodologies make comparisons of the two studies difficult, but problems in the design of Cavallo *et al.*'s (1987) report raise questions about the validity of the findings.

Given the limited literature regarding children and adolescents, it is difficult to determine the significance of the retino–hypothalamic–pineal axis in this population. Nevertheless, recent trends in the adult literature seem to question previous hypotheses of a 'low melatonin syndrome' in relation to noradrenergic hypoactivity in depression in well-controlled studies. Clearly more rigorously controlled studies need to be performed in the adolescent population as well.

NON-SYSTEM SPECIFIC CHALLENGE TESTS

A number of studies in adult depressives, using a variety of probes, have evaluated a multiple hormone response to CNS stimulation (Checkley, 1980; Siever & Uhde, 1984; Lopez-Ibor, Saiz-Ruiz & Iglesias, 1989;). Although Ryan *et al.* (1992) have demonstrated decreased cortisol and increased prolactin responses to L-5-hydroxytryptophan in children with major depressive disorder compared to normal controls, no similar studies have been reported in adolescents. Ryan *et al.* (1992) argue that their findings are consistent with CNS serotonin dysregulation in this population.

Cholinergic system challenges have been only rarely reported in the depressed adolescent population. Sitaram *et al.*, (1987) found that some young family members of depressed adults, particularly those with a history of depression themselves, showed a supersensitive REM sleep response to cholinergic stimulation that was similar to that found in adults with major depressions. However, Dahl *et al.* (1989), using an arecholine challenge, failed to note this response in depressed children, while McCracken *et al.* (1991) reported an exaggerated REM response to scopolamine in depressed adolescents. Given the confusing state of reported results in baseline REM sleep measures of adolescent depressives (Kutcher & Williamson, 1992), however these findings are difficult to evaluate.

OTHER PERIPHERAL MARKERS

Rogeness *et al.* (1985) measured whole blood serotonin and platelet monoamine oxidase activity in depressed children and found no differences in comparison to normal controls. In an uncontrolled study of inpatient adolescents, Modai *et al.* (1989), reported lower serotonin platelet uptake V_{max} values in affectively disordered teenagers compared to other psychiatric disorders including schizophrenia. Imipramine binding studies conducted in depressed adolescents have shown increased B_{max} of imipramine binding (Carstens *et al.*, 1988). Furthermore, Carstens *et al.* (1988) have reported increased alpha[2] and beta adrenoceptors on platelets and lymphocytes respectively in depressed teens and children. The difficulties with these studies, apart from lack of replication, is that the peripheral models (platelet and lymphocyte) may not accurately reflect CNS receptor functioning and studies of these parameters in adult

213

depressives are inconsistent and contradictory (Elliott, 1991). Thus the interpretation of these studies awaits further investigations.

Studies of peripheral metabolites of noradrenaline, which is thought to be implicated in the aetiology of depression, have been few. Kahn (1987) and de Villiers, Russell & Carstens (1989) found no differences in peripheral measures of MHPG (a metabolite of noadrenaline) in depressed teens compared to normal controls. However, since only about 10 to 30% of peripheral MHPG may have its origin in the CNS, measurement of peripheral MHPG is unlikely to accurately reflect possible subtle changes that may be occurring centrally.

Thus, the various studies of peripheral measures noted above stand in relative isolation and at this time contribute little towards our understanding of the neurobiology of adolescent depression. Obviously, further systematic assessment of these aspects is necessary.

CONCLUSIONS

Neuroendocrine studies of adolescent depression are still in their early formative years. They developed from similar approaches which had been utilised in studies of depressed adults and have moved from a simple attempt to replicate adult findings to a systematic study of the uniquely adolescent neuroendocrine aspects of depression. As such, they are still in the pioneering stage and require much further detailed investigation of a variety of neuroendocrine systems before their utility in determining aetiology or defining state or trait markers of the disorder are realised. However, to date, the accumulated evidence suggests that neurobiologically at least, adolescent and adult depressions are not identical. The neuroendocrine perturbations which have been identified in adolescent depressives have generally been consistent with dysregulations within CNS serotonin system functioning, with less evidence of noradrenergic system dysfunctioning. Cholinergic system function, however, has not really been addressed. This suggests, in part, that depressions onsetting in the adolescent years may primarily reflect dysregulation of the indolamine system with noradrenergic and possibly cholinergic disturbances arising later in the course of the illness, as a result of repeated episodes, or a reflection of the CNS effect of antidepressant medications, or a result of CNS regulated homeostatic activity. While the serotonin hypothesis of depression is not new (Coppen et al., 1972; Murphy, Campbell & Costa, 1978), it may be best studied in the adolescent population at the time when the disorder first occurs, and the subjects and the psychopathology are relatively free from the confounds noted above. Further research into the multiple aspects of serotonergic functioning should be a priority in the future development of neuroendocrine strategies in the assessment of adolescent depression.

REFERENCES

Agren, H. Lundqvist ,G. (1984). Low levels of somatostatin in human CSF mark depressive episodes. *Psychoneuroendocrinology*, **9**, 233–48.

Aguilera, G., Millan, M. A., Hauger, R. L. *et al.* (1987). Corticotropin-releasing factor receptors: Distribution and regulation in brain, pituitary, and peripheral tissues. *Annals of the New York Academy of Science*, **12**, 48–66.

Ahren, B. (1986). Thyroid neuroendocrinology: neural regulation of thyroid hormone secretions. *Endocrine Reviews*, **7**, 149–55.

Amsterdam, J. D. & Maislin, G. (1991). Hormonal responses during insulin-induced hypoglycemia in manic-depressed, unipolar depressed, and healthy control subjects. *Journal of Clinical Endocrinology and Metabolism*, **73**, 541–8.

Amsterdam, J. D., Maislin, G., Winokur, A. *et al.* (1987a). Pituitary and adrenocortical responses to the ovine corticotropin releasing hormone in depressed patients and healthy volunteers. *Archives of General Psychiatry*, **44**, 775–81.

Amsterdam, J. D., Schweizer, E. & Winokur, A. (1987b) Multiple hormonal responses to insulin induced hypoglycemia in depressed patients and normal volunteers. *American Journal of Psychiatry*, **144**, 170–5.

Appleboom-Fondu, J., Kerkhofs, M. & Mendlewicz, J. (1988). Depression in adolescents and young adults: Polysomnographic and neuroendocrine aspects. *Journal of Affective Disorders*, **14**, 35–40.

Axelrod, J. & Reisine, T. D. (1984). Stress hormones: Their interaction and regulation. *Science*, **224**, 452.

Banki, C. M., Bissette, G. Arato, M. & Nemeroff, C. B. (1988). Elevation of immunoreactive CSF TRH in depressed patients. *American Journal of Psychiatry*, **145**, 1526–31.

Bauer, M. S. & Whybrow, P. C. (1988). Thyroid hormones and the central nervous system in affective illness: interactions that may have clinical significance. *Integrated Psychiatry*, **6**, 75–100.

Baumgartner, A. (1986). Central thyroid stimulation in severely ill depressed, manic and schizophrenic patients. *Biological Psychiatry*, **21**, 417–21.

Baumgartner, A., Graf, K. J., Kurten, I. & Meinhold, H. (1988). The hypothalamic–pituitary–thyroid axis in psychiatric patients and healthy subjects: parts 1–4. *Psychiatry Research*, **24**, 271–331.

Beck-Friis, J., Kjellman, B. F., Aperia, B. *et al.* (1985). Serum melatonin in relation to clinical variables in patients with major depressive disorder and a hypothesis of a low melatonin syndrome. *Acta Psychiatrica Scandinavica*, **71**, 319–30.

Birmaher, B., Dahl, R.E., Ryan, N.D. *et al.* (1992). Dexamethasone suppression test in adolescent outpatients with major depressive disorder. *American Journal of Psychiatry*, **149**, 1040–5.

Brambilla, F., Musetti, C., Tacchini, C. *et al.* (1989). Neuroendocrine investigation in children and adolescents with dysthymic disorders: the DST, TRH and clonidine tests. *Journal of Affective Disorders*, **17**, 279–84.

Brown, W. (1984). Use of dexamethasone suppression test in depression. In

Neurobiology of Mood Disorder (ed. R. Post & O. Ballanger). Williams & Wilkins, London,

Brown, W. A. & Shuey, I. (1980). Response to dexamethasone and subtype of depression. *Archives of General Psychiatry*, **37**, 747–51.

Carman, J. S., Post, R. M., Buswell, R. & Goodwin, F. K. (1976). Negative effects of melatonin on depression. *American Journal of Psychiatry*, **133**, 1181–6.

Carroll, B. J., Curtis, G. C. & Mendels, J. (1976). Neuroendocrine regulation in depression. II. Discrimination of depressed from non-depressed patients. *Archives of General Psychiatry*, **33**, 1051–8.

Carroll, B. J., Feinberg, M., Greden, J. F. *et al.* (1981). A specific laboratory test for the diagnosis of melancholia. Standardization, validation, and clinical utility. *Archives of General Psychiatry*, **38**, 15–22.

Carstens, M. E., Engelbrecht, A. H., Russell, V. A. *et al.* (1988). Biological markers in juvenile depression. *Psychiatry Research*, **23**, 77–88.

Carstens, M. E., Taljaard, J. F. F. & Van Zyl, A. M. (1990). The adrenoceptor and endocrine abnormalities in juvenile depression. *South African Medical Journal*, **77**, 360–3.

Casat, C. & Powell, K. (1988). Utility of the dexamethasone suppression test in children and adolescents with major depressive disorder. *Journal of Clinical Psychiatry*, **49**, 390–3.

Cavallo, A., Holt, K. G., Hejazi, M. S. *et al.* (1987). Melatonin circadian rhythm in childhood depression. *Journal of American Academy of Child Adolescent Psychiatry*, **26**, 395–9.

Chabrol, H., Claverie, J. & Moron, P. (1983). DST, TRH test, and adolescent suicide attempts. *American Journal of Psychiatry*, **140**, 265.

Charles, G. A, Schittecatte, M., Rush, A. J. *et al.* (1989). Persistent cortisol non-suppression after clinical recovery predicts symptomatic relapse in unipolar depression. *Journal of Affective Disorders*, **17**, 271–8.

Charney, D. S., Heninger, G. R. & Ternberg, D. E. (1982). Adrenergic receptor sensitivity in depression: Effects of clonidine in depressed patients and healthy subjects. *Archives of General Psychiatry*, **39**, 290–4.

Charney, D., Southwick, S., Delgado, P. *et al.* (1990). Current status of the receptor sensitivity hypothesis of antidepression action: Implications for the treatment of severe depression. In *Pharmacotherapy of depression* (ed. J. Amsterdam), pp. 13–34. M. Dekker, Basal.

Checkley, S. A. (1980) A neuroendocrine study of adrenoceptor function in endogenous depression. *Acta Psychiatrica Scandinavica* (Suppl 280) **61**, 211–17.

Checkley, S. A., Slade, A. P. & Shur, E. (1981) Growth hormone and other responses to clonidine in patients with endogenous depression. *British Journal of Psychiatry*, **138**, 51–5.

Christie, K., Burke, J., Reiger, D. *et al.* (1989). Epidemiologic evidence for early onset of mental disorders and higher risk of drug abuse in young adults. *American Journal of Psychiatry*, **145**, 971–5.

Claustrat, B., Chazot, G., Brun, J. *et al.* (1984). A chronobiological study of melatonin and cortisol secretion in depressed subjects: plasma melatonin, a biochemical marker in major depression. *Biological Psychiatry*, **19**, 1215–28.

Coppen, A. (1967) The biochemistry of affective disorders. *British Journal of Psychiatry*, **113**, 1237–64.

Coppen, A., Prange, A. J., Whybrow, P. C. & Noguera, R. (1972). Abnormalities of indoleamines in affective disorder. *Archives of General Psychiatry*, **26**, 474–8.

Coryell, W. (1990). DST abnormality as a predictor of course in major depression. *Journal of Affective Disorders*, **19**, 163–9.

Dahl, R., Kaufman, J., Ryan, N. *et al.* (1992). The Dexamethasone Suppression Test in children and adolescents: A review and a controlled study. *Biological Psychiatry*, **32**, 109–26.

Dahl, R. E., Puig-Antich, J., Ryan, N. D. *et al.* (1989) Cortisol secretion in adolescents with major depressive disorder. *Acta Psychiatrica Scandinavica*, **80**, 18–26.

Dahl, R. E., Ryan, R., Puig-Antich, J. *et al.* (1991). 24 hour cortisol measures in adolescents with major depression: a controlled study. *Biological Psychiatry*, **30**, 25–36.

Dahl, R., Ryan, N., Williamson, D. *et al.* (1992). Regulation of sleep and growth hormone in depressed adolescents. *Journal of the American Academy of Child and Adolescent Psychiatry*, **31**, 615–21.

Daughaday, O. O. & Trivedi, O. O. (1991). Clinical aspects of GH binding proteins. *Acta Endocrinologica*, **124**, 27–32.

De Villiers, A., Russell, V. & Carstens, M. (1989). Noradrenergic function and hypothalamic–pituitary–adrenal axis activity in adolescents with major depressive disorder. *Psychiatry Research*, **27**, 101–9.

Dewhurst, K. E., El Kabir, D. T., Exley, D. *et al.* (1968). Blood levels of TSH, protein-bound iodine and cortisol in schizophrenia and affective states. *Lancet*, **ii**, 1160–2.

Dieguez, C., Page, M. D. & Scanlon, M. F. (1987). Growth hormone neuroregulation and its alteration in disease states. *Clinical Endocrinology*, **27**, 109–43.

Doig, R. J., Mummery, R. V., Wills, M. R. & Elkes, A. (1966). Plasma cortisol levels in depression. *British Journal of Psychiatry*, **112**, 1263–7.

Elliott, J. M. (1991). Peripheral markers in affective disorders. In *Biological aspects of affective disorders*, pp. 95–144. Plenum, New York.

Emslie, G., Weinberg, W., Rush, A.J. *et al.* (1987). Depression and dexamethasone suppression testing in children and adolescents. *Journal of Child Neurology*, **2**, 31–7.

Eriksson, E., Balldin, J., Linstedt, G. & Modigh, K. (1988). Growth hormone responses to the alpha 2 adrenoceptors against guanifacine and to growth hormone releasing hormone in depressed patients and controls. *Psychiatry Research*, **26**, 59–67.

Evans, D., Nemeroff, C., Haggerty, J. & Perdersen, C. (1987). Use of the dexamethasone suppression test with DSM-III criteria in psychiatrically hospitalized adolescents. *Psychoneuroendocrinology*, **12**, 203–9.

Extein, I., Rosenberg, G., Pottash, A. & Gold, M. (1982). The dexamethasone suppression test in depressed adolescents. *American Journal of Psychiatry*, **139**, 1617–19.

Finkelstein, J. W., Roffwarg, H. P., Boyar, R. M. *et al.* (1972). Age related change in the twenty-four-hour spontaneous secretion of growth hormone. *Journal of Clinical Endocrinology and Metabolism*, **35**, 665–70.

Follenius, M., Simon, C., Brandenberger, G. & Lenzi, P. (1987). Ultradian plasma corticotropin and cortisol rhythms. Time series analysis. *Journal of Endocrinological Investigations*, **10**, 261–6.

Freeman, L., Pozanski, E., Grossman, J. *et al.* (1985). Psychotic and depressed children: a new entity. *Journal of American Academy of Child Psychiatry*, **24**, 195–202.

Garbutt, J. C., Loosen, P. T., Tipermas, A. & Prange, A. J., Jr (1983). The TRH test in patients with borderline personality disorder. *Psychiatry Research*, **9**, 107–13.

Garcia, M. R., Ryan, N. D., Rabinovitch, H. *et al.* (1991). Thyroid stimulating hormone response to thyrotropin in prepubertal depression. *Journal of American Academy of Child Adolescent Psychiatry*, **30**, 398–406.

Gelato, M. C. & Merriam, G. R. (1986). Growth hormone releasing hormone. *Annual Review of Physiology* **48**, 569–91.

Gold, M. S., Pottash, A. L. & Extein, I. (1981). Hypothyroidism and depression.

S. Kutcher & S. Sokolov

Evidence from complete thyroid function evaluation. *Journal of American Academy of Child and Adolescent Psychiatry*, **245**, 1919–22.

Gold, M. S., Pottash, A. L. & Martin, D. *et al.* (1980). Thyroid stimulating hormone and growth hormone responses to thyrotropin-releasing hormone in anorexia nervosa. *Journal of Psychiatric Medicine*, **10**, 51–7.

Gold, P. W., Chrousos, G., Kellner, C. *et al.* (1984). Psychiatric implications of basic and clinical studies with corticotropin-releasing factor. *American Journal of Psychiatry*, **141**, 619–27.

Gold, P. W., Goodwin, F. K. & Chrousos, G. P. (1988). Clinical and biochemical manifestations of depression. *New England Journal of Medicine*, **319**, 348–420.

Goodyer, I., Herbert, J., Moor, S. & Altham, P. (1991) Cortisol hypersecretion in depressed school-aged children and adolescents. *Psychiatry Research*, **37**, 237–44.

Greden, J. F., Gardner, R., King, D. *et al.* (1983). Dexamethasone suppression tests in antidepressant treatment of melancholia – the process of normalization and test–retest reproducibility. *Archives of General Psychiatry*, **40**, 493–500.

Gregoire, F., Branman, G., DeBuck, R. & Corvilain, J. (1977). Hormone release in depressed patients before and after recovery. *Psychoneuroendocrinology*, **2**, 303–12.

Grunhaus, L., Zelnik ,T., Albala, A. A. *et al.* (1987). Serial dexamethasone suppression tests in depressed patients treated only with electroconvulsive therapy. *Journal of Affective Disorders*, **13**, 233–40.

Ha, H., Kaplan, S. & Foley, C. (1984). The dexamethasone suppression test in adolescent psychiatric patients. *American Journal of Psychiatry*, **141**, 421–3.

Halbreich, U., Asnis, G. M,. Zumoff, B. *et al.* (1984) Effect of age and sex on cortisol secretion in depressives and normals. *Psychiatry Research*, **13**, 221–9.

Halbreich, U., Sachar, E., Asnis, G. *et al.* (1982). Growth hormone response to dextroamphetamine in depressed patients and normal subjects. *Archives of General Psychiatry*, **39**, 189–92.

Halbreich, U., Weinberg, U., Stewart, J. *et al.* (1981). An inverse correlation between serum levels of desmethylimipramine and melatonin-like immunoreactivity in DMI-responsive depressives. *Psychiatry Research*, **4**, 109–13.

Hatotami, N., Nomura, J., Yamaguchi, T. *et al.*: (1974). Clinical and experimental studies of the pathogenesis of depression. *Psychoneuroendocrinology*, **2**, 115–30.

Hattori, N., Kurahachi, H., Ikekubo, K. *et al.* (1991). Effects of sex and age on serum GH binding protein levels in normal adults. *Clinical Endocrinology*, **35**, 295–7.

Hauger, R. L. Risch, S. C. & Millan, M. *et al.* (1989). Corticotropin-releasing factor regulation of the pituitary–adrenal axis and the central nervous system. In *Psychiatry: Psychobiological Foundations of Clinical Psychiatry* (Vol 3) (ed. R. Michels), pp. 1–22. J. B. Lippincott, New York.

Heninger, G. & Charney, D. (1987). Mechanism of action of antidepressant treatments: Implications for the etiology and treatment of depressive disorders. In *Psychopharmacology: the third generation of progress* (ed. H. Meltzer), pp. 535–44. Raven Press, New York.

Holaday, J. W., Martinez, H. M. & Natelson, B. H. (1977). Synchronized ultradian cortisol rhythms in monkeys: persistence during corticotropin infusion. *Science*, **198**, 56–8.

Holsboer, F., Gerken, A. & Stalla, G. K. (1987). Blunted aldosterone and ACTH release after human CRH administration in depressed patients. *American Journal of Psychiatry*, **144**, 229–31.

Holsboer, F., Phillip, M., Steiger, A. & Gerken, A. (1986). Multisteriod analysis after DST in depressed patients – a controlled study. *Journal of Affective Disorders*, **10**, 241–9.

Holsboer, F., Steiger, A. & Maier, W. (1983). Four cases of reversion to abnormal

218

dexamethasone suppression test response as indicator of clinical relapse: A preliminary report. *Biological Psychiatry*, **18**, 911–6.

Jarrett, D. B., Miewald, J. M. & Kupfer, D. J. (1990). Recurrent depression is associated with a persistent reduction in sleep-related growth hormone secretion. *Archives of General Psychiatry*, **47**, 113–118.

Jensen, J. B. & Garfinkel, B. D. (1990). Growth hormone dysregulation in children with major depressive disorder. *Journal of the American Academy of Child and Adolescent Psychiatry*, **29**, 295–301.

Jimmerson, D. C., Post, R. M., von Kommen, D. P. *et al.* (1980). Cerebrospinal fluid cortisol levels in depression and schizophrenia. *American Journal of Psychiatry*, **137**, 979–80.

Joffe, R. T. (1990). A perspective on the thyroid and depression. *Canadian Journal of Psychiatry*, **35**, 754–8.

Joffe, R. T. & Singer, W. (1990). The effect of tricyclic antidepressants on basal thyroid hormone levels in depressed patients. *Pharmacopsychiatry*, **23**, 67–9.

Joffe, R. T. & Sokolov, S.T.H. (1994). Thyroid hormones, the brain and affective illness. *Critical Reviews in Neurobiology*, in press.

Joshi, B. N., Troiani, M. E., Milin, J. *et al.* (1986). Adrenal–mediated depression of N-acetyltransferase activity and melatonin levels in the rat pineal gland. *Life Science*, **38**, 1573–80.

Johnson, O. E., Kamilaris, T. C., Chrousos, G. P. & Gold, P. W. (1992). Mechanisms of stress: A dynamic overview of hormonal and behavioural homeostatis. *Neuroscience and Biobehavioural Reviews*, **16**, 115–30.

Kahn, A. U. (1987). Biochemical profile of depressed adolescents. *Journal of American Academy of Child and Adolescent Psychiatry*, **26**, 873–8.

Kahn, A. U. (1988). Sensitivity and specificity of TRH stimulation test in depressed and nondepressed adolescents. *Psychiatry Research*, **25**, 11–7.

Kalin, N. H. & Takahashi, L. K. (1988). Altered hypothalamic–pituitary–adrenal regulation in animal models of depression. In *The Hypothalamic–Pituitary–Adrenal Axis* (ed. P. W. Gild, G. Chrousos), pp. 67–70. Raven Press, New York.

Kennedy, S. H. & Brown, G. M. (1992). Effect of chronic antidepressant treatment with adinazolam and desipramine on melatonin output. *Psychiatry Research*, **43**, 177–85.

Kirkegaard, C. (1981). The thyrotropin response to thyrotropin-releasing hormone in endogenous depression. *Psychoneuroendocrinology*, **6**, 189–212.

Kirkegaard, C., Bjorum, N., Cohn, D. *et al.* (1977). Studies in the influence of biogenic amines and psychoactive drugs on the prognostic value of the TRH stimulation test in endogenous depression. *Psychoneuroendocrinology*, **2**, 131–6.

Kirkegaard, C. & Carroll, B. J. (1980) Dissociation of TSH adrenocortical disturbances in endogenous depression. *Psychiatry Research*, **3**, 253–64.

Kirkegaard, C. & Faber, J. (1981). Altered serum levels of thyroxine, triiodothyronines and diiodothyronines in endogenous depression. *Acta Endocrinologica (Copenhagen)*, **96**, 199–207.

Kirkegaard, C. & Faber, J. (1991). Free thyroxine and 3,3',5'-triiodothyronine levels in cerebrospinal fluid in patients with endogenous depression. *Acta Endocrinologica (Copenhagen)*, **124**, 166–7.

Kirkegaard, C., Faber, J., Hummer, L. & Rogowski, P. (1979). Increased levels of TRH in cerebrospinal fluid from patients with edogenous depression. *Psychoneuroendocrinology*, **4**, 227–35.

Kirkegaard, C., Korner, A. & Faber, J. (1990). Increased production of thyroxine and inappropriately elevated serum thyrotropin in levels in endogenous depression. *Biological Psychiatry*, **27**, 472–6.

Kirkegaard, C., Norlern, N., Lauridsen, U. B. *et al.* (1975). Protirelin stimulation test and thyroid function during treatment of depression. *Archives of General Psychiatry*, **32**, 1115–8.

Klee, S. & Garfinkel, B. (1984). Identification of depression in children and adolescents: The role of the dexamethasone suppression test. *Journal of the American Academy of Child Psychiatry*, **23**, 410–5.

Kopin, I. J., Gordon, E. K. & Jimmerson, D. (1983). Relation between plasma and cerebrospinal fluid levels of 3-methoxy-4-hydroxyphenethyl-eneglycol. *Science*, **291**, 73–6.

Koslow, S. H., Stokes, P. E., Mendels, J. *et al.* (1982). Insulin Tolerance Test: human growth hormone response and insulin resistance in primary unipolar depressed, bipolar depressed and control subjects. *Psychological Medicine*, **12**, 45–55.

Krieger, D. T., Allen, W., Rizzo, F. & Krieger, H. P. (1971). Characterization of the normal temporal pattern of plasma corticosteroid levels. *Journal of Clinical Endocrinology and Metabolism*, **32**, 266–84.

Krishnan, K. R. R. Ritchie, J. C. Saunders, W. *et al.* (1990). Nocturnal and early morning secretion of ACTH and cortisol in humans. *Biological Psychiatry*, **38**, 47–57.

Krulich, L. (1982). Neurotransmitter control of thyrotropin secretion. *Neuroendocrinology*, **35**, 139–47.

Kutcher, S. P., Malkin, D., Silverberg, J. *et al.* (1991). Nocturnal cortisol, thyroid stimulating hormone and growth hormone secreting properties in depressed adolescents. *Journal of American Academy of Child Adolescent Psychiatry*, **30**, 407–14.

Kutcher, S. P. & Marton, P. (1989). Parameters of adolescent depression. *Psychiatric Clinics of North America*, **12**, 895–918.

Kutcher, S. & Shulman, K. (1985). Dexamethasone suppression test normalization and treatment outcome in elderly depressives. *British Journal of Psychiatry*, **147**, 453–4.

Kutcher, S. P. & Williamson, P. (1992) REM latency in endogenously depressed adolescents. *British Journal of Psychiatry*, **161**, 399–402.

Kutcher, S. P., Williamson, P., Silverberg, J. *et al.* (1989) Nocturnal growth hormone secretion in depressed older adolescents. *Journal of the American Academy of Child and Adolescent Psychiatry*, **27**, 751–4.

Larsen, P. & Ingbar, S. (1992). The thyroid gland. In *Williams textbook of endocrinology* (ed. J. Wilson & D. Foster), pp. 257–287. W.B. Saunders Company, Philadelphia.

Lerner, A. B., Case, J. D., Takahashi, Y. *et al.* (1958). Isolation of melatonin, the pineal gland factor that lightens melanocytes. *Journal of American Chemistry Society*, **80**, 2587.

Lesch, K. P., Erb, A., Pfuller, H. *et al.* (1987) Attenuated growth hormone response to growth hormone-releasing hormone in major depressive disorder. *Biological Psychiatry*, **22**, 1495–9.

Linkowski, P., Mendlewicz, J., Kerkhofs, M. *et al.* (1987a). 24-hour profile of adrenocorticotropin, cortisol and growth hormone in major depressive illness: Effect of antidepressant treatment. *Journal of Clinical Endocrinology and Metabolism*, **65**, 141–51.

Linkowski, P., Mendlewicz, J., LeClerq, R. *et al.* (1987b). The 24-hour profile of ACTH and cortisol in major depressive illness. *Journal of Clinical Endocrinology and Metabolism*, **61**, 429–38.

Linnoila, M., Lamberg, B. A., Rosberg, G. *et al.* (1979). Thyroid hormones and TSH, prolactin and LH responses to repeated TRH and LRH injections in depressed patients. *Acta Psychiatrica Scandinavica*, **59**, 536–44.

Loosen, P. T. (1986). Thyroid function in affective disorders and alcoholism. *Endocrinology Metabolic Clinics North America* **17**, 55–82.

Lopez-Ibor, J. J., Saiz-Ruiz, J. & Iglesias, L. M. (1989). Neuroendocrine challenges in the diagnosis of depressive disorders. *British Journal of Psychiatry*, **154** (suppl. 4), 73–6.

McCracken, J.T., Poland, R.E. & Tondo, L. *et al.* (1991). Cholinergic dysregulation in adolescent depression: Preliminary comparisons with adult depression. *Proceedings of the 144th Annual Meeting of the American Psychiatric Association*, New Orleans.

McIntyre, I. M., Judd, F. K., Norman, T. R. & Burrows, G. D. (1986). Plasma melatonin concentrations in depression. *Australian and New Zealand Journal of Psychiatry*, **20**, 381–3.

Mendlewicz, J., Branchey, L., Weinberg, U. *et al.* (1980). The 24 hour pattern of plasma melatonin in depressed patients before and after treatment. *Community Psychopharmacology*, **4**, 49–55.

Mendlewicz, J., Linkowski, P., Kerhofs, M. *et al.* (1985). Diurnal hypersecretion of growth hormone in depression. *Journal of Clinical Endocrinology & Metabolism*, **60**, 505–12.

Miller, A., Spencer, R., Palera *et al.* (1992) Adrenal steroid receptor activation in rat brain and pituitary following dexamethasone: implications for the dexamethasone suppression test. *Biological Psychiatry*, **32**, 850–69.

Modai, I., Apter, A., Meltzer, M. *et al.* (1989). Serotinin uptake by platelets of suicidal and aggressive adolescent psychiatric inpatients. *Neuropsychobiology*, **21**, 9–13.

Moore, R. Y. & Eichler, V. B. (1972). Loss of a circadian adrenal corticosterone rhythm following suprachiasmatic lesions in the rat. *Brain Research*, **42**, 201–6.

Mortola, J. F., Liu, J. H., Gillin, J. C. *et al.* (1987). Pulsatile rhythms of adrenocorticotropin (ACTH) and cortisol in women with endogenous depression: evidence for increased ACTH pulse frequency. *Journal of Endocrinology and Metabolism*, **65**, 962–8.

Murphy, D. L., Campbell, I. C. & Costa, J. L. (1978). The brain serotonergic system in the affective disorders. *Progress in Neuropsychopharmacology*, **2**, 5–31.

Nair, N. P., Hariharasubramanian, N. & Pilapil, C. (1984). Circadian rhythm of plasma melatonin in endogenous depression. *Progress in Neuropsychopharmacology and Biological Psychiatry*, **8**, 715–8.

Nasr, S. J., Pandey, G., Altman, E. G. *et al.* (1983). Symptom profile of patients with positive DST: a pilot study. *Biological Psychiatry*, **18**, 571–4.

Nemeroff, C. B., Widerlov, E., Bissett, G. *et al.* (1984). Elevated concentrations of CSF corticotropin-releasing factor-like immunoreactivity in depressed patients. *Science*, **226**, 1342–4.

Pepper, G. M. & Krieger, D. T. (1984). Hypothalamic–pituitary–adrenal abnormalities in depression: Their possible relation to central mechanisms regulating ACTH release. *Neurobiology of Mood Disorders*, **16**, 245–70.

Pfeffer, C., Stokes, P. & Shindledecker, R. (1991). Suicidal behaviour and hypothalamic–pituitary–adrenocortical axis indices in child psychiatric inpatients. *Biological Psychiatry*, **29**, 909–17.

Puig-Antich, J., Goetz, R., Davies, M. *et al.* (1984*a*). Growth hormone secretion in prepubertal major depressive children. II. Sleep related plasma concentrations during a depressive episode. *Archives of General Psychiatry*, **41**, 463–6.

Puig-Antich, J., Novacenko, H., Davies, M. *et al.* (1984*b*). Growth hormone secretion in prepubertal children with major depression. III. Response to insulin-induced hypoglycemia after recovery from a depressive episode and in a drug-free state. *Archives of General Psychiatry*, **41**, 471–5.

Puig-Antich, J., Novancenko, H., Davies, M., *et al.* (1984*c*). Growth hormone secretion in prepubertal major depressive children: I. *Archives General Psychiatry*, **41**, 455–60.

Reichlin, S., (1992) Neuroendocrinology. In *Williams textbook of endocrinology* (8th edn) (ed. J. D. Wilson & D. W. Foster), pp. 135–220. W.B. Saunders Company, Philadelphia.

Reiter, R. J. (1989). The pineal and its indole products: basic aspects and clinical applications. In *The brain as an endocrine organ* (ed. M. P. Cohen & P. P. Foa), pp. 96–149. Springer-Verlag, New York.

Riddle, M. A., Anderson, G. M. & McIntosh, S. (1986). Cerebrospinal fluid monoamine precursor and metabolitic levels in children treated for leukemia: age and sex effects and individual variability. *Biological Psychiatry*, **21**, 69–72.

Risch, S. C., Ehlers, C. & Janowsky, D. S. (1988). Human growth hormone releasing factor infusion effects on plasma growth hormone in affective disorder patients and normal controls. *Peptides*, **9**, 45–8.

Rivier, C. & Plotsky, P. M. (1986). Mediation by corticotropin releasing factor (CRF) or adenohypophysial hormone secretion. *Annual Review of Physiology*, **48**, 475.

Robbins, D. & Alessi, N. (1985). Suicide and the dexamethasone suppression test in adolescence. *Biological Psychiatry*, **20**, 107–10.

Robbins, D., Alessi, N., Yanchyshyn, G. & Colfer, M. (1982). Preliminary report on the dexamethasone suppression test in adolescents. *American Journal of Psychiatry*, **22**, 467–9.

Robbins, D., Alessi, N., Yanchyshyn, G. & Colfer, M. (1983). The dexamethasone suppression test in psychiatrically hospitalized adolescents. *Journal of the American Academy of Child and Adolescent Psychiatry*, **22**, 467–9.

Rogeness, G. A., Mitchell, E .L., Custer, G. J. & Harris, W. R. (1985). Comparison of whole blood serotonin and platelet MAO in children with schizophrenia and major depressive disorder. *Biological Psychiatry*, **20**, 270–5.

Rubin, R. T., Heist, E. K., McGeoy, S. S. *et al.* (1992). Neuroendocrine aspects of primary endogenous depression. XI. Serum melatonin measures in patients and matched control subjects. *Archives of General Psychiatry*, **49**, 558–67.

Rubin, R. T., Poland, R. E., Lesser, I. M. *et al.* (1987) Neuroendocrine aspects of primary endogenous depression. *Archives of General Psychiatry*, **44**, 328–36.

Rubin, R., Poland, R. & Lesser, I. (1990). Neuroendocrine aspects of primary endogenous depression X: serum growth hormone measures in patients and matched control subjects. *Biological Psychiatry*, **27**, 1065–82.

Rubinow, D. R., Gold, P. W. & Post, R. M. (1983). CSF somatostatin in affective illness. *Archives of General Psychiatry*, **40**, 403–12.

Ryan, N., Birmaher, B. & Perel, J. *et al.* (1992). Neuroendocrine response to L-5-hydroxytryptophan challenge in prepubertal major depression. *Archives of General Psychiatry*, **49**, 843–51.

Ryan, N. D., Puig-Antich, J. & Rabinovich, H. (1988). Growth hormone response to desmethylimipramine in depressed and suicidal adolescents. *Journal of Affective Disorders,* **15**, 323–37.

Sachar, E. J., Finkelstein, J. & Hellman, L. (1971). Growth hormone responses in depressive illness. I. Response to insulin tolerance test. *Archives of General Psychiatry*, **25**, 263–9.

Sachar, E. J., Hellman, L., Roffwarg, H. P. *et al.* (1973). Disrupted 24-hour patterns of cortisol secretion in psychiatric depression. *Archives of General Psychiatry*, **28**, 19–24.

Scanlon, M. R. (1991). Neuroendocrine control of thyrotropin secretion. In *Werner and Ingbar's The thyroid: a fundamental and clinical text* (6th edn) (ed. L. E. Braverman & R. D. Utiger), pp. 230–56. J.B. Lippincott Company, Philadelphia.

Schilkrut, R., Chandra, D. & Oswald, M. (1975). Growth hormone release during sleep and with thermal stimulation in depressed patients. *Neuropsychobiology*, **1**, 70–4.

Siever, L. & Davis, K. (1985). Overview: towards a dysregulation hypothesis of depression. *American Journal of Psychiatry*, **142**, 1017–31.

Siever, L. J. & Uhde, T. W. (1984). New studies and perspectives on the noradrenergic receptor system in depression: Effects of the alpha-adrenergic agonist clonidine. *Biological Psychiatry*, **19**, 131–56.

Siever, L. J., Uhde, T. W., Silberman, L. K. *et al.* (1982). Growth hormone response to clonidine as a probe of noradrenergic receptor responsiveness in affective disorder patients and controls. *Psychiatry Research*, **6**, 171–83.

Sitaram, N. Dube, S., Keshavan, M. *et al.*: (1987). The association of supersensitive cholinergic REM-induction and affective illness within pedigrees. *Journal of Psychiatric Research*, **21**, 487–97.

Sokolov, S. T. H., Kutcher, S. P. & Joffe, R. T. (1994). Baseline thyroid indices in adolescent depression and bipolar disorder. *Journal of the American Academy of Child and Adolescent Psychiatry*, **33**, 469–75.

Souetre, E., Salvati, E., Belugou, J. L. *et al.* (1989) Circadian rhythms in depression and recovery: evidence for blunted amplitude as the main chronobiological abnormality. *Psychiatry Research*, **3**, 263–78.

Stokes, P. E. & Sikes, C. R. (1987). Hypothalamic–pituitary–adrenal axis in affective disorders. *Psychopharmacology*, The Third Generation of Progress, Raven Press, New York. **59**, 589–607.

Stokes, P. E., Stoll, P. M., Koslow, S. H. *et al.* (1984). Pretreatment DST and hypothalamic–pituitary–adrenocortical function in depressed patients and comparison groups. *Archives of General. Psychiatry*, **41**, 257–67.

Styra, R., Joffe, R. & Singer, W. (1991). Hyperthyroxinemia in major affective disorders. *Acta Psychiatrica Scandinavica*, **83**, 61–3.

Targum, S. & Capodanno, A. (1983). The dexamethasone suppression test in adolescent psychiatric inpatients. *American Journal of Psychiatry*, **140**, 589–91.

Thomas, E. B., Levine, S. & Arnold, W. J. (1968). Effects of maternal deprivation and incubator rearing on adrenocortical activity in the adult rat. *Developmental Psychobiology*, **1**, 21–23.

Thomas, R., Beer, R., Harris, B. *et al.* (1989). GH responses to growth hormone releasing factor in depression. *Journal of Affective Disorders*, **16**, 133–7.

Thompson, C., Franey, C., Arendt, J. & Checkley, S. A. (1988). A comparison of melatonin secretion in depressed patients and normal subjects. *British Journal of Psychiatry*, **152**, 260–5.

Thompson, C., Mezey, G., Corn, T. *et al.* (1985). The effect of desipramine upon melatonin and cortisol secretion in depressed and normal subjects. *British Journal of Psychiatry*, **147**, 389–93.

Traskman, L., Tybring, G., Asberg, M. *et al.* (1980). Cortisol in the CSF of depressed and suicidal patients. *Archives of General Psychiatry*, **37**, 761–7.

Troiani, M. E., Oaknin, S., Reiter, R. J. *et al.* (1987). Depression in rat pineal N-acetyltransferase activity and melatonin content produced by a hind leg saline injection is time and darkness dependent. *Journal of Pineal Research*, **4**, 185–95.

Troiani, M. E., Reiter, R. J., Vaughan, M. K. *et al.* (1998). The depression in rat pineal melatonin production after saline injection at night may be elicited by corticosterone. *Brain Research*, **450**, 18–24.

von Bardeleben, U. & Holsboer. F. (1991). Effect of age on the cortisol response to human CRH in depressed patients pretreated with dexamethasone. *Biological Psychiatry*, **29**, 1042–50.

Waterman, G. S., Ryan, N. D., Puig-Antich, J. *et al.* (1991). Hormonal responses to dextroamphetamine in depressed and normal adolescents. *Journal of the American Academy of Child and Adolescent Psychiatry*, **30**, 415–22.

Waterman, G., Ryan, N. & Percel, J. *et al.* (1992). Nocturnal urinary excretion of 6–hydroxy melatonin sulphate in prepubertal major depressive disorder. *Biological Psychiatry*, **31**, 582–90.

Weissman, M. & Klerman, G. (1992). Depression: current understanding and changing trends. *American Review of Public Health*, **13**, 319–39.

Wetterberg, L., Aperia, B., Beck–Friis, J. *et al.* (1982). Melatonin and cortisol levels in psychiatric illness [letter] *Lancet*, **2**, 100.

Wetterberg, L., Beck-Friis, J., Aperia, B. & Petterson, U. (1979). Melatonin/cortisol ratio in depression [letter] *Lancet*, **2**, 1361.

Wetterberg, L., Beck-Friis, J., Kjellman, B. F. & Ljunggren, J. G. (1984). Circadian rhythms in melatonin and cortisol secretion in depression. *Advances in Biochemical Psychopharmacology* **39**, 197–205.

Whybrow, P. C., Coppen, A., Prange, A. J. Jr *et al.* (1972). Thyroid function and the response to liothyronine in depression. *Archives of General Psychiatry*, **26**, 242–5.

Wilson, B. W. (1988). Chronic exposure to ELF fields may induce depression. *Bioelectromagnetics*, **9**, 195–205.

Winokur, A., Caroff, S. N., Amsterdam, A. J. & Maislin, G. (1984). Administration of thyrotropin-releasing hormone at weekly intervals in a diminished thyrotropin response. *Biological Psychiatry*, **19**, 695–702.

Woodside, B., Brownstone, D. & Fisman, S. (1987). The dexamethasone suppression test and the children's depression inventory in psychiatric disorders in children. *Canadian Journal of Psychiatry*, **32**, 2–4.

Zadik, Z., Chalew, S. A., McCarter, R. *et al.* (1985). The influence of age on the 24-hour integrated concentration of growth hormone in normal individuals. *Journal of Clinical Endocrinology and Metabolism*, **60**, 513–16.

10

Suicidal behaviour in adolescents

C. W. M. Kienhorst, E. J. de Wilde and R. F. W. Diekstra

INTRODUCTION

Depression demonstrates its most severe consequences when it merges with suicidality (see e.g. Crumley, 1982; Friedman *et al.*, 1984; Chabrol & Moron, 1988; Kienhorst *et al.*, 1990*a*). Therefore, the study of depression concerns the study of suicidal behaviour and vice versa. Both phenomena are overlapping but distinct, since the majority of depressed adolescents do not attempt or commit suicide, and not every suicidal adolescent is depressed. Understanding the interrelationships between depression and suicidal behaviour may improve current intervention strategies for suicidal adolescents.

The words **suicide** and **suicidal** in everyday life are used to refer to self-chosen behaviour that is intended to bring about one's own death. However, of all the behaviours and experiences to which these words are attached, many are or might not be motivated by a wish to die or to do away with oneself for good. Often they are not even meant to harm oneself, but only to express or communicate complex emotions such as despair, hopelessness and anger. Contemporary literature, therefore, usually defines suicidal behaviour into three classes or categories.

Suicidal ideation refers to cognitions that can vary from fleeting thoughts that life is not worth living, via very concrete well-thought out plans for killing oneself to an intense delusional preoccupation with self-destruction (Goldney *et al.*, 1989). **Attempted suicide** (sometimes also referred to as **parasuicide**) covers behaviours that can vary from what sometimes is called suicidal gestures and manipulative attempts to seri-

225

ous but unsuccessful attempts to kill oneself. **Suicide** refers to death that is the direct or indirect result of an act accomplished by the victim him/herself which he or she knows or believes will produce this result.

EPIDEMIOLOGY

Suicides

Suicide statistics consist of official data only, which are known to be underestimates of the phenomenon (e.g. Jobes, Berman & Josselsen, 1986). Within the member states of the United Nations that reported mortality statistics (WHO, 1989), a considerable number of suicidal deaths, estimates vary from 30 to 200%, are not recorded as such. Suicide is underreported as a cause of death. Studies on the reliability of suicide statistics clearly indicate that errors of reporting are randomised, at least to an extent that allows epidemiologists profitably to compare rates between countries, within them and over time (Diekstra et al. (1994).

In many European countries, as well as in highly industrialised countries in other parts of the world, the overall suicides rates have risen to their current status during the past two decades. The range of suicide rates spans from a low of 6 per million females in Malta to a high of 581 per million males in Hungary (WHO, 1989).

According to several authors (see Vaillant & Blumenthal, 1990) one of the most basic facts about suicide is that its risk increases as a function of age. Indeed, completed suicide is extremely rare in children under the age of 12 (see, e.g. Shaffer & Fisher, 1981; Brooksbank, 1985; Kienhorst et al., 1987) but becomes more common after puberty, with its incidence increasing in each of the adolescent years. Also, the proportion of young suicides from all suicidal deaths has become larger (Diekstra, 1989). In fact, the rise in the overall suicide rates in many countries is to a large extent due to the increase in suicides in the younger age groups and even countries with a stable or decreasing overall suicide rate, still witness increasing rates in the young.

In 1989, 9 to 21% (varying in different countries) of all deaths among adolescent males in these countries aged 15 to 24 were caused by suicides, and the figure was 6 to 28% for females. Among adolescents, suicide ranked among the first three causes of death. The magnitude becomes even more evident if one considers that today in many industrialised countries the number of people dying through suicide (according to official statistics) is significantly higher than the number of people dying on the road through motor traffic accidents. Over the last two decades motor traffic mortality rates have been decreasing while at the same time suicide rates, particularly among adolescents and young adults, have been sharply increasing. However, in all countries, without a single exception, the resources being made available for preventive interventions regarding suicidal behaviour constitute only a very tiny fraction of what is available for the prevention of motor traffic deaths.

Correlates of suicide trends

Diekstra and coworkers, within the framework of the WHO programme on Preventive Strategies on Suicide (WHO, 1988), carried out an analysis of suicide rates among 15 to 29-year-olds in 18 European countries. They found that increases in suicides were related to increases of unemployment, the size of the population under 15, the number of women employed, the divorce rate, the homicide rate, alcohol use, and decrease in church affiliation. In a multiple regression equation, this combination of variables showed a 0.84 correlation with the change in suicide rates.

Holinger, Offer & Zola (1988) found that, in the US, between 1956 and 1977 fluctuations in adolescent (15 to 24 years) suicide rates corresponded positively with the proportion of adolescents in the population at large. On the basis of future American population characteristics, they predicted that the adolescent suicide rates *in the United States* will continue to decrease until the mid-1990s. These findings are in accord with Diekstra and colleagues' European study (WHO, 1988).

The prognosis for the world suicide rates among adolescents are rather different. On the basis of their results and given the current and future overurbanisation, demographic explosion of young people in the developing countries and its concomitants of un- or underemployment, further instability of traditional family structure and increase of substance abuse, Diekstra *et al.* (1994) estimate that, contrary to the American trend and owing to the expansion in adolescent numbers worldwide, the *world* suicide rates will continue to rise until the year 2000.

Suicide attempts

No country in the world collects statistics that reflect the number of suicide attempts or parasuicidal acts. Data from several countries

(Diekstra, 1982; WHO, 1982) indicate that hospital discharge rates for attempted suicide in adults is linked strongly to the suicide rates, which have been rising during the recent decades. Only a fraction of all para-suicidal acts are, however, followed by hospital admissions. Investigators in North America estimate that the proportion of suicide-attempters range from 8 to 18% for high-school and college students (Smith & Crawford, 1986; Garrison, 1989). By contrast, Choquet (1981) reported an attempted-suicide rate of 2.3% in a sample of 2000 French 'Lycéens' (high-school students). Kienhorst *et al.* (1990*b*) estimated a similar 2.2% in a population of 9393 Dutch students of secondary education. This would imply that respectively 1600 female (95% C.I. 1330–1870) and 685 male (95% C.I. 525–845) students per 100 000 aged 14 to 20 attempted suicide at some time in their lives. Approximately one out of each 150 students aged 14 to 20 attempts suicide *each year* (Kienhorst, 1988). In a similar survey, Garnefski & Diekstra (1993) arrive at a lifetime prevalence of 4.6% in Dutch secondary education students: one out of 20 Dutch adolescents reports to have *ever* attempted suicide. Although there are some methodological differences between this latter investigation and the one by Kienhorst *et al.* (1990*b*) there is a suggestion of increasing rates of attempted suicide in the few years between both studies. In various at risk groups of youngsters the reported lifetime rates for attempted suicide are even higher (e.g. Stiffman (1989), in runaway youth, estimated 30%).

It is undoubtedly true that the number of suicide attempts far surpasses the number of suicides in adolescents, more than in any other (older) group. Therefore, and because the majority of clinical and research activities have to do with *attempted* suicide, this will be the main topic throughout the rest of this chapter.

Suicidal thoughts

As was stated before, the concept of suicidal thoughts or ideation has been operationalised in very different ways, often concerning different time periods.

Studies that use complete scales for suicidal ideation arrive at high percentages, probably because the respondents have more items to respond to, thereby increasing the chance that they respond positively to any single item. Two studies (Schotte & Clum, 1982; Strang & Orlofsky, 1990) suggest that up to 61% of adolescents have 'some' *recent* suicidal ideation. Rudd (1989) reports that 43.7% of 737 university students experienced some suicidal ideation *during the previous year.* Smith & Crawford, (1986) report 62.6% of high-school students experienced some degree of suicidal ideation or action *during their lifetime.* In the Netherlands, Garnefski & Diekstra (1993) reported prevalence of 19% in the preceding year, and Kienhorst (1988) found that 3.5% of those adolescents reported *recent* suicidal thoughts, i.e. in the weeks preceding the interview. In a recent study of 4157 Mexican and Texan adolescents, 23% of the Texas youth and 12% of the Mexican youth admitted that they had thought about killing themselves *during the past week* (Swanson *et al.*, 1992)

Continuum of suicidality: from ideation to completion?

Suicidal ideation, attempted suicide and completed suicide are behaviours that are hierarchically related: suicidal thoughts generally precede suicidal acts, and many completed suicides were preceded by attempts. Although this may not apply for everyone, it is tempting to see these successive behaviours as part of a continuum of suicidality.

The studies that address this issue study the differences and similarities between groups that display these different behaviours. Brent *et al.* (1988) compare adolescent suicide victims ($n = 27$) with suicidal psychiatric in-patients, who had either seriously considered ($n = 18$) or actually attempted suicide ($n = 38$). There were no differences between rates of affective disorder and family history of affective disorder, antisocial disorder and suicide. However, four putative risk factors were more prevalent among the suicide victims: diagnosis of bipolar disorder; affective disorder with comorbidity; lack of previous mental health treatment, and availability of firearms in the homes. Kosky, Silburn & Zubrick (1990) were not able to differentiate adolescent suicide attempters ($n = 82$) from ideators ($n = 258$) with respect to clinical symptoms such as level of depression, anxiety, sleep disorders and irritability. However, suicide attempts were more likely to be associated with chronic family discord and substance abuse. For boys, the odds of suicide attempts were substantially increased if the subject had experienced loss.

In a high school sample ($n = 380$) Harkavy Friedman *et al.* (1987) suggested that suicidal ideators and suicide attempters represent overlapping groups. On the other hand, Carlson & Cantwell (1982), in a

229

sample of 102 psychiatrically referred children and adolescents, concluded that 'suicide attempts did not reflect a continuum of suicidal ideation' (p. 361). Also, attempters tend to be younger and more often women. Completers are more often male, older, and use more lethal methods for self-destruction (Blumenthal, 1990).

The contradictions in these results may very well be explained by the possibility that in some persons suicidal behaviour has emerged in a hierarchical way and in others it did not, but strictly speaking, one can neither confirm nor deny the existence of a continuum of suicidality from the results of these cross-sectional studies. This can only be done by employing a longitudinal study that follows suicide ideators during a period of time.

CORRELATES OF SUICIDAL BEHAVIOUR

Concepts and methods

There is no single answer to the question 'why do adolescents attempt or commit suicide?' Research findings concerning correlates of suicidal behaviour are complicated by (a) the lack of adequate, widely accepted definitions and (b) the limitations of data collection (in most cases data can only be collected *ex post facto*: after the suicide or suicide attempt has taken place). As well as these methodological problems no general causes have been determined that explain suicidal behaviour. *The* suicidal adolescent does not exist, since the path to a suicide (attempt) is different for everyone. A complex conglomeration of factors precedes the behaviour and *in specific individuals* different combinations of elements may play a role. Nevertheless adolescents who have to deal with a combination of problematic elements are more at risk. Mostly, these characteristics are identified by comparing adolescents who displayed suicidal behaviour with adolescents who did not. Although the interrelationship of some of the characteristics has been demonstrated (Kienhorst *et al.,* 1990*a*, 1991), they have been predominantly described as separate correlates (e.g. Herjanic & Welner, 1980; Petzel & Riddle, 1981; Spirito *et al.,* 1989; Blumenthal, 1990; Kienhorst *et al.,* 1990*b*, 1991; De Wilde, Kienhorst, Diekstra & Wolters, 1992, 1994). Here, a distinction is made between four categories: environmental factors, psychological or psychopathological factors, behavioural factors and physiological changes. Before doing so, characteristics of the suicide (attempt), such as method and intent, will be discussed as well as the adolescents' *own* reasons.

Method, intent and reasons

The majority of suicide attempts by adolescents are by self-poisoning, such as drug overdose (Hawton & Goldacre, 1982; Hawton, 1986; Kienhorst et al., 1991). Other methods include self-mutilation, hanging, jumping from a height and jumping in front of a moving vehicle. No differences in the degree of suicidal intent have been reported between British and Dutch adolescents, or between adolescents and adults (Hawton et al., 1982; Kerkhof, 1985; Kienhorst et al., 1991). Despite these findings it has often been said that a suicide attempt by an adolescent is predominantly an effort to draw attention from others. Apart from the fact that this would be a very dramatic way of focusing attention upon oneself, which in our opinion should be heard at any time, some empirical evidence seems to contradict this. A few studies have focused on the attempters' own reported motivation for attempting suicide. Bancroft and colleagues (Bancroft, Skrimshire & Simkin, 1976; Bancroft et al., 1979) formulated a number of reasons that describe why suicide was attempted. The endorsements by 50 British (Hawton et al., 1982) and 48 Dutch adolescents (Kienhorst, De Wilde, Diekstra & Wolters, 1995) were rather congruent: all frequently endorsed items refer to either the stopping of a certain state of mind or the escape from a painful situation. All items concerning the appeal-motive ('drawing attention'), and the revenge-motive were only endorsed by a minority of the adolescents. Interestingly, clinicians gave far more weight to the appeal items (Hawton et al., 1982).

Furthermore, there is evidence that the items ' I wanted to stop feeling pain', 'I wanted to die', 'I wanted to get relief from a terrible state of mind', are all verbalisations of the same construct: 'to die' also meant 'to stop an unbearable consciousness' (Kienhorst et al., 1995). Possibly, death, in this context, is the pathway to relief.

Four groups of correlates

The separate description of a correlate of suicidal behaviour often leads to the (wrong) interpretation that this single correlate is in itself predictive of suicidal behaviour. The actual situation is far more complicated: a single event may precede various different kinds of morbidity and the effects can be mediated by psychological, psychopathological, social, or physiological circumstances, which are also interrelated. On the other

231

hand, the very complex prodromes of suicidal behaviour can hardly be described in any other way than by isolating the various aspects. By doing so, one must remain aware of the fact that the description is simplified.

Environmental factors

The study of environmental factors in relation to suicidal behaviour is extremely difficult, because of the impossibility of controlling for all other events and personal characteristics when studying a single factor. Nevertheless, a lot of effort has been made to demonstrate relations between suicidal behaviour and environmental factors. For instance, in Europe as well as in the United States, the current unemployment rates among youngsters are very high. Several studies have suggested that the increase in (adolescent) suicide rates are associated with an increase in unemployment rates (Filby & Eicher, 1983; Meares, Kraiuhin, & Benfield, 1983; Cormier & Klerman, 1985; Diekstra, 1989; Snyder, 1992). Comparison of suicidal groups with nonsuicidal 'normal' groups indicates that other life events such as physical illness, previous accidents, etc. seem to be associated with suicidal behaviour. These differences are not apparent, however, when a comparison is made between a suicidal group and a depressed non-suicidal group. Some extreme and traumatic events appear to discriminate these latter groups from each other. Thus sexual and physical abuse, unwanted pregnancies and abortus provocatus appear more common in the suicidal group. The association between exposure to physical and sexual abuse and suicidal behaviour has been noted in a high-school sample of 600 adolescents (Riggs, Alario & McHorney, 1990). In a recent study among pregnant adolescents, a positive history of physical or sexual abuse delineated a subgroup that was at high risk for self destructive behaviour (Bayatpour, Wells & Holford, 1992).

Moreover, suicide attempters report knowing more (significant) others who attempted or committed suicide (Kienhorst et al., 1992; Pfeffer, 1985; see also, below Imitation).

Generally, attempters seem to grow up in families with more turmoil than other groups of adolescents do (see, e.g. McKenry, Tishler & Kelly, 1982; Topol & Reznikoff, 1982; Spirito et al., 1989; Blumenthal, 1990). These adolescents more often come from *broken homes* (by death or divorce), experience more changes in living situation, unemployment of father, psychopathology, drug addiction and suicidality of parents (Friedman *et al.*, 1984; Kienhorst *et al.*, 1987, 1990*a*, 1992). Many of these family problems are already present in childhood and do not stabilise in adolescence (De Wilde *et al.*, 1992).

So, besides the type of event, the accumulation of events is also of importance. Jacobs (1971) reported an escalation of stressful life events, from the onset of puberty, in the lives of adolescent suicide attempters, more than in normal adolescents. De Wilde *et al.* (1992) found similar results, even in comparison with a depressed group. Especially during the year preceding the attempt, the differences were substantial, predominantly on characteristics related to social isolation.

Adolescent suicide attempters reported less perceived support and understanding from their parents than depressed adolescents (Kienhorst *et al.*, 1992), although this was not true for other persons in their social network, such as friends, other family members, and peers. Accordingly, most of the adolescents who attempted suicide reported problems in the relationship with their parents to be the primary reason for attempting suicide (Mansmann & Schenck, 1983; Kienhorst *et al.*, 1987). Miller *et al.* (1992) found that suicidal adolescents, in comparison with psychiatric and normal controls, rated their families as the least cohesive and most rigid.

Tishler & McKenry (1982) found an interesting difference between fathers and mothers of adolescent suicide attempters: mothers of these youngsters were significantly more anxious, whereas fathers were significantly more depressed (than parents of adolescent non-attempters). In a small group of adolescent attempters, Friedman *et al.* (1984) found a 56% prevalence of parental affective disorders, compared to a prevalence of 39% in a nonattempter group. Contrary to the findings of Pfeffer (1985) and Kienhorst *et al.* (1990*a*), occurrence of suicide attempts or deaths in the family did not discriminate between the two groups.

Psychological and psychopathological factors

A lifetime perspective is essential when one tries to understand suicidal behaviour (see also Leenaars, 1989). Especially with psychological or psychopathological factors, the developmental stage should be taken into consideration. So, before addressing the main psychological and psychopathological factors, the relation between the adolescents' developmental stage and suicidal behaviour will be discussed.

C. W. M. Kienhorst, E. J. de Wilde & R. F. W. Diekstra

Developmental stage and suicidal behaviour

From a psychoanalytic background, Tabachnick (1981) delineated certain aspects of the psychology of adolescence and certain aspects of the psychology of suicide in terms of object loss, loneliness, hopelessness and helplessness. Maris (1985) emphasised adolescence as a contemporary developmental life stage:

Adolescence tends to be a time marked by marginality, confusion and ambiguity. In fact, some have contended that the major problem of adolescence is that adolescents are freed from the responsibilities and rights of adults. As Paul Goodman put it long ago in the classic *Growing Up Absurd* (1960), the greatest problem that young people have today is their own *uselessness* (Maris, 1985, p. 100).

In our opinion, the interlocking psychologies of suicidal behaviour and the developmental stage of adolescence can become visible by taking into account the main developmental tasks of adolescents: achieving an adult (sexual) identity and learning new relationships to their age mates (including performing sex roles), achieving independence (from parents and economically), and an own system of values.

Remschmidt (1975) comments on these tasks as follows:

When such tasks have to be accomplished by a person, who at the same time has to deal with profound physical changes, the realization of a balance between the 'sense of oneself', the 'sense of the other' and adaptation to social norms, is extremely difficult (Remschmidt, 1975, p. 317).

Looking more specifically at the above-mentioned tasks, it becomes clear that they involve psychological abilities that still have to be obtained. For example, achieving independence from parents may involve the achievement of an adult, social and economic status which requires, for example, self-confidence. So, if in this process something falters it has a direct (negative) influence on the accomplishment of the other developmental tasks. In this sense, there seems to be an intermingling of developmental and psychological aspects, which may even lead to some degree of psychopathology. Considering their relative lack of power and the absence of a fully acquired ability for self-control (Diekstra & Methorst, 1986), the developmental tasks may become a difficult mission. Although most of the adolescents seem to accomplish these tasks rather well, an element of distress cannot be excluded. For example Rutter (Rutter, 1979) noted that feelings of misery and self depreciation are frequently reported by normal 14 and 15-year-olds.

The demand of developmental tasks may be greater than the capacities of adolescents. Under these circumstances despair and helplessness may occur (Tabachnick, 1981). A suicide attempt may be a way to communicate these feelings. From a developmental point of view, this can be considered as an implicit request for help to achieve an adult identity and position, which will provide the desired, although sometimes so feared independence. This desire for independence may explain the relatively low number of suicides in comparison with the high numbers of suicide attempts. In spite of the risk the suicide attempt has an adaptive developmental, rather than fatal outcome. In fact, disturbances in the above-mentioned developmental tasks (such as sexual and identity formation, evolution of friendships and self-esteem) are associated with suicidal behaviour (Mansmann & Schenck, 1983).

Cognitive factors

In this section a distinction is made between cognitive components (such as cognitive distortions and coping, impulsiveness and imitation) and emotional states (such as depression and anxiety). In the paragraph on depression, hopelessness will be considered as well, although this concept could also be considered as a cognitive factor.

Central to these factors is that suicidal behaviour is mediated or facilitated by certain thoughts or patterns of thoughts. These may reflect differences in the general normal cognitive style of dealing with social problems or difficult emotions, or they may be due to the presence of abnormal cognitive distortions. Another, but separate, theme is that of 'skipping' thoughts, that is, attempting or committing suicide in an 'impulsive' manner. Also, the imitation of suicides and suicide attempts will be discussed at the end of this section.

Cognitive distortions and coping

Suicidal persons are reported as having a limited number of ways to deal with problems. Orbach, Rosenheim & Hary (1987) established that suicidal children could think of less alternative solutions in a predefined dilemma about life and death than a chronically ill and a normal group. Cohen-Sandler (1982) also observed the relative inability of suicidal children to generate alternative solutions to common interpersonal problems. This quantitative aspect of problem solving is often referred to as *inflexibility* or rigidity. Suicidal adolescents (like suicidal adults)

235

seem to be less fortunate in this respect (Neuringer & Lettieri, 1982). For instance, Puskar, Hoover & Miewald (1992) found that adolescent suicide attempters, contrary to a non-suicidal group, used only affected-oriented coping methods, whereas the others used problem-oriented methods as well. It is unclear if this characteristic is specific for suicidal persons or also found in individuals with depression and/or psychiatric disorders. For example Schmidtke (1992) concluded, in an adult sample, that cognitive rigidity is a common feature of persons in crisis and those with depressive states. It is unclear if this also true in adolescence.

Hart, Williams & Davidson (1988) found that adolescent suicide attempters displayed more attributional errors as compared to psychiatric controls. Kahn (1987) found that many suicidal adolescents, compared to non-suicidal adolescents, experienced difficulties in coping with their emotions and could not think through the consequences of their actions. Topol & Reznikoff (1982) reported a significantly more external locus of control in hospitalised adolescent suicide attempters than control adolescents. De Wilde et al. (1994) confirmed these results but added that the locus of control was not more external than that of a comparable depressed group of adolescents.

However, Kienhorst et al. (1992) found that adolescents who attempted suicide evaluated comparable events as more negative than depressed adolescents. This suggests that suicide attempters may have a more negative style than depressed adolescents. It remains unclear if such a cognitive style is state or trait dependent (Perrah & Wichman, 1987).

Apart from distortions or limitations of cognitive processes of suicidal persons, adolescents are said not to think at all about or plan a suicide attempt, in most cases. That this conclusion may be premature will be considered next.

Impulsiveness

In the suicide literature, impulsiveness in relation to suicidal behaviour has been conceptualised in two ways; as a trait-like characteristic of personality and as lack of planning. Although it is possible to see the latter as a consequence of the former, most often both concepts have been studied separately. As an example of the first concept, Withers & Kaplan (1987) reported in a study of 173 adolescents suicide attempters that 54% of the male and 39% of the female subjects had an 'impulsive' personality characteristic. Other studies consider impulsiveness as lack of reflection and planning before the suicide or suicide attempt takes place. Conceptually, the idea of an impulsive suicidal act is difficult to grasp. Having no reflection or planning implies that there is no or just a short timespan between evolving the idea to attempt suicide and the actual behaviour. The problem does not primarily concern the 'planning' element, since planning implies all kind of decisions with respect to *enacting* the behaviour (like, for example, the method that will be used). This implies that there has already been some kind of *reflection* with respect to performing the behaviour; in other words, planning follows reflection. So, the core of the conceptual problem lies in the word 'reflection'. Strictly speaking, impulsivity (in the sense of 'no reflection') implies that an individual (for the first time) must have the notion that the potential of mankind to commit suicide can be applied to oneself and crucially, this thought must lead to the action (almost) immediately. That this is a doubtful assumption, is supported by the finding that suicidal ideation (sometimes existing for years) is one of the most powerful predictors of (future) attempts, also in adolescents.

Despite these theoretical complexities, some authors have investigated the relation between impulsiveness and adolescent suicidal behaviour. Hawton & Catalan (1987) found that two-thirds of their subjects in two studies ($n = 48$; $n = 50$) thought about attempting suicide only within one hour before the attempt. They also report doubts about these findings by suggesting that at some time in the development of the crisis there must have been earlier thoughts about a suicide attempt. Stiffman (1989) concluded that 80% of the attempts (from 291 adolescent runaway youth) were not planned, not even a day in advance. Somewhat surprising are her contradictory reports that one in every five had thought of a suicide plan within the last 2 days, and one in every three had considered such a plan within the last week, whereas only 3% planned the attempt more than a week ahead of time. Hoberman & Garfinkel (1988) report that in their sample of 229 adolescent suicides it appeared that: 'in only 28% of the cases there was credible evidence of a plan to commit suicide and this typically appeared of brief duration' (p.691). As Spirito *et al.* (1989) also stated, given the frequent reference to teenage suicide attempts as impulsive, it is surprising how few studies have been conducted on the relation between impulsivity and adolescent development. Summarising from the above findings, despite the commonsense idea that adolescent suicidal behaviour is impulsive, the operationalisation of the concept seems quite diverse and the scientific verification of it is still unclear. Perhaps the frequent reference to the (supposed) relation between impulsivity and suicide attempts of adolescents serves as a belief that assumes that suicide attempts by adolescents are carried out without a rationale. As such, this belief may become a prejudice, which may inhibit reflections about the actual factors involved.

Imitation

Although no study has yet clearly demonstrated a causal relation between exposure to suicide and suicidal behaviour itself, there are various ways to comprehend this process: individuals can learn to react with suicidal acts under specific conditions. This can be done by direct learning (a person's own previous suicidal gestures or attempts, see above), or by vicarious or observational learning (for example, observing a significant other attempting or committing suicide while being depressed or after a severe personal loss). Regarding this latter process, the role of media exposure has also been investigated.

In the field of observational learning, attention was focused on the direct environment of suicidal persons. Adolescent suicide attempters report more (significant) others who attempted or committed suicide than ideating, depressed or non-suicidal adolescents (see e.g. Jacobs, 1971; Smith & Crawford, 1986; Conrad, 1992; Kienhorst et al, 1992). There is, however, another explanation for this concurrence than that of learned behaviour: It is also possible that adolescent suicide attempters are situated in more difficult circumstances, since they are more likely to be living with suicidal persons (and more often went through a mourning process of a beloved person who committed suicide) in their direct environment than the controls are.

The imitation effect may also occur in a (high-school) community. Several studies (e.g. Robbins & Conroy, 1983; Gould & Shaffer, 1986; Philips & Carstensen, 1986; Brent et al., 1989; Davidson et al., 1989) describe clustering of teenage suicides or suicide attempts. Although Robbins & Conroy suggested 'contagion' as a possible cause for suicide attempts, Davidson et al. (1989) found that the adolescents who committed suicide ($n = 14$) were not more likely than the control subjects ($n = 42$) to have had direct exposure to suicide as measured by their acquaintance with a person who committed suicide.

Even more indirect is learning of suicidal behaviour through media exposure. Kessler *et al.* (1988) could not find a (direct) relation between exposure to three fictional films and television newscasts about suicide and an increase in adolescent suicide afterwards. However, some studies do demonstrate an increase in this respect (Philips & Carstensen 1986; Ostroff, Boyd & Jeffrey, 1987). Not only an increase in adolescent suicides, but also an imitation of the exhibited method is observed (Ostroff *et al.*, 1987; Schmidtke & Häfner, 1988). Moreover, there is some evidence that adolescent suicides increase more than adult suicides (Schmidtke & Häfner, 1988), even if the 'model' was not an adolescent (Philips & Carstensen, 1986).

Still, since these studies are purely correlational, an increase in suicides after (media) exposure of suicide does not demonstrate the existence of imitation. Imitation effects have to be established in controlled experiments. By exposing 116 high-school students to different video-simulated conditions, Steede & Range (1989) concluded that adolescents may not be influenced by news about suicide or may just deny such influence. In another experimental study, Range, Goggin & Steede (1988) reported that their 142 subjects acknowledged the existence of behavioural contagion after suicide is reported, and that they perceived themselves to be influenced by such information. Overall the findings suggest that exposure to suicide increases current levels of personal distress but does not predict an inevitable increase in subsequent suicidal thinking.

In conclusion, the literature in this field is rather ambiguous. Therefore, important implications for preventive strategies are still unclear.

Emotional states

Similar to the other factors related to adolescent suicidal behaviour, describing various emotional states separately does not do justice to the complexities and co-occurrence of these phenomena. For instance, Brady & Kendall (1992) reported that a substantial part of the group of children and adolescents that were identified as anxious or depressed, had comorbid anxiety and depressive disorders. Measures of anxiety and depression were highly correlated. In the following paragraphs, depression (and hopelessness) and anxiety are discussed in relation to adolescent suicidal behaviour.

Depression and hopelessness

Depression is clearly one of the strongest correlates of suicidal behaviour (see e.g. Crumley, 1982; Chabrol & Moron, 1988; Friedman *et al.*, 1984; Kienhorst *et al.*, 1990*a*). Also, depression is related to the various psychological and behavioural characteristics that also correlate with adolescent suicidal behaviour, such as self-esteem, locus of control, alcohol and drug abuse, negative life events, etc. Support was found for the conclusion that various previously reported differences between suicide attempters and non-attempters may have to be attributed to affective disorders or depressed mood present in most of the suicide attempters (Kienhorst *et al.*, 1992; De Wilde *et al.*, 1994). In this respect, the cognitive triad of Beck (1976) describes some of these processes in suicidal persons.

The first component of the triad refers to a negative view of oneself. This low self-esteem was demonstrated in adolescent suicide attempters (Yanish & Battle, 1985; Kienhorst *et al.*, 1990*a*). The second component of the triad concerns a negative view of their situation. As stated before, suicide attempters rate comparable events as more negative. The triad is completed by a negative view of one's future. In this respect, hopelessness is frequently investigated in relation to adolescent suicidal behaviour. The correlation between suicidal intent and depression is influenced by hopelessness, among adults (Minkoff *et al.*, 1973; Salter & Platt, 1990; Wetzel *et al.*, 1980) and children (Kazdin *et al.*, 1983), and hopelessness is a significant predictor of completed suicide, in (psychiatric) adults (Beck *et al.*, 1985). For adolescents, the picture is less clear. On the one hand, Topol & Reznikoff (1982) found a significant difference in hopelessness between hospitalised suicidal adolescents and hospitalised non-suicidal adolescents. On the other hand, Asarnow, Carlson & Guthrie (1987) saw the correlation between hopelessness and suicide diminish when controlling for depression in children and young adolescents. Rotherham-Borus & Trautman (1988) found no significant difference comparing minority adolescent female suicide attempters and a matched group of psychiatrically disturbed adolescents. Therefore, the relation between hopelessness and suicidal behaviour needs more clarification.

The majority of depressed adolescents do not attempt or commit suicide and since not all suicide attempters are depressed, a distinction remains necessary. Therefore an exploration of different subgroups of depressed and suicidal adolescents is needed. For instance, Kovacs, Goldston & Gatsonis (1993) described higher rates of suicidal behaviours in out-patient youth with major depressive and dysthymic disorders than those with adjustment disorders with depressed mood and non-depressive disorders. Further comparisons should be made between, for example, bipolar and unipolar depressed adolescents in relation to different types of suicidal behaviour.

Anxiety

Given the comorbidity of anxiety and depression and the non-discriminability of life events in this respect (e.g. Goodyer, Wright & Altham, 1990), it is surprising how little research is done about the relation between anxiety and suicidal behaviour in adolescents. A recent study (Marttunen *et al.*, 1991) showed a relatively low occurrence of anxiety disorders in adolescent who died by suicide. In adults some studies indicate that suicidal persons have a higher level of anxiety than non-suicidal controls (Kreitman, 1977; Diekstra, 1973, 1981). Schmidtke & Schaller (1992) were unable to find any difference on both state and trait anxiety between suicidal and non-suicidal psychiatric patients, although differences on these dimensions were reported between their patient groups and normal controls. De Wilde *et al.* (1993) report no difference in trait and state anxiety between the adolescent suicide attempters, and depressed adolescents who never attempted suicide. However, both these groups reported more state and trait anxiety than a group of 'normal' adolescents. Furthermore, state anxiety was higher than trait anxiety in the depressed as well as the suicidal adolescents. Only 7% and 3% of the suicidal subjects of the same study respectively reported feelings of anxiety in the last days and hours before the attempt (Kienhorst *et al.*, 1994*b*).

Behavioural factors

In adults there are no characteristics, neither antecedent events or problems, nor personality characteristics (as measured by standard psychological tests), that are as powerful in predicting a suicide attempt or suicide, as behavioural characteristics. This was shown by Diekstra (1973, 1981) and Schmidtke (1988), where the most powerful predictors of a suicide attempt were (in the following order): (1) previous suicide attempt(s), (2) previous threats with suicide or suicidal ideation,

241

(3) alcohol, psychopharmaca- or hard drug abuse and (4) suicide or suicide attempt(s) and alcohol or drug addiction among significant others.

In adolescents, as was shown in two studies, this picture seems the same: previous suicidal behaviour and use of drugs and alcohol are ranking in the top of the most powerful predictive factors, but contrary to adults, disruptions in the family are the next in importance (Kienhorst *et al.*, 1990*a*).

Drug addiction or toxicomania, both of the person himself or of significant others, is also predictive of suicidal behaviour (e.g. McKenry, Tishler & Kelley, 1983). Most suicidal acts are performed by using poisoning substances and can be considered as a form of abuse of drugs. Once a person is accustomed to the use of drugs, the intake of an overdose (which then often is defined as a suicide attempt or a suicide) becomes more likely. The same applies to alcohol abuse. Chronic and/or excessive alcohol use is associated with severe personal and social problems. Coping with these problems through the intake of a mind-changing chemical substance (i.e. alcohol) increases the risk of use of other chemical substances in high doses. Suicidal behaviour and drug dependency may both be indicative of a palliative response pattern. There is some evidence that suicidal behaviour in adolescents is part of a general problematic reaction style (including the use of mind-changing chemical substances) towards problematic circumstances (Kienhorst, 1988; Kienhorst *et al.*, 1992).

Physiological changes

In the highly industrialised countries of Europe and North America a remarkable biological-developmental change has taken place over the course of the past 150 years. Around 1850 the average age of the menarche was 16 years; today in most countries the average age is around 12.5 years. A similar trend seems to have taken place in boys (age of spermarche) but is harder to document. A number of authors have tried to attribute the increases in secular changes in emotional disturbances in early adolescence to this change (Hamburg, 1989; Fombonne, 1992). The assumption that physiological changes at puberty directly contribute to risk remains unclear (Angold & Rutter 1992) and early onset puberty does not automatically explain higher prevalence rates of depression or suicidal behaviour.

A more plausible explanation seems to be that the lowering of puberty has caused a disjunction of biological development on the one hand and psychological development and social development on the other. The brain still does not reach a fully adult state of development until the end of the teenage years (Hamburg, 1989) and social changes during two centuries and particulary during the last century have postponed the end of adolescence – and of social dependence – until much later. This phenomenon of **bio-psycho-social dysbalance** is a distinctly human evolutionary novelty (Hamburg, 1989). This might pose stresses and strains on many youngsters that overtax their own coping repertoires as well as that of their families and other educators, at least for a number of years. Besides, in most countries the present average age of puberty coincides with another developmental task for the early adolescent, i.e. the transition from elementary to secondary or high school (Petersen *et al.*, 1993).

Some researchers hypothesise (Fombonne, 1992) that these processes particularly affect girls. This hypothesis is supported by the fact that depressive disorders, suicidal ideation and parasuicide are more prevalent in girls than in boys. The rise in number of suicides is, however, greater among boys than among girls. In our opinion, the sex difference in adolescence (as well as in adults) may be understood from the perspective that many suicide attempts and helplessness and hopelesseness accompanying depression can be considered as help-seeking behaviours. Girls, more than boys, are socialised to depend on the help of others in our society. Boys are educated to be more independent and to find their own solutions for their problems. This may explain the difference in suicide and suicide attempt rates between the sexes. The fact that boys, more than girls, suffer from conduct disorders, and girls, more than boys, from depression seems related in this respect.

PREVENTION

Although there is a rich and scholarly literature on sociological, psychological and biological aspects of suicide there is a scarcity of studies on the development and evaluation of well-structured programmes and schemes for treatment and prevention. This also applies to adolescent suicidal behaviour, although there is an exception for curriculum-based programmes or education programmes. The number of such programmes introduced into schools in the USA between 1984 and 1989 increased by 200% (Garland, Shaffer & Whittle, 1989), and continues to grow. Briefly, the main goals are: (1) to raise awareness of the problem of adolescent suicide, (2) to train participants to identify adolescents at risk for suicide, and (3) to educate participants about community mental health resources and referral techniques. The programmes are presented by mental health professionals or educators and are most commonly directed to secondary school students, their parents, and educators. The mean duration of the programmes is approximately 2 hours.

Unfortunately, most suicide prevention programmes have fallen short on both of these requirements. Although many curriculum-based suicide prevention programmes have been operating since 1981 (Garland et al., 1989), there are only a few published evaluation studies, and most of these are poorly designed in that there is no control group (Nelson, 1987; Ross, 1980), with exceptions such as the Spirito et al. (1988) evaluation of a suicide awareness programme for ninth graders or the New Jersey study of Shaffer et al. (1990). The first study concluded that the programme was minimally effective in imparting knowledge, and ineffective in changing attitudes. The latter found few positive effects of three suicide prevention curriculum programmes and some possible negative effects.

Further evaluation is clearly needed, with an emphasis on the assessment of behavioural variables including suicidal behaviour and help-seeking behaviour.

Another way of preventing suicides and suicide attempts lies in the interventions when dealing with a suicidal adolescent. To our knowledge, there are no well-controlled efficacy studies in this field. Kienhorst et al. (1992) empirically derived some intervention strategies when dealing with a suicidal depressed adolescent. They should focus on three main areas: (1) attacking the suicidal adolescent's problematic life situation, which may include family therapy. Attention should be given to the treatment of possible traumatic experiences such as sexual abuse, unwanted pregnancies and induced abortions, (2) changing a negative cognitive style with a special focus on hopelessness, (3) changing the problem solving-and/or coping strategies with special attention on replacing withdrawal reactions by more adequate strategies.

CONCLUDING REMARKS

The epidemiology of suicidal behaviour is well documented and the least puzzling aspect of the problem. As far as Europe and the United

States are concerned, suicidal behaviour has been increasing in recent years. Correlational studies on adolescent suicide are few and little new information has been forthcoming. This may be due to methodological shortcomings and the fact that within the general group of suicide attempters, different patterns of behaviours are likely to reflect different subtypes. Determining the association between suicidal behaviour and other problematic behaviours, psychological states and psychiatrical disturbances, such as depression, is therefore difficult. For example, the concept of depression covers a whole realm, ranging from depressed mood to unipolar and bipolar depressive disturbances. In clinical practice, this is reflected in the complicated recognition of suicidal risk in the various subtypes of depressed patients. This is certainly an important field for further study.

Maybe, a shift in objective from suicidal behaviour as a single dependent variable to suicidal behaviour as part of a larger concept, such as a style concerning problematic reactions to problematic situations, can be of help here. Such a reconceptualisation would also be valuable in designing intervention strategies and programmes. Although there is undoubtedly research going on in this field, there is far less in the clinical and public health direction (especially regarding the effectiveness of interventions) than the endeavours made regarding epidemiology and discriminating characteristics. Despite continuous scientific and clinical efforts, it is clear that there is still a long way to go in preventing suicidal behaviour in adolescence.

REFERENCES

Angold, A. & Rutter, M. (1992). The effects of age and pubertal status on depression in a large clinical sample. *Development and Psychopathology*, **4**, 5–29.

Asarnow, J., Carlson, G. & Guthrie, D. (1987). Coping strategies, self-perceptions, hopelessness, and perceived family environments in depressed and suicidal children. *Journal of Consulting and Clinical Psychology*, **55**, 361–6.

Bancroft, J., Hawton, K., Simkin, S. & Kingston, B. (1979). The reasons people give for taking overdoses: A further inquiry. *British Journal of Medical Psychiatry*, **52**, 353–65.

Bancroft, J. H. J., Skrimshire, A. M. & Simkin, S. (1976). The reasons people give for taking overdoses. *British Journal of Psychiatry*, **128**, 538–48.

Bayatpour, M., Wells, R. D. & Holford, S. (1992). Physical and sexual abuse as predictors of substance use and suicide among pregnant teenagers. *Journal of Adolescent Health*, **13**, 128–32.

Beck, A. T. (1976). *Cognitive therapy and the emotional disorders.* International Universities Press, New York.

Beck, A., Steer, R., Kovacs, M. & Garrison, B. (1985). Hopelessness and eventual suicide: a 10-year prospective study of patients hospitalized with suicidal ideation. *American Journal of Psychiatry*, **142**, 559–63.

Blumenthal, S. J. (1990). Youth suicide: Risk factors, assessment, and treatment of adolescent and young adult suicidal patients. Adolescence: Psychopathology, normality, and creativity. *Psychiatric Clinics of North America*, **13**, 511–56.

Brady, E. U. & Kendall, P. C. (1992). Comorbidity of anxiety and depression in children and adolescents. *Psychological Bulletin*, **111**, 244–55.

Brent, D. A., Kerr, M. M., Goldstein, C. *et al.* (1989). An Outbreak of suicide and suicidal behavior in a high school. *Journal of the American Academy of Child and Adolescent Psychiatry*, **28**, 918–24.

Brent, D., Perper, J., Goldstein, C. *et al.* (1988). Risk factors for adolescent suicide A comparison of adolescent suicide victims with suicidal inpatients. *Archives of General Psychiatry*, **45**, 581–8.

Brooksbank, D. (1985). Suicide and parasuicide in childhood and early adolescence. *British Journal of Psychiatry*, **146**, 459–63.

Carlson, G. A. & Cantwell, D. P. (1982). Suicidal behavior and depression in children and adolescents. *Journal of the American Academy of Child Psychiatry*, **21**, 361–8.

Chabrol, H. & Moron, P. (1988). Depressive disorders in 100 adolescents who attempted suicide [letter]. *American Journal of Psychiatry*, **145**, 379.

Choquet, M. (1981). Tentatives de suicide en milieu scolaire Unpublished manuscript.

Cohen, E., Motto, J. A. & Seiden, R. H. (1966). An instrument for evaluating suicide potential: A preliminary study. *American Journal of Psychiatry*, **122**, 886–91.

Cohen-Sandler, R. (1982). Interpersonal problem-solving skills of suicidal and non-suicidal children: assessment and treatment. *Dissertation Abstracts International*, **43**, 17.

Conrad, N. (1992). Stress and knowledge of suicidal others as factors in suicidal behavior of high school adolescents. *Issues in Mental Health Nursing*, **13**, 95–104.

Cormier, H. & Klerman, G. (1985). Unemployment and male-female labor force participation as determinants of changing suicide rates of males and females in Quebec. *Social Psychiatry*, **20**, 109–14.

Crumley, F. E. (1982). Adolescent suicide attempts and melancholia. *Texas Medicine*, **78**, 62–5.

Davidson, L. E., Rosenberg, M. L., Mercy, J. A. *et al.* (1989). An epidemiologic study of risk factors in two teenage suicide clusters. *Journal of the American Medical Association*, **262**, 2687–92.

Diekstra, R. F. W. (1973). *Crisis en Gedragskeuze*. Swets & Zeitlinger, Amsterdam.

Diekstra, R. F. W. (1981). *Over suïcide. [About suicide]*. Samsom, Alphen aan den Rijn.

Diekstra, R. F. W. (1982). Epidemiology of attempted suicide in the EEC. In *New trends in suicide prevention* (ed. P. Wilmotte & J. Mendlewicz), pp. 1–16. Karger, New York.

Diekstra, R. F. W. (1989). Suicidal behavior and depressive disorders in adolescents and young adults. *Neuropsychobiology*, **22**, 194–207.

Diekstra, R. F. W., Kienhurst, C. W. M. & De Wilde, E. J. (1994). Suicide and suicidal behaviour among adolescents. In *Psychosocial disorders in young people, time trends and their causes* (ed. M. Rutter & D. J. Smith). Wiley, London, in press.

Diekstra, R. F. W. & Methorst, G. J. (1986). De samenleving als verslaver: leefstijl, geestelijke gezonheid en verslavingsrisico bij jongeren. *Gedrag en Gezondheid*, **14**, 145–52.

Filby, R. & Eicher, G. (1983). Unemployment and the suicide rate. *Ohio State Medical Journal*, **79**, 837–9, 848.

Fombonne, E. (1992). Depressive disorders. Paper prepared for the Academia Study Group on Youth Problems.

Friedman R.C., Corn, R., Hurt, S. W. *et al.* (1984). Family history of illness in the seriously suicidal adolescent. *American Journal of Orthopsychiatry*, **54**, 390–7.

Garland, A., Shaffer, D. & Whittle, B. (1989). A national survey of school-based, adolescent suicide prevention programs. *Journal of the American Academy of Child and Adolescent Psychiatry*, **28**, 931–4.

Garnefski, N. & Diekstra, R. F. W. (1993). *Scholierenonderzoek 1992: landelijke uitkomsten rond een orderzoek naar gedrag en gezondheid van ca. 11000 scholieren van het voortgezet orderwijs.* Vangroep Klinische-en Gezondheid spsychologie, RUL, Leiden.

Garrison, C. Z. (1989). The study of suicidal behavior in the schools. *Suicide and Life-Threatening Behavior*, **19**, 120–30.

Goldney, R. D., Winefield, A. H., Tiggemann, M., *e tal.* (1989). Suicidal ideation in a young adult population. *Acta Psychiatrica Scandinavia*, **79**, 481–9.

Goodyer, I., Wright, C. & Altham, P. (1990). The friendships and recent life events of anxious and depressed school-aged children. *British Journal of Psychiatry*, **156**, 689–98.

Gould, M. & Shaffer, D. (1986). The impact of suicide in television movies. Evidence of imitation. *New England Journal of Medicine*, **315**, 690–4.

Hamburg, D. (1989). Preparing for life: the critical transition of adolescence. In *Preventive interventions in adolescence* (ed. R. F. W. Diekstra), (pp. 4–15). Hogrefe & Huber, Toronto/Bern.

Harkavy Friedman, J. M., Asnis, G. M., Boeck, M. & DiFiore, J. (1987). Prevalence of specific suicidal behaviors in a high school sample. *American Journal of Psychiatry*, **144**, 1203–6.

Hart, E. E., Williams, C. L. & Davidson, J. A. (1988). Suicidal behavior, social networks and psychiatric diagnosis. *Social Psychiatry and Psychiatric Epidemiology*, **23**, 222–8.

Hawton, K. (1986). *Suicide and attempted suicide among children and adolescents.* Sage Publications, Beverly Hills.

Hawton, K. & Catalan, J. (1987). *Attempted suicide: a practical guide to its nature and management.* Oxford University Press, Oxford.

Hawton, K., Cole, D., O'Grady, J. & Osborn, M. (1982). Motivational aspects of deliberate self-poisoning in adolescents. *British Journal of Psychiatry*, **141**, 286–91.

Hawton, K. & Goldacre, M. (1982). Hospital admissions for adverse effects of medicinal agents (mainly self-poisoning) among adolescents in the Oxford region. *British Journal of Psychiatry*, **141**, 166-170.

Herjanic, B. & Welner, Z. (1980). Adolescent suicide. *Advances in Behavioral Pediatrics*, **1**, 195–223.

Hoberman, H. & Garfinkel, B. (1988). Completed suicide in children and adolescents. *Journal of the American Academy of Child and Adolescent Psychiatry*, **27**, 689–95.

Holinger, P., Offer, D. & Zola, M. (1988). A prediction model of suicide among youth. *Journal of Nervous and Mental Disease*, **176**, 275–9.

Jacobs, J. (1971). *Adolescent suicide.* Wiley Interscience, London.

Jobes, D. A., Berman, A. L. & Josselsen, A. R. (1986). The impact of psychosocial autopsies on medical examiner's determination of manner of death. *Journal of Forensic Science*, **31**, 177–89.

Kahn, A. U. (1987). Heterogeneity of suicidal adolescents. *Journal of the American Academy of Child and Adolescent Psychiatry*, **1**, 92–6.

Kazdin, A., Esveldt, D. K., Unis, A. & Rancurello, M. (1983). Child and parent

C. W. M. Kienhorst, E. J. de Wilde & R. F. W. Diekstra

evaluations of depression and aggression in psychiatric inpatient children. *Journal of Abnormal Child Psychology*, **11**, 401–13.

Kerkhof, A. J. F. M. (1985). *Suicide en de geestelijke gezondheidszorg*. Swets & Zeitlinger, Amsterdam.

Kessler, R., Downey, G., Milavsky, J. & Stipp, H. (1988). Clustering of teenage suicides after television news stories about suicides: a reconsideration. *American Journal of Psychiatry*, **145**, 1379–83.

Kienhorst, C. W. M. (1988). Suicidaal gedrag bij jongeren. Onderzoek naar omvang en kenmerken. [Suicidal behaviour among adolescents. A study of the frequency and characteristics.] *Thesis)*. Ambo, Baarn.

Kienhorst, C. W. M., De Wilde, E. J., Diekstra, R.F.W. & Wolters, W. H. G. (1990*a*). Characteristics of suicide attempters in a population-based sample of Dutch adolescents. *British Journal of Psychiatry*, **156**, 243–8.

Kienhorst, C. W. M., De Wilde, E. J., Diekstra, R. F. W. & Wolters, W. H. G. (1991). Construction of an index for predicting suicide attempts in depressed adolescents. *British Journal of Psychiatry*, **159**, 676–82.

Kienhorst, C. W. M., De Wilde, E. J., Diekstra, R. F. W. & Wolters, W. H. G. (1992). Differences between adolescent suicide attempters and depressed adolescents. *Acta Psychiatrica Scandinavica*, **85**, 222–8.

Kienhorst, C. W. M., De Wilde, E. J., Diekstra, R. F. W. & Wolters, W. H. G. (1995). The adolescents' image of their suicide attempt. *Journal of the American Academy of Child and Adolescent Psychiatry*, in press.

Kienhorst, C. W. M., De Wilde, E. J., Van den Bout, J. *et al.* (1990*b*). Self-reported suicidal behavior in Dutch secondary education students. *Suicide and Life-Threatening Behavior*, **20**, 101–12.

Kienhorst, C. W. M., Wolters, W. H. G., Diekstra, R. F. W. & Otte, E. (1987). A study of the frequency of suicidal behaviour in children aged 5 to 14. *Journal of Child Psychology and Psychiatry*, **28**, 153–65.

Kosky, R., Silburn, S. & Zubrick, S. (1990). Are children and adolescents who have suicidal thoughts different from those who attempt suicide? *Journal of Nervous and Mental Disease*, **178**, 38–43.

Kovacs, M., Goldston, D. & Gatsonis, C. (1993). Suicidal behaviors and childhood onset depressive disorders. *Journal of the American Academy of Child and Adolescent Psychiatry*, **32**, 8–20.

Kreitman, N. (1977). *Parasuicide*. Wiley & Sons, London.

Leenaars, A. (1989). Are young adults' suicides psychologically different from those of other adults? (the Schneidman Lecture). *Suicide and Life-Threatening Behavior*, **19**, 249–63.

Mansmann, V. & Schenck, K. (1983). Vordergrundige Motive und langfristige Tendenzen zum Suiczid bei Kindern und Jugendlichen. In *Suizid bei Kindern und Jugendlichen*. (ed. I. Jochmus & E. Forster), pp. 38–44. Enke, Stuttgart.

Maris, R. (1985). The adolescent suicide problem. *Suicide and Life-Threatening Behavior*, **15**, 91–109.

Marttunen, M. J., Aro, H. M., Henriksson, M. M. & Lönnqvist, J. K. (1991). Mental disorders in adolescent suicide. *Archives of General Psychiatry*, **48**, 834–9.

McKenry, P. C., Tishler, C. L. & Kelley, C. (1982). Adolescent suicide – a comparison of attempters and nonattempters in an emergeny room population. *Clinical Pediatrics*, **5**, 266–70.

McKenry, P., Tishler, C. & Kelley, C. (1983). The role of drugs in adolescent suicide attempts. *Suicide and Life-Threatening Behavior*, **13**, 166–75.

Meares, R., Kraiuhin, C. & Benfield, J. (1983). Adolescent suicide. *Australian Family Physician*, **12**, 614–16.

248

Miller, K. E., King, C. A., Shain, B. N. & Naylor, M. W. (1992). Suicidal adolescents perceptions of their family enviroment. *Suicide and Life-Threatening Behavior*, **22**, 226–39.

Minkoff, K., Bergman, E., Beck, A. T. & Beck, R. (1973). Hopelessness, depression and attempted suicide. *American Journal of Psychiatry*, **130**, 455–9.

Motto, J., Heilbron, D. & Juster, R. (1985). Development of a clinical instrument to estimate suicide risk. *American Journal of Psychiatry*, **142**, 680–6.

Nelson, F. (1987). Evaluation of a youth suicide prevention school program. *Adolescence*, **22**, 813–25.

Neuringer, C. & Lettieri, D. (1982). *Suicidal women. Their thinking and feeling patterns*. Gardner Press, New York.

Orbach, I., Rosenheim, E. & Hary, E. (1987). Some aspects of cognitive functioning in suicidal children. *Journal of the American Academy of Child and Adolescent Psychiatry*, **26**, 181–5.

Ostroff, R. B., Boyd & Jeffrey H. (1987). Television and suicide. *New England Journal of Medicine*, **316**, 877–9.

Perrah, M. & Wichman, H. (1987). Cognitive rigidity in suicide attempters. *Suicide and Life-Threatening Behavior*, **17**(3), 251–5.

Petersen, A. C., Compas, B., Brooks-Gunn, J. *et al.* (1993). Depression in adolescence. *American Psychologist*, **48**, 155–68.

Petzel, S. V. & Riddle, M. (1981). Adolescent suicide: psychological and cognitive aspects. *Adolescent Psychiatry*, **9**, 343–98.

Pfeffer, C. R. (1985). Self-destructive behavior in children and adolescents. *Psychiatric Clinics of North America*, **8**, 215–26.

Philips, D. P. & Carstensen, L. L. (1986). Clustering of teenage suicides after television news. Stories about suicide. *New England Journal of Medicine*, **315**, 685–9.

Puskar, K., Hoover, C. & Miewald, C. (1992). Suicidal and nonsuicidal coping methods of adolescents. *Perspectives in Psychiatric Care*, **28**, 15–20.

Range, L., Goggin, W. & Steede, K. (1988). Perception of behavioral contagion of adolescent suicide. *Suicide and Life-Threatening Behavior*, **18**, 334–41.

Remschmidt, H. (1975). Psychologie und Psychopathologie der Adoleszenz. *Medischer Kinderheilkunde*, **123**, 316–23.

Riggs, S., Alario, A. & McHorney, C. (1990). Health risk behaviors and attempted suicide in adolescents who report prior maltreatment. *Journal of Paediatrics*, **116**, 815–21.

Robbins D. & Conroy, R. C. (1983). A cluster of adolescent suicide attempts: Is suicide contagious? *Journal of Adolescent Health Care*, **3**, 253–5.

Ross, C. P. (1980). Mobilizing schools for suicide prevention. *Suicice and Life-Threatening Behavior*, **10**, 239–43.

Rotheram-Borus, M. & Trautman, P. (1988). Hopelessness, depression, and suicidal intent among adolescent suicide attempters. *Journal of the American Academy of Child and Adolescent Psychiatry*, **27**, 700–4.

Rudd, M. (1989). The prevalence of suicidal ideation among college students. *Suicide and Life-Threatening Behavior*, **19**, 173–83.

Rutter, M. (1979). *Changing youth in a changing society*. London: Nuffield Provincial Hospitals Trust, London.

Salter, D. & Platt, S. (1990). Suicidal intent, hopelessness and depression in a parasuicide population: the influence of social desirability and elapsed time. *British Journal of Clinical Child Psychology*, **29**, 361–71.

Schmidtke, A. (1988). *Verhaltenstheoretisches Erklärungsmodell Suizidalen Verhalten*. Roderer, Regensburg.

Schmidtke, A. (1992). The influence of mood factors on cognitive styles, Paper presented on the Silver Anniversary Conference of the American Association of Suicidology, Chicago, April 1–4, 1992.

Schmidtke, A. & Häfner, H. (1988). The Werther effect after television films: new evidence for an old hypothesis. *Psychological Medicine*, **18**, 665–76.

Schmidtke, A. & Schaller, D. (1992). Covariation of cognitive styles and mood factors during crisis. In *Suicidal behavior in Europe* (ed. P. Crepet, G. Ferrari, S. Platt & M. Bellini), pp. 225–32. Wiley, Rome and New York.

Schotte, D. E. & Clum, G. A. (1982). Suicide ideation in a college population: a test of a model. *Journal of Consulting and Clinical Psychology*, **50**, 690–6.

Shaffer, D. & Fisher, P. (1981). The epidemiology of suicide in children and young adolescents. *Journal of the American Academy of Child Psychiatry*, **20**, 545–65.

Shaffer, D., Vieland, V., Garland, A. *et al.* (1990). Adolescent suicide attempters. Response to suicide-prevention programs. *Journal of the American Medical Association*, **264**, 3151–5.

Smith, K. & Crawford, S. (1986). Suicidal behavior among 'normal' high school students. *Suicide and Life-Threatening Behavior*, **16**, 313–25.

Snyder, M. L. (1992). Unemployment and suicide in Northern Ireland. *Psychological Reports*, **70**, 1116–18.

Spirito, A., Brown, L., Overholser, J. & Fritz, G. (1989). Attempted suicide in adolescence: a review and critique of the literature. *Clinical Psychology Review*, **9**, 335–63.

Spirito, A., Overholser, J., Ashworth, S. *et al.* (1988). Evaluation of a suicide awareness curriculum for high school students. *Journal of the American Academy of Child and Adolescent Psychiatry*, **27**, 705–11.

Steede, K. K. & Range, L. K. (1989). Does television induce suicidal contagion with adolescents? *Journal of Community Psychology*, **17**, 166–72.

Stiffman, A. (1989). Suicide attempts in runaway youths. *Suicide and Life-Threatening Behavior*, **19**, 147–59.

Strang, S. & Orlofsky, J. (1990). Factors underlying suicidal ideation among college students: a test of Teicher and Jacobs' model. *Journal of Adolescence*, **13**, 39–52.

Swanson, J. W., Linskey, A. O., Quintero-Salinas, R. *et al.* (1992). A binational school survey of depressive symptoms, drug use, and suicidal ideation. *Journal of the American Academy of Child and Adolescent Psychiatry*, **31**, 669–78.

Tabachnick, N. (1981). The interlocking psychologies of suicide and adolescence. *Adolescent Psychiatry*, **10**, 399–410.

Tishler, C. L. & McKenry, P. C. (1982). Parental negative self and adolescent suicide attempts. *Journal of the American Academy of Child Psychiatry*, **21**, 404–8.

Topol, P. & Reznikoff, M. (1982). Perceived peer and family relationships, hopelessness and locus of control as factors in adolescent suicide attempts. *Suicide and Life-Threatening Behavior*, **12**, 141–50.

Vaillant, G. E. & Blumenthal, S. J. (1990). *Suicide over the life cycle: Risk factors and life span development*. American Psychiatrists Press, Washington DC.

Wetzel, R. D., Margulies, T., Davies, R. & Karam, E. (1980). Hopelessness, depression, and suicide intent. *Journal of Clinical Psychiatry*, **41**, 159–67.

WHO (1982). *Changing patterns in suicide behaviour*. World Health Organization/Euro, reports and studies, Copenhagen, Denmark.

WHO (1988). *Correlates of youth suicide. Division of Mental Health*. World Health Organization, Geneva.

WHO (1989). *World health statistic annual*. World Health Organization, Geneva.

Wilde, E. J. de (1992). *Specific characteristics of adolescent suicide attempters thesis*. Thesis publishers, Amsterdam.

Wilde, E. J. de, Kienhorst, C. W. M., Diekstra, R. F. W. & Wolters, W. H. G.

(1992). The relationship of life events in childhood and adolescence with adolescent suicidal behavior. *American Journal of Psychiatry*, **1**, 45–51.

Wilde, E. J. de, Kienhorst, C. W. M., Diekstra, R. F. W. & Wolters, W. H. G. (1994). Social support, life events and behavioral characteristics in psychologically distressed adolescents with high risk for attempting suicide. *Adolescence*, **29**, 49–60.

Wilde, E. J. de, Kienhorst, C. W. M., Diekstra, R. F. W. & Wolters, W. H. G. (1993). The specificity of psychological characteristics of adolescent suicide attempters. *Journal of the American Academy of Child and Adolescent Psychiatry*, **3**, 51–9.

Withers, L. E. & Kaplan, D. W. (1987). Adolescents who attempt suicide: A retrospective clinical chart review of hospitalized patients. *Professional Psychology: Research & Practice*, **18**, 391–3.

Yanish, D. & Battle, J. (1985). Relationship between self-esteem, depression and alcohol consumption among adolescents. *Psychological Reports*, **57**, 331–4.

11

Psychopharmacology of depressive states in childhood and adolescence

Helmut Remschmidt and Eberhard Schulz

INTRODUCTION

Over the past 50 years there has been a controversial debate concerning the issue of depression in childhood and adolescence. According to Carlson & Garber (1986), *five historical phases* of thinking can be distinguished: (1) The *first* one was represented by psychoanalysts who doubted the existence of depressive syndromes in children because children were said not to have a fully developed and well organised superego regarded as a precondition for depressive symptomatology. (2) The *second phase* can be characterised as the phase of **masked depression** meaning that children show behavioural equivalents rather than pronounced and observable depressive symptoms. (3) In the *third phase* the notion was put forward that childhood depression includes the core symptomatology of adult depression, combined with additional symptoms such as somatic complaints, social withdrawal, conduct disorders and aggression. (4) The *fourth perspective* states a complete isomorphism with adult depression according to DSM-III and DSM-III-R criteria. (5) Finally, the *fifth* phase states that isomorphism between childhood and adult depression must be unrealistic from a developmental point of view: 'This viewpoint suggests that the classification of childhood psychopathology should go beyond the simple categorisation of symptoms and behaviours and should include the broader notions of patterns of adaptation and competence' (Carlson & Garber, 1986, p. 402).

If we look at mood states and depressive syndromes in children and adolescents from a psychopharmacological point of view, we find remarkable differences, but also similarities between childhood/adolescence and adulthood. They are included in this chapter which gives an overview over the present state of pharmacological treatment of depressive syndromes in young people.

THE EVALUATION OF TRICYCLIC ANTIDEPRESSANTS

Comparable with other fields of child psychopharmacology, the treatment of children and adolescents with major depressive disorder is characterised by the paucity of empirical studies evaluating the efficacy and safety of applied drugs. In the light of investigations performed during the last decade, early enthusiasm for the efficacy of tricyclic antidepressants has waned. None of these double-blind studies of tricyclic antidepressants in prepubertal or adolescent major depressive disorder found the drugs superior to placebo. Ambrosini (1987) has published a review of the collective results from past placebo controlled studies, namely those of Kramer & Feiguine, 1981; Petti & Law, 1982; Preskorn, Weller & Weller, 1982; Kashani, Shekin & Reid, 1984; Puig-Antich *et al.*, 1987. In prepuberty, of 52 children on tricyclic medication 62% showed improvement, whereas a surprising 55% of 29 children reacted positively to placebo. Overall, approximately 60% of prepubertal depressives improved within 4 to 6 weeks regardless of the medication received. Of 44 adolescents on medication, 52% recovered, whereas 60% of 10 adolescents improved after having received only a treatment with placebos. Similar to the pre-pubertal group, 55% of adolescent depressives responded within 4 to 6 weeks regardless of their medication regimen. Recently performed controlled trials with nortriptyline in prepubertal (Geller *et al.*, 1989) or adolescent major depression (Geller *et al.*, 1990), as well as in an uncontrolled study of imipramine in adolescents (Strober, Freeman & Rigali, 1990), confirmed the previous conflicting results. Table 11.1 focuses on some of the special features attributed to the underlying causes of tricyclic antidepressant non-response.

Plasma level monitoring in young depressives treated with tricyclic antidepressant drugs

Notably, the plasma levels of tricyclic antidepressants show age-dependent variations (Nies, Robinson & Friedman, 1977; Ryan *et al.*, 1986;

Table 11.1. *Supposed factors associated with tricyclic non-response in children and adolescents with depressive disorder*

Heterogeneity in the age group of young depressives – although meeting research diagnostic criteria for major depression

Developmental functional characteristics with special features in neurotrasmitter-receptor status different from adult brain

Strong inter- and intraindividual variability in tricyclic drug metabolism and plasma level status with less knowledge about age-dependent influences on pharmacokinetics and pharmacodynamics

Neuroendocrine factors with possibly different neuro-modulator functions on transmitter–receptor interactions as compared with adult brain

Sample size and selectivity in the recruitment of young depressives for TCA clinical trials

Wilens *et al.*, 1992). This is partially due to pharmacokinetic and pharmacodynamic special characteristics of the child to end of adolescence age group. In general, the child has an increased hepatic surface area and body weight relative to the adult. In childhood, many drugs including tricyclics are eliminated via hepatic metabolism at greater rates than in adults. Consequently, there are relatively higher steady-state drug concentrations of tricyclic antidepressants in plasma of children, although it must be noted that the variation between the child and adult hepatic surface areas is not the only reason for the increased concentrations.

Additionally, the antidepressants were found to be less highly protein bound in children as compared with adults (for review, see Ereshefsky *et al.*, 1988). Wilens and coworkers (1992) recently reported findings that there are essential developmental changes in serum concentrations of desipramine and its major metabolite between three main age groupings; the study involved 40 children (6 to 12 yrs), 36 adolescents (13 to 18 years), and 27 adult (19 to 67 years) patients. One of the study's main findings is that serum concentrations of desipramine, the metabolite 2-hydroxydesipramine, and the sum of the two concentrations were all found to be lowest in children, moderate in adolescents, and highest in adults. Contrary to expectations, children appeared to be more efficient in clearing both the parent drug, and its metabolite, than adult patients. For all practical purposes, this study supports an ever-growing body of evidence that with respect to dosage regimens, children and adolescents, on average, require higher weight-corrected daily doses of desipramine than adults to achieve similar serum concentrations.

Besides the pharmacokinetic particularities, there are also possible pharmacodynamic influences, resulting from hormonal status and other potential biological variables within the age group of young depressives, which are regarded as responsible for the relatively unsuccessful outcome of patients who have been treated with tricyclic antidepressants (Ryan *et al.*, 1986). To date, studies of tricyclic antidepressants in prepubertal and adolescent depressives have shown inconsistent correlations between plasma drug concentrations and responder versus nonresponder status. In this connection, Puig-Antich and coworkers (1987) described a linear relationship between imipramine plasma level and clinical response in prepubertal depressives. In support of this finding, two independent groups of investigators (Preskorn *et al.*, 1982 and Geller *et al.*, 1986) showed that plasma level monitoring is a better predictor of response than dosage regimens of the tricyclic drug alone. Other studies have failed to find a positive correlation between the plasma levels and clinical improvement (Ryan *et al.*, 1986; Geller *et al.*, 1992). Despite the controversial connections between plasma level and response patterns, drug level monitoring is still considered to be a useful tool in drug safety management. Plasma level measurement enables the physican to better cope with potential differences in drug metabolism (e.g. genetic polymorphisms), to avoid toxicity by means of dosage-side effects correlations, and to adapt dosage regimens to the individual needs of the patient (for a review, see Preskorn *et al.*, 1988*a*). In this regard, the empirically based data of developmental age-dependent and pharmacological defined characteristics in drug metabolism of the child–adolescent age group are of special relevance for the practical employment of antidepressant drug management.

Dosage regimens for tricyclic antidepressant drugs

As a result of the recent insights gained from plasma-level monitoring, recommendations for antidepressant drug dosage should be based on the measurement of the drugs and their major metabolites. Preskorn and colleagues (1988*b*, 1989) demonstrated the interindividual variability of a fixed dose of 75 mg of imipramine in 68 children. On this dosage, 78% of the children fell outside the recommended therapeutic range (125–250 ng/ml). Of the 78% group, 66% were below the recommended range, and 12% were above. The authors recommend that, based on their plasma level data, the dosage should be adjusted using

Table 11.2. *Dosage and plasma level receommendations for tricyclic antidepressants used with young depressives*

Drug	Daily dosage < 14 years	Daily dosage > 14 years	Plasma level range
Amitriptyline	50–75 mg	75–150 mg	Amitripyline + nortriptyline level: 80–200 ng/ml
Imipramine	50–75 mg	75–150 mg	Imipramine + desipramine level: 130–250 ng/ml
Desipramine	50–75 mg	75–100 mg	–
Clomipramine	50–75 mg	75–100 mg	Clomipramine + desmethyl–clomipramine level: 70–200 ng/ml
Maprotiline	50–100 mg	75–150 mg	75–200 ng/ml

the formula: **new dose = (initial dose/initial level) x desired level**. If this dosage recommendation is properly followed, results indicate that 84% of the patients will stay within the desired therapeutic range. The remaining 16% with plasma levels below the recommended range will then simply require only an additional increase in dosage (Preskorn *et al.*, 1989). CNS toxicity exhibits a strong concentration-dependency to the plasma level (even with fixed doses within recommended dosage ranges), and therefore, regular measurement and management of concentration levels appears to be the only acceptably safe and predictable strategy to avoid iatrogenic damage of the treated patients (Preskorn *et al.*, 1988). Table 11.2 shows the recommended, combined dosage and plasma level ranges for the most common tricyclic antidepressants in child and adolescent psychiatry.

Side-effects of tricyclic antidepressants

The most common side-effects of tricyclic antidepressants are consequences of their blockade at different receptor systems (for a review, see Richelson, 1991). Cardiovascular toxicity of tricyclic antidepressants has attracted most attention because of sudden death in children receiving imipramine or desipramine (Saraf *et al.*, 1974; Biederman, 1991; Riddle *et al.*, 1991). The tricyclic antidepressant related cardiotoxicity can be divided in five categories (Warrington, 1988):

1. arrhythmias or atrioventricular extrasystoles
2. sudden death
3. reduced left ventricular performace
4. orthostatic (postural) hypotension
5. accidental or deliberate overdose with intractable arrhythmia or hypotension.

According to Warrington (1988) the classical tricyclic antidepressants could be expected to cause sudden deaths on rare occasions because their quinidine-like activity might provoke a lethal arrhythmia. Electrocardiographic abnormalities, tachycardia, orthostatic hypotension, T-wave abnormalities, ventricular extrasystoles and bundle branch block are potenital risks described in clinical trials with children and adolescents using tricyclic medication (Gittelman-Klein & Klein, 1971; Hayes, Panitch & Barker, 1975; Winsberg *et al.*, 1975; Saraf *et al.*, 1978; Ryan *et al.*, 1986).

Additionally, it should be noted that under careful clinical monitoring (including not only baseline but also dosage adjustment EKGs combined with plasma level monitoring and physical examination), most clinical investigators find only few and minor changes in cardiovascular function (Biederman *et al.*, 1989*a*; Schroeder *et al.*, 1989; Bartels *et al.*, 1991). Other potenial risks with tricyclic antidepressants result from their possible seizure induction (Petti & Campbell, 1975), which necessitates baseline and follow-up EEG monitoring. Blockade of histaminergic and muscarinic receptors is a common side-effect of tricyclic compounds.In a dose-dependent manner this receptor antagonism may provoke side effects such as sedation drowsiness, blurred vision, dry mouth, constipation, urinary retention and impaired cognitive function. Additionally, weight loss and growth deficits in children treated with tricyclic compounds such as desipramine and imipramine have been reported (Biedermann *et al.*, 1989*b*; Spencer *et al.*, 1992).

LITHIUM SALTS IN THE TREATMENT OF YOUNG DEPRESSIVES

Strober and colleagues (1992), in a 3-week open trial involving 24 adolescents (mean 15.4 years), assessed usage-results of lithium carbonate in co-medication with imipramine. All of the patients had previously remained highly depressive after a 6-week treatment of imipramine alone while receiving a mean daily dose of 229 mg of the drug. Through drug monitoring, a mean steady state concentration of 251 ng imipramine/ml plus desipramine plasma level was found. After addition of lithium, two patients had a dramatically positive response and eight other patients showed partial improvement. The study suggests the beneficial use of lithium carbonate adjunct to tricyclic medication in primary non-responding adolescents, in spite of the fact that the co-medication treatment strategy appears less efficacious overall in this age group than in similar studies done on adults (for review of adult studies with antidepressants potentiated by lithium see Kramlinger & Post, 1989).

ALTERNATIVE TREATMENT STRATEGIES WITH SEROTONIN-SPECIFIC DRUGS

Recent developments in molecular biology offer new insights into the heterogeneity of the serotonin (5-HT) receptor family and its functional equivalents.

Serotonin is synthesised within neurons by two enzymatic steps: (1) the amino acid tryptophan is first converted to 5-hydroxytryptophan (5-HTP) by the enzyme tryptophan hydroxylase, and (2) is subsequently decarboxylated to 5-hydroxytryptamine (serotonin) by aromatic acid decarboxylase. Released serotonin is inactivated primarily through reuptake via the serotonin transporter (a sodium-dependent transmembrane carrier). Within neurons or glial cells this transmitter is metabolised by monoamine oxidase (MAO) type-A (for details see below) and aldehyde reductase to the major metabolite 5-hydroxyindoleaceticacid (5-HIAA) (Boadle-Biber, 1982; Youdim & Ashkenazi, 1982; Hamon et al., 1974). In the serotoninergic system there are pre-synaptic autoreceptors that regulate activity in a negative feedback fashion by inhibiting the activity of serotonergic neurons in the somatic regions, and thus inhibiting the release of the transmitter in the terminal regions. At the post-synaptic site, one finds an integral element in the chemical signal transduction called the 5-HT receptors. Results from recent studies in molecular genetics have led to a reclassification of these receptors based on receptor structural homologies in DNA and amino acid sequences, rather than receptor affinity for ligands (for a review, see Zemlan & Garver, 1990). Four serotonin receptor clones have now been isolated and characterised. All monoamine receptor subtypes identified to date fall into either of two gene superfamilies: the G protein-coupled receptor super-

Table 11.3. *Classification of monoamine receptors based on DNA structural homologies of receptors and their functional expression systems*

G-Protein receptor superfamily
(I) Adenylate cyclase-coupled receptors
5-HT$_1$ receptor subtypes(1$_A$, 1$_B$, 1$_D$, 1$_E$, 1$_F$)
5-HT$_4$ receptor
Beta-1 receptors
Beta-2 receptors
Alpha-2 receptor subtypes
Dopamine receptor subtypes

(II) Phosphoinositide-coupled receptors
5-HT$_2$ receptors
5-HT$_{1C}$ receptor
Alpha-2 receptor subtypes

Ligand-gated ion channel superfamily
5-HT$_3$ receptor subtypes

Modified according to Zemlan & Garver (1990) and Hartig et al. (1992).

family or the ligand-gated ion channel superfamily (for a review, see Hartig *et al.*, 1992). The 5-HT$_4$ receptor is also positively linked to an adenylate cyclase (Bockaert, Sebben & Dummuis, 1990; Chaput, Araneda & Andrade, 1990), although it should be noted that it is still under debate whether this subtype may be classified as a 5-HT$_1$ site or not (Leonard, 1992; Humphrey, Hartig & Hoyer, 1993). With respect to a recently proposed new nomenclature for 5-HT receptors, the 5-HT$_{1C}$ receptor subtype should be classified in the 5-HT$_2$ receptor group and could be labelled as 5-HT$_{2C}$ receptor (Humphrey *et al.*, 1993).

The serotonin receptor subtypes can be ultimately classified according to Table 11.3. The 5-HT$_{1A}$ agonists represent the first major class of drugs to treat anxiety since the discovery of the benzodiazepines. Buspirone, flesinoxan, ipsapirone and gepirone all show antidepressant-like activity in a range of animal models, examples of which are the forced swim test, learned helplessness and forced restraint (Lucki, 1990, 1991). Also, recent clinical studies have found that buspirone, gepirone, and ipsapirone are effective antidepressants (for a review, see Robertson & Fuller, 1991).

The possibility of a future practical clinical relevance of these current findings concerning serotonin receptors comes from varying lines of evidence all suggesting that the usage of 5-HT specfic agents may prove to be favourable tools in the treatment of depressive states. According to Zemlan & Garver (1990) the central findings can be summarised as follows:

Table 11.4. *Three primary mechanisms by which antidepressants facilitate 5-HT$_1$ neural transmission*

(A) Somatodendritic 5-HT$_{1A}$ autoreceptors
Postsynaptic 5-HT transmission is facilitated by chronic application of 5-HT$_{1A}$ agonists (buspirone and gepirone) by down-regulating inhibitory 5-HT$_{1A}$ autoreceptors

(B) Presynaptic 5-HT$_{1B}$ autoreceptor
Postsynaptic 5-HT transmission is facilitated by chronic reuptake pump blockade (floxetine) by down-regulating inhibitory 5-HT$_{1B}$ autoreceptors

(C) Postsynaptic 5-HT receptor complex
Postsynaptic 5-HT transmission is facilitated by chronic application of tricyclics (e.g. imipramine) by acting on post-receptor coupling mechanisms like the G-protein and adenylate cyclase linked processes

---

1. Electrophysiological studies in rats suggest that 5-HT$_1$ receptor function is facilitated by chronic antidepressant treatment.
2. Preclinical studies employing a range of 5-HT$_1$ mediated behavioral models also suggest that chronic antidepressant treatment facilitates trasmission at central 5-HT$_1$ receptors.
3. Patient studies, employing a 5-HT$_1$ mediated neuroendocrine model, suggest that depression is associated with decreased transmission at 5-HT$_1$ receptors, and that chronic antidepressant treatment facilitates 5-HT$_1$ receptor responsiveness in depressed adult patients.
4. New 5-HT$_1$ selective agonists have been developed and found to be effective antidepressants.
5. The above clinical and preclinical data suggest that some forms of depression are related to a decreased responsiveness of 5-HT$_1$ receptors which is reversed by chronic antidepressant treatment.
6. 5-HT$_2$ receptor binding studies and initial studies of 5-HT$_2$ receptor coupled phosphoinositide turnover suggest that chronic antidepressant treatment decreases 5-HT$_2$ receptor number and function.
7. The development of new atypical antidepressants with 5-HT$_2$ receptor related mechanisms of action suggest that 5-HT$_2$ receptors may be associated with certain types of depression and their clinical treatment.

For clinical purposes three primary mechanisms (Table 11.4) can be used to classify the action by which antidepressive agents facilitate 5-HT$_1$ neural transmission (Zemlan & Garver, 1990).

Fluoxetine belongs to a class of drugs characterised by selective *in vivo* and *in vitro* inhibition of serotonin uptake. Table 11.5 lists the most important selective inhibitors of serotonin uptake with clinical relevance. Within the spectrum of 5-HT-specific uptake inhibitors, fluoxetine, fluvoxamine, sertraline and paroxetine have been described as antidepressants with fewer anti-adrenergic, anticholinergic and antihistaminergic

Table 11.5. *Selective serotonin uptake inhibitors*

Fluoxetine	Wong *et al.*, 1974
Paroxetine	Buus Lassen, 1978
Zimelidine	Ross *et al.*, 1981
Fluvoxamine	Claassen *et al.*, 1977
Femoxetine	Buus Lassen *et al.*, 1975
Citalopram	Hyttel, 1977
Indalpine	Le Fur *et al.*, 1978
Sertraline	Koe *et al.*, 1983

side-effects compared to tricyclic antidepressive drugs (for a review, see Kerr, Sherwood & Hindrarch, 1991; Robertson & Fuller, 1991). The risk to benefit ratio in prescribing 5-HT-specific uptake inhibitors like fluoxetine to children is still under debate since exacerbation of self-destructive behaviour, mania or suicidality as potential risks have been reported (King *et al.*, 1991; Power & Cowen 1992; Venkataraman, Naylor & King, 1992).

Figure 11.1 illustrates the primary mechanisms by which antidepressants are supposed to interact with serotoninergic transmission. Serotonin-specific substances like fluoxetine do not directly affect the postsynaptic 5-HT_1 receptor complex but facilitate 5-HT transmission at 5-HT_1 receptors by presynaptic disinhibition. Presynaptic 5-HT_1 receptors decrease the amount of serotonin released per action potential. Fluoxetin acts by blocking presynaptic 5-HT inhibition of 5-HT release. The 5-HT_{1A} receptors are autoreceptors in the cell body region and regulate activity of 5-HT neurons, and are also located postsynaptically. Buspirone, gepirone and ipsapirone are agonists at 5-HT_{1A} receptors. TCA are typically reuptake blockers of different biogenic amines. Tricyclic antidepressants like imipramine, amitripyline and mianserine are also potent antagonists of 5-HT_2 receptors.

Regulation of postsynaptic activity involves the linkage of the activated receptor with its transmembrane second messenger system. The second messengers include adenylate cyclase and phosphoinositate and the activity of phosphorylated kinases which phosphorylate membrane proteins, thus altering membrane potentials and therefore facilitating or inhibiting neuronal activity. According to Figure 11.1 the 5-HT-1A linked second messenger system decreases cAMP, the 5-HT_2 receptor is coupled to phosphatidyl inositol hydrolysis, whereas 5-HT_2 receptors are supposed to increase cAMP.

In general, antidepressant treatment increases the amount of trans-

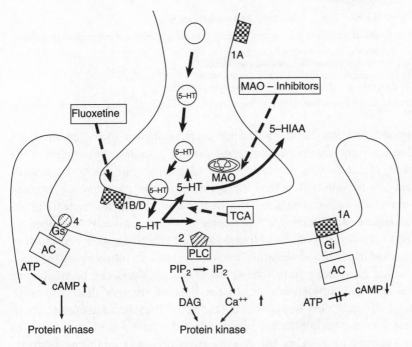

Figure 11.1. Synaptic transmission and drug interactions – 5-HT model.

mitter substance, thereby altering the balance between neurotransmitter levels and their receptors. The specific transmitter receptors are able to change their conformational state by regulation of affinity and/or maximal number of binding sites through interaction with the transmitter molecules. Linkage of the receptor complex to postsynaptic second messenger systems decides whether receptor binding results in facilitation or inhibition of the activated systems.

PSYCHOPHARMACOLOGICAL ASPECTS OF MONOAMINE OXIDASE INHIBITION

Neurochemistry of monoamine oxidase

The first support for the involvement of biogenic amines in depressive syndromes came from a series of observations done in the early fifties, which suggested that reserpine – a Rauwolfia alkaloid – used in the treatment of hypertension, caused depressive states in some of the

Table 11.6. *Four basic steps of neurotransmission*

---

(1) Synthesis of transmitter substance
(2) **Storage and release of transmitter substance**
(3) Post-synaptic receptor–transmitter interaction
(4) Reuptake of the transmitter from the synaptic cleft

---

treated patients. In the following years, animal studies demonstrated that reserpine inactivates aminergic storage granules, thus depleting the brain primarily of serotonin and noradrenaline. The released transmitters are unprotected within the cytoplasma and consequently become vulnerable as substrates to the degradation by monoamine oxidase. Iproniazid, an inhibitor of monoamine oxidase, initially developed to treat tuberculosis, was later found to be an effective antidepressant drug because of its mood-elevating action observed in tuberculosis patients. From a historical point of view, the MAO inhibitors can be labelled as the first true antidepressants. In the light of the fact that until now, none of controlled double-blind studies of tricyclic antidepressants in prepubertal or adolescent depressive disorder have found medication to be superior to placebo, the re-evaluation of MAO inhibitors as treatment strategy for initial tricyclic nonresponse will have to be conducted in the future. The following section describes some of the basic biochemical actions of monoamine oxidase and the neurotransmitter systems involved.

For simplicity, a general scheme (Table 11.6) can be used to describe the basic steps of chemical transmission. The storage and release of neurotransmitters (Table 11.6) are mediated by synaptic vesicles that accumulate the transmitter and release it at the synapse by the process of exocytosis. In the nerve terminal, these vesicles are called synaptic vesicles. In the other regions of the neuron, the vesicles that store transmitter substances are called transmitter storage granules (Schwartz, 1985). If free in the cytoplasma, neurotransmitters would be subject to intracellular degradative enzymes such as the monoamine oxidases, which are situated in the outer membrane of mitochondria.

Neurochemical research has revealed that monoamine oxidase (MAO) occurs in two subforms, MAO-A and MAO-B, with distinct distribution and different primary structures, each of which are coded by separate genes. The genes for the two enzyme forms are both located on the short arm of the human X chromosome. MAO-A and MAO-B genes are closely linked and have been assigned to the Xp11.23-p11 and

Table 11.7. *Major characteristics of monoamine oxidases and their genes*

Primary structure (Human)	MAO-A: 527 amino acids (59.7 kDa)
	MAO-B: 520 amino acids (58.8 kDa)
	Amino acid identity: approximately 70%
Subunit composition	Uncertain
Cofactor	Flavin-adenine diphosphate (FAD)
	1 FAD per subunit
Subcellular localisation	Outer mitochondrial membrane
Gene location	Chromosome X
(Human)	MAO-A: Xp11.23–p11
	MAO-B: Xp22.1
Gene organisation	15 exons- 14 introns (60–70 kb)
mRNA transcript	
(human)	MAO-A: 5 kb and 2 kb
	MAO-B: 3 kb

Xp22.1 regions respectively (for a review, see Cesura & Pletscher, 1992). Table 11.7 summarises the major characteristics of monoamine oxidases and their genes.

MAO-A and MAO-B are distributed in most tissues found in both the CNS and in peripheral organs. Despite the widespread distribution of both simultaneously occuring MAO sub-types, some tissues express exclusively or predominantly only one form of the enzyme: The human placenta mainly expresses MAO-A activity, whereas human lymphocytes, blood platelets and chromaffin cells contain only the MAO-B subtype (Cesura & Pletscher, 1992).

As Table 11.8 demonstrates, MAO-A and MAO-B are distributed in distinct functional neurotransmitter systems and occur within glial cells According to Table 11.8 serotoninergic neurons express MAO-B activity, whereas noradrenergic neurons contain predominantly the MAO-A subform of the enzyme. Dopaminergic neurons of the substantia nigra exhibit only in a subpopulation of approximately 10% MAO-A activity (Moll *et al.*, 1990).

Studies with human brain obtained from autopsy specimens demonstrate that, in contrast to rat brain data, MAO-B is globally the predominant enzyme. Findings derived from [^{3}H]pargyline binding experiments, in the presence and absence of known MAO inhibitors, demonstrated that in human basal ganglia structures (caudate, putamen, globus pallidus and substantia nigra), and in hippocampus, the levels of MAO had approximately twice the concentrations that were present in the cerebral cortex and cerebellum. In addition, the choroid plexus,

Table 11.8. *Distribution of MAO-A and MAO-B in the CNS*

	MAO-A	MAO-B
Neurons		
Serotonin	No	Yes
Noradrenaline	Yes	No
Adrenaline	Yes	?
Dopamine	(Yes)	No
Histamine	?	Yes
Glial cells	Yes	Yes

According to Cesura & Pletscher, 1992.

which constitutes the blood–cerebrospinal fluid barrier, had higher MAO levels than any brain region. The vast majority of MAO (80–95 %) in these tissues was of the B-type of the enzyme (Kalaria, Mitchell & Harik, 1988).

Interestingly, the neuronal distribution of the two MAO subtypes does not entirely correspond to that of their preferred substrates. Recent research data has revealed that there is no definite subdivision into substrates which are highly specific for one or the other form of MAO. In contrast to earlier expectations, these empirically based studies showed clearly that most natural substrates can be metabolised by both subforms of MAO (Dostert, Strolin Benedetti & Tipton, 1989). Table 11.9 demonstrates the current knowledge about the endogenous substrates deaminated by human MAO types A and B. Table 11.9 shows that serotonin is exclusively deaminated by MAO-A, whereas serotoninergic neurons contain predominantly the MAO B of the enzyme (see Table 11.8). According to Cesura & Pletscher (1992), this discrepancy may suggest that MAO-B has a role in the regulation of the intraneuronal concentrations of cytosolic 5-HT as 5-HT precursor and/or in the inactivation of other amines. Furthermore, MAO-A in other compartments might be involved in the catabolism of serotonin released from neurons.

Classification and pharmacology of monoamine oxidase inhibitors

MAO inhibitors can be classified according to their relative specificity for the two subtypes of the enzyme, and with respect to the so called 'new generation' of these drugs by the reversibility of their actions (Table 11.10).

Table 11.9. *Endogenous substrates of MAO-A and MAO-B in human CNS*

Substrate	*In vivo*	*In vitro*
Serotonin	A	A
Noradrenaline	A (B)	A+B
Adrenaline	A	A+B
Dopamine	B(A)	A+B
Phenylethylamine	B	B
Tyramine	A+B	A+B

According to Waldmeier 1987; Dostert *et al.*, 1989.

Table 11.10. *Classification of MAO inhibitors according to specificity for the enzymes and reversibility of their actions*

Non selective MAO inhibitors
Iproniazid (I)
Isocarboxazid (I)
Phenelzine (I)
Traylcypromine (I)

MAO-A selective inhibitors
Clorgyline (I)
Moclobemide (R)
Brofaromine (R)
Toloxatone (R)
Cimoxatone (R)
Amiflamine (R)

MAO-B selective inhibitors
Pargyline (I)
L-Deprenyl (I)
Almoxatone (R?)

(I), Irreversible mode of action; (R), Reversible mode of action.

Irreversible MAO inhibitors are recognised by the enzyme as substrates and interact during the first phase of the reaction in a competitive fashion through non-covalent bonds. Thereafter the drug will be converted into reactive intermediates that can then form, in the following reactions, a stable covalent and therefore 'irreversible' complex (Dostert *et al.*, 1989). After formation of such an irreversible complex (consisting of a stable covalent adduct) the recovery of catalytic activity depends on the synthesis of a new enzyme. For clinical purposes this irreversible blockade of the enzyme implicates that new MAO enzyme has to be resynthesised, thus accounting for the long duration of MAO inhibition, with a time span of up to 2 weeks after discontinuation of drug treatment. Out of the above mentioned spectrum of MAO inhibitors, in the following only those compounds with relevance to child and adolescent psychopharmacotherapy will be discussed.

Clinical studies performed with MAO inhibitors in children and adolescents

The study led by Frommer (1967) was the first controlled double-blind study with crossover design of antidepressant medication in prepubertal depression to be conducted. She compared the irreversible non-selective MAO inhibitor **phenelzine** in combination with chlordiazepoxide to phenobarbital in a 2 week trial. Of 32 depressed children, 25 (78%) improved on the new combination of medications. It is difficult to interpret the results of this study because of (1) the combination treatment and (2) the short duration of the trial period – a time span far below the latency of MAO inhibitors to obtain antidepressive response.

Interestingly, the relatively incomplete body of data dealing with the application of MAO inhibitors in child and adolescent psychiatry came primarily from clinical trials with hyperkinetic children. Because of the suspected involvement of MAO in both externalising symptoms and in ADDH (Young *et al.*, 1980; Shekim *et al.*, 1982; Browden, Deutsch & Swanson, 1988; Stoff *et al.*, 1989), a few clinical trials with MAO inhibitors were conducted: Zametkin and coworkers, after observing a group of 14 children with ADDH under treatment with **clorgyline** ($n = 6$) and **tranylcypromine** ($n = 8$) found similar response patterns to those resulting from the dextroamphetamine-treated group (Zametkin *et al.*, 1985). Recently, Trott *et al.* (1991, 1992) demonstrated the safe and efficient use of the 'new generation' MAO inhibitor **moclobemide**, exhibiting short-lasting and reversible effects in 17 hyperkinetic children aged 6 to 12 years old. With respect to depressive disorder, only one retrospective chart review, including 23 adolescent patients, has been conducted (Ryan *et al.*, 1988). Ryan's study assessed the outcome from 11 males and 12 females, aged 11 to 18 years (mean age 15 ± 2 years) with major depression who had minimal or only partial response to tricyclic antidepressants. Because of the non-response, the patients were thereafter treated with one or the other MAO inhibitors **tranylcypromine** and

phenelzine, both alone and in combination with tricylic antidepressants. From this group, 74% of the adolescents, regardless of dietary compliance, showed fair or good clinical improvement, but 57% who also showed fair to good improvement, had good dietary compliance. Except for dietary non-compliance, the side-effects resulting from the usage of the two irreversible MAO inhibitors were similar in intensity and frequency to that with tricyclic antidepressants.

Side-effects of irreversible MAO inhibitors

Tranylcypromine (2-phenylcyclopropylamine (Parnate[R]), a non-selective MAO inhibitor, is chemically similar to amphetamine. This drug potentiates the blood pressure effect of tyramine and shows indirect sympathomimetic effects, either directly or indirectly through a supposed conversion to amphetamine. It should, however, be noted that this metabolic route has been disputed (Reynolds, Rausch & Riederer, 1980; Baker & Coutts 1989).

Ryan *et al.* (1988) even reported that one patient complained of withdrawal symptoms such as frequent nightmares for two weeks after tranylcypromine discontinuation. Dilsaver (1988) summarised these withdrawal symptoms connected to tranylcypromine cessation.

Phenelzine (Nardil[R]) belongs to the hydrazine derivatives with iproniazid as prototype. This class of irreversible inhibitors were mostly discredited because of adverse side-effects, such as blood pressure-raising due to strong interactions with food amines (e.g. tyramine), and the induction of liver damage (for reviews, see Larsen 1988; Remick, Froese & Keller, 1989). Table 11.11 summarises the most common adverse side-effects observed in studies with irreversible MAO inhibitors predominatly involving phenelzine and tranylcypromine.

Moclobemide (Aurorix[R]), a substituted benzamide, has been shown to be a reversible inhibitor of MAO-A under different experimental conditions (for a review, see Cesura & Pletscher, 1992). Reversible MAO inhibitors appear to have fundamental advantages over irreversible ones. Table 11.12 demonstrates some of the major advantages of moclobemide in comparison with the first generation of MAO inhibitors.

Nutt & Glue (1989) labelled MAO inhibitors as the 'Cinderella drugs of psychopharmacy'. In adult psychiatry the re-evaluation of monoamine oxidase inhibition as a treatment strategy for tricyclic-resis-

Table 11.11. *The most common adverse effects of irreversible monoamine oxidase inhibitors*

Orthostatic hypotension
Hypertensive crisis precipitated by food amines
Flushing and chills
Insomnia
Hypomania/mania
Sedation
Blurred vision
Urinary retention
Constipation
Weight gain
Sexual dysfunction
Oedema
Headache
Myoclonic jerking

Table 11.12. *Clinical profile of moclobemide*

Reduced degree of tyramine potentiation

Absence of cumulative effects

Short duration of action (moclobemide half-life of approximately 12 h)

Side-effects less pronounced or comparable to tricyclic antidepressants

Co-administration with tricyclic antidepressnats has been thus far well tolerated by patients

Superiority over placebo and marked effectiveness against depressive syndromes in several adult clinical trials

For reviews, see Angst & Stabl, 1992; Cesura & Pletscher, 1992.

tant depression and anxiety disorders (especially social phobia) is still ongoing. In the light of the new generation of reversible MAO inhibitors, it must be proven by careful clinical monitoring that these substances will be suitable for safe and practical usage in the age group of depressed prepubertal and adolescent patients.

PRACTICAL GUIDE TO ANTIDEPRESSANT TREATMENT

Antidepressant medication in childhood and adolescence is indicated in cases of severe depressive symptomatology, unresponsive to psychotherapeutic interventions. In particular, the persistence of functional impairments in school, social or family domain and/or the continuing risk of suicidal behaviour are clinical indicators for pharmacological interventions (Remschmidt 1992; Ambrosini *et al.*, 1993).

Based on the data obtained from a meta-analysis of 63 randomized controlled trials comparing the efficacy and acceptability of selective serotonin reuptake inhibitors (including, for example, fluoxetine, fluvoxamine, sertraline, paroxetine) with those of tricyclic antidepressants (namely imipramine, amitriptyline, clomipramine), Song *et al.* (1993) came to the conclusion that there is no statistically or clinically significant difference in the acceptability of serotonin specific drugs and the tricyclic compounds in patients with major depression. In addition, the serotonin reuptake inhibitors seem to have similar efficacy to the tricyclic and related antidepressants. One major advantage over tricyclic and related antidepressants came from a constant line of evidence suggesting that selective serotonin reuptake inhibitors may be low-toxicity antidepressants. In this connection it is claimed that the serotonin-specific antidepressants have a lower toxicity in the event of a drug overdose (Kasper, Fuger & Mîller, 1992; Mann *et al.*, 1993). According to the consensus statement of the American College of Neuropsychopharmacology (Mann *et al.*, 1993), there is, to date, no evidence that serotonin reuptake inhibitors such as fluoxetine may trigger emergent suicidal ideation over and above rates that may be associated with other antidepressants or the underlying depressive illness. According to our clinical practice, the use of selective serotonin reuptake inhibitors in the treatment of depressive states in children or adolescents remain a second line treatment strategy to cope with initial nonresponse to tricyclic compounds. In addition, they offer together with the selective monoamine oxidase inhibitors an enrichment of the antidepressant treatment in cases of contraindications for tricyclic drugs. The main contraindications for the administration of tricyclic antidepressants are the following: cardiac conduction abnormalities, known hypersensitivity to tricyclic antidepressants and manifest seizure disorders. Prior to the initiation of antidepressant medication the following routine assessments should be performed (Schulz & Remschmidt, 1988; Green, 1991): (1) careful physical examination; (2) baseline electrocardiogram (ECG); (3) baseline electroencephalogram (EEG); (4) laboratory tests including complete blood count (CBC), differential and haematocrit; serum electrolyte levels, blood urea nirogen level, bilirubin and the basic liver function tests (AST, SGOT, ALT, SGPT, alkaline phosphatase and LDH). In addition thyroid function tests (thyroxine (T_4), triiodothyrosine resin uptake (T_3RU) and thyroid stimulating hormone (TSH)) are recommended, because abnormal thyroid function can aggravate abnormal cardiac function (arrhythmias) as possible untoward effect of tricyclic antidepressants (Green, 1991). With respect to lithium carbonate administration, thyroid function tests and kidney function tests (baseline serum creatinine and urinalysis) are generally recommended. Lithium carbonate is known to cause hypothyroidism and to alter kidney function.

Derived from a prospective study of the electrocardiographic effects of imipramine in children (Fletcher *et al.*, 1993) the following recommendations are given: a resting corrected QT interval greater than 450 ms or a bundle-branch heart block should be contraindications to beginning or continuing therapy with a tricyclic drug. The authors recommend that patients with a family history of sudden death, a baseline PR interval greater than the 90th percentile for age, or any degree of intraventricular conduction delay, undergo further careful monitoring.

During tricyclic antidepressant medication, plasma levels in children and adolescents show strong interindividual variabilities with the potential risk of toxic concentrations. A therapeutic plasma/serum level monitoring of the applied drug is still recommended. In addition to the well known variabilities in plasma level concentrations, genetic polymorphisms in the hepatic enzyme cytochrome P4502D6 may play a causal role in clinical non-response and untoward effects owing to inadequate dosage regimens. Both tricyclic antidepressants and the specific serotonin reuptake inhibitors are substrates for this enzyme (Crewe *et al.*, 1992; Van Harten, 1993). For practical purposes, therapeutic drug monitoring of antidepressant drugs should be performed according to the following recommendations (Riederer & Laux, 1992): blood samples (serum collected in polypropylene tubes) should generally be taken prior to the morning dose, about 12 h after the last administration. Blood sampling should be performed under strict steady-state conditions, i.e. when four or five half-life intervals have elapsed. As a result of the recent insights gained from plasma-level monitoring, recommendations for antidepressant drug dosage should be based on the measurement of the applicated drugs and their major metabolites. According to Ambrosini *et al.* (1993), oral tricyclic dosing should provide plasma levels in the 200 ng/ml range, although for nortriptyline somewhat lower plasma levels of approximately 100 ng/ml are recommended. In cases of initial non-response and sufficient plasma levels of the tricyclic drug, lithium augmentation as a safe alternative should be performed. In patients unresponsive to this strategy a monotherapy with moclobemide as a reversible inhibitor of monoamine oxidase type A could be promising. Recently published studies, including children (Trott *et al.*, 1991, 1992) demonstrate that moclobemide can safely be administered without the risk of toxic interactions well known from the irreversible inhibitors of monoamine oxidase (Amrein *et al.*, 1992; Dingemanse 1993; Hollister & Claghorn, 1993). Alternatively, specific serotonin reuptake inhibitors can be used as a second line indication for initial non-response. In this regard further investigations should be performed to decide whether these compounds (due to their lower toxicity) should preferably be administered (Ambrosini *et al.*, 1993) in cases with suicidal and/or impulsive tendencies or not.

CONCLUSIONS

Though the beginning of pharmacological treatment of depressive states in childhood started with the notion of non-response to tricyclic antidepressants, the further development in the field was successful in several respects: (1) In relation to a better knowledge of pharmacological pecularities of tricyclic and other antidepressants in children and adolescents, a more rational therapeutic regime led to remarkable improvements of therapy and to a reduction of side-effects. (2) Lithium salts in combination with tricyclic antidepressants seem to be an effective therapeutic tool also in cases who are resistant to a tricyclic medication alone. (3) Alternative treatment strategies with serotonin-specific drugs (especially serotonin-specific reuptake inhibitors) seem to be a promising way of treatment, though exacerbation of self-destructive behaviour, mania, and suicidality have been reported. (4) Finally, new reversible MAO-inhibiting drugs have been useful in the treatment of hyperkinetic children and children with major depressive disorder.

The results are encouraging, but nevertheless, the whole field of psychopharmacology in childhood and adolescent depression is still underdeveloped and huge efforts are necessary in order to understand the basic mechanisms of drug actions and to establish rational and safe therapeutic regimes.

REFERENCES

Ambrosini, P. J. (1987). Pharmacotherapy in child and adolescent major depressive disorder. In *Psychopharmacology. The third generation of progress* (ed. H. Y. Meltzer), pp. 1247–54. Raven Press, New York.

Ambrosini, P. J., Bianchi, M. D., Rabinovich, H. & Elia, J. (1993). Antidepressant treatments in children and adolescents. I. Affective disorders. *Journal of the American Academy of Child and Adolescent Psychiatry*, **32**, 1–6.

Amrein, R., Hetzel, W., Stabl, M. & Schmidt-Burgk, W. (1992). RIMA: a safe concept in the treatment of depression with moclobemide. *Canadian Journal of Psychiatry*, **37**, (Suppl. 1), 7–11

Angst, J. & Stabl, M. (1992). Efficacy of moclobemide in different patient groups: a meta analysis of studies. *Psychopharmacology, (Suppl.)*, **106**, 109–13.

Baker, G. B. & Coutts, R. T. (1989). Metabolism of monoamine oxidase inhibitors. *Progress in Neuro-Psychopharmacology and Biological Psychiatry*, **13**, 395–403.

Bartels, M. G., Varley, C. K., Mitchell, J. & Stamm, S. J. (1991). Pediatric cardiovascular effects of imipramine and desipramine. *Journal of the American Academy of Child and Adolescent Psychiatry*, **30**, 100–3.

Biederman, J. (1991). Sudden death in children treated with a tricyclic antidepressant. *Journal of the American Academy of Child and Adolescent Psychiatry*, **30**, 495–8.

Biederman, J., Baldessarini, R. J., Wright, V. *et al.* (1989*a*). A double-blind placebo controlled study of desipramine in the treatment of ADD: II. Serum drug levels and cardiovascular findings. *Journal of the American Academy of Child and Adolescent Psychiatry*, **28**, 903–11.

Biederman, J., Baldessarini, R. J., Wright, V. *et al.* (1989*b*). A double-blind placebo controlled study of desipramine in the treatment of ADD: I. Efficacy. *Journal of the American Academy of Child and Adolescent Psychiatry*, **28**, 777–84.

Boadle-Biber, M. C. (1982). Biosynthesis of serotonin. In *Biology of serotonergic transmission* (ed. N. N. Osborne), pp. 63–94. Wiley, New York.

Bockaert, J., Sebben, M. & Dumuis, A. (1990). Pharmacological characterization of 5-hydroxytryptamine(5-HT-4-) receptors positively coupled to adenylate cyclase in adult guinea pig hippocampal membranes: effect of substituted benzamide derivatives. *Molecular Pharmacology*, **37**, 408–11.

Browden, C. L., Deutsch, C. K. & Swanson, J. M. (1988). Plasma dopamine-beta-hydroxylase and platelet monoamine oxidase in attention deficit disorder and conduct disorder. *Journal of the American Academy of Child and Adolescent Psychiatry*, **27**, 171–4.

Buus Lassen, J. (1978). Influence of the new 5-HT-uptake inhibitor paroxetine on hypermotility in rats produced by *p*-chloroamphetamine (PCA) and 4-alpha-dimethyl-*m*-tyramine (H77/77). *Psychopharmacology*, **57**, 151–3.

Buus Lassen, J., Squires, R. F., Christensen, J. A. & Molander, L. (1975). Neurochemical and pharmacological studies on a new 5-HT-uptake inhibitor, FG4963, with potential antidepressant properties. *Psychopharmacology*, **42**, 21–6.

Carlson, G. A. & Garber, J. (1986). Developmental issues in the classification of depression in children. In *Depression in young people. Developmental and clinical perspectives* (ed. M. Rutter, C. E. Izard, & P. E. Read). Guilford Press, New York–London.

Cesura, A. M. & Pletscher, A. (1992). The new generation of monoamine oxidase inhibitors. *Progress in Drug Research* **38**, 171–297.

Chaput, Y., Araneda, R. C. & Andrade, R. (1990). Pharmacological and functional analysis of a novel serotonin receptor in the rat hippocampus. *European Journal of Pharmacology*, **182**, 441–56.

Claassen, V., Davies, J. E., Hertting, G. & Placheta, P. (1977). Fluvoxamine, a specific 5-hydroxytryptamine uptake inhibitor. *British Journal of Pharmacology*, **60**, 505–16.

Crewe, H. K., Lennard, M. S., Tucker, G. T. *et al.* (1992). The effect of selective serotonin re-uptake inhibitors on cytochrome P4502D6 (CYP2D6) activity in human liver microsomes. *British Journal of Clinical Pharmacology*, **34**, 262–5.

Dilsaver, S.C. (1988). Monoamine oxidase inhibitor withdrawal phenomena: symptoms and pathophysiology. *Acta Psychiatrica Scandinavica*, **78**, 1–7.

Dingemanse, J. (1993). An update of recent moclobemide interaction data. *International Clinical Psychopharmacology*, **7**, 167–80.

Dostert, P., Strolin Benedetti, M. & Tipton, K. F. (1989). Interactions of monoamine oxidase with substrates and inhibitors. *Medicinal Research Reviews*, **9**, 45–89.

Ereshefsky, L., Tran-Johnson, T., Davis, C. M. & LeRoy, A. (1988). Pharmacokinetic factors affecting antidepressant drug clearance and clinical effect: evaluation of doxepin and imipramine – new data and review. *Clinical Chemistry*, **34**, 863–80.

Fletcher, S. E., Case, C. L., Sallee, F. R. *et al.* (1993). Prospective study of the electrocardiographic effects of imipramine in children. *Journal of Pediatrics*, **122**, 652–4.

Frommer, E. A. (1967). Treatment of childhood depression with antidepressant drugs. *British Medical Journal*, **1**, 729–32.

Geller, B., Cooper, T. B., Chesnut, E. C. *et al.* (1986). Preliminary data on the relationship between nortriptyline plasma level and response in depressed children. *American Journal of Psychiatry*, **143**, 1283–6.

Geller, B., Cooper, T. B., Graham, D. L. *et al.* (1990). Double-blind placebo-controlled study of nortriptyline in depressed adolescents using a 'fixed plasma level' design. *Psychopharmacology Bulletin*, **26**, 85–90.

Geller, B., Cooper, T. B., Graham, D. L. *et al.* (1992). Pharmacokinetically designed double-blind placebo-controlled study of nortriptyline in 6- to 12-year-olds with major depressive disorder. *Journal of the American Academy of Child and Adolescent Psychiatry*, **31**, 34–44.

Geller, G., Cooper, T. B., McCombs, H. G. *et al.* (1989). Double-blind placebo-controlled study of nortriptyline in depressed children using a 'fixed plasma level' design. *Psychopharmacology Bulletin*, **25**, 101–8.

Gittelman-Klein, R. & Klein, D. F. (1971). Controlled imipramine treatment of school phobia. *Archives of General Psychiatry*, **25**, 204–7.

Green, W.H. (1991). *Child and adolescent clinical psychopharmacology*. Williams & Wilkins, Baltimore.

Hamon, M., Bourgoin, S., Morot-Gaudry, Y. *et al.* (1974). Role of active transport of tryptophan in the control of 5-hydroxytryptamine biosynthesis. *Advances in Biochemical Psychopharmacology*, **11**, 153–62.

Hartig, P. R., Adham, N., Zgombick, J. *et al.* (1992). Molecular biology of the 5-HT-1-receptor subfamily. *Drug Development Research*, **26**, 215–24.

Hayes, T. A., Panitch, M. L. & Barker, E. (1975). Imipramine dosage in children: a comment on 'imipramine and electrocardiographic abnormalities in hyperactive children'. *American Journal of Psychiatry*, **132**, 546–7.

Hollister, L. E. & Claghorn, J. L. (1993). New antidepressants. *Annual Reviews of Pharmacology and Toxicology*, **32**, 165–77.

Humphrey, P. P. A., Hartig, P. & Hoyer, D. (1993). A proposed new nomenclature for 5-HT receptors. *Trends in Pharmacological Sciences*, **14**, 233–6.

Hyttel, J. (1977). Neurochemical characterization of a new potent and selective serotonin uptake inhibitor: LU10-171. *Psychopharmacology*, **51**, 225–33.

H. Remschmidt & E. Schulz

Kalaria, R. N., Mitchell, M. J. & Harik, S. I. (1988). Monoamine oxidases of the human brain and liver. *Brain*, **111**, 1441–51.

Kashani, J. H., Shekin, W. O. & Reid, J. C. (1984). Amitriptyline in children with major depressive disorder: a double-blind crossover pilot study. *Journal of the American Academy of Child Psychiatry*, **23**, 348–51.

Kasper, S., Fuger, J. & Mîller, H.J. (1992). Comparative efficacy of antidepressants. *Drugs*, **43**, (Suppl. 2), 11–23.

Kerr, J. S., Sherwood, N. & Hindmarch, I. (1991). The comparative psychopharmacology of 5-HT reuptake inhibitors. *Human Psychopharmacology – Clinical and Experimental*, **6**, 313–17.

King, R. A., Riddle, M. A., Chappell, P. B. *et al.* (1991). Emergence of self-destructive phenomena in children and adolescents during fluoxetine treatment. *Journal of the American Academy of Child and Adolescent Psychiatry*, **30**, 179–86.

Koe, B. K., Weissman, A., Welch, W. M. & Browne, R. G. (1983). Sertraline, 1S,4S-n-methyl-4-(3,4-dichlorophenyl)-1,2,3,4-tetrahydro-1-naphthylamine, a new uptake inhibitor with selectivity for serotonin. *Journal of Pharmacology and Experimental Therapeutics*, **226**, 686–700.

Kramer, A. D. & Feiguine, R. J. (1981). Clinical effects of amitriptyline in adolescent depression: a pilot study. *Journal of the American Academy of Child Psychiatry*, **20**, 636–44.

Kramlinger, K. G. & Post, R. M. (1989). The addition of lithium to carbamazepine. Antidepressant efficacy in treatment-resistant depression. *Archives of General Psychiatry*, **46**, 794–800.

Larsen, J. K. (1988). MAO inhibitors: pharmacodynamic aspects and clinical implications. *Acta Psychiatrica Scandinavica*, (Suppl. 78) **345**, 74–80.

Le Fur, G., Kabouche, M. & Uzan, A. (1978). On the regional and specific serotonin uptake inhibition by LM 5008. *Life Sciences*, **23**, 1959–66.

Leonard, B.E. (1992). Sub-types of serotonin receptors: biochemical changes and pharmacological consequences. *International Clinical Psychopharmacology*, **7**, 13–21.

Lucki, I. (1990). Behavioral responses associated with serotonin receptors. In *Advances in Behavioral Pharmacology*, **Vol. 7** (ed. J. E. Barrett, T. Thompson, P. B. Dews), pp. 119–48. Lawrence Erlbaum, Hillsdale, NJ.

Lucki, I. (1991). Behavioral studies of serotonin receptor agonists as antidepressant drugs. *Journal of Clinical Psychiatry*, **52**, Suppl, 24–31.

Mann, J. J., Goodwin, F. K., O'Brien, C. P. & Robinson, D. S. (1993). Suicidal behavior and psychotropic medication. *Neuropsychopharmacology*, **8**, 177–83.

Moll, G., Moll, R., Riederer, P. *et al.* (1990). Immunofluorescence cytochemistry on thin frozen sections of human substantia nigra for staining of monoamine oxidase A and monoamine oxidase B: a pilot study. *Journal of Neural Transmission* (Suppl.) **32**, 67–77.

Nies, A., Robinson, D. S. & Friedman, M. J. (1977). Relationship between age and tricyclic antidepressant plasma levels. *American Journal of Psychiatry*, **134**, 790–3.

Nutt, D. & Glue, P. (1989). Monoamine oxidase inhibitors: rehabilitation from recent research? *British Journal of Psychiatry*, **154**, 287–91.

Petti, T. A. & Campbell, M. (1975). Imipramine and seizures. *American Journal of Psychiatry*, **132**, 538–40.

Petti, T. A. & Law, W. (1982). Imipramine treatment of depressed children: a double-blind pilot study. *Journal of Clinical Psychopharmacology*, **2**, 107–10.

Power, A. C. & Cowen, P. J. (1992). Fluoxetine and suicidal behavior. Some clinical and theoretical aspects of a controversy. *British Journal of Psychiatry*, **161**, 735–41.

Preskorn, S. H., Weller, E. B. & Weller, R. A. (1982). Depression in children: relationship between plasma imipramine levels and response. *Journal of Clinical Psychiatry*, **43**, 450–3.

Preskorn, S. H., Dorey, R. C. & Jerkovich, G. S. (1988a). Therapeutic drug monitoring of tricyclic antidepressants. *Clinical Chemistry*, **34**, 822–8.

Preskorn, S. H., Weller, E., Jerkovich, G. *et al.* (1988b). Depression in children: concentration-dependent CNS toxicity of tricyclic antidepressants. *Psychopharmacology Bulletin*, **24**, 140–2.

Preskorn, S. H., Bupp, S. J., Weller, E. B. & Weller, R. A. (1989). Plasma levels of imipramine and metabolites in 68 hospitalized children. *Journal of the American Academy of Child and Adolescent Psychiatry*, **28**, 373–5.

Puig-Antich, J., Perel, J. M., Lupatkin, W. *et al.* (1987). Imipramine in prepubertal major depressive disorders. *Archives of General Psychiatry*, **44**, 81–9.

Remick, R. A., Froese, C. & Keller, F. D. (1989). Common side effects associated with monoamine oxidase inhibitors. *Progress in Neuro-Psychopharmacology and Biological Psychiatry*, **13**, 497–504.

Remschmidt, H. (1992). *Psychiatrie der Adoleszenz*. Thieme Verlag, Stuttgart–New York.

Reynolds, G. P., Rausch, W. G. & Riederer, P. (1980). Effects of tranylcypromine stereoisomers on monoamine oxidation in man. *British Journal of Clinical Pharmacology*, **9**, 521–3.

Reynolds, G. P., Rausch, W. G. & Riederer, P. (1980). Effects of tranylcypromine stereoisomers on monoamine oxidation in man. *British Journal of Clinical Pharmacology*, **9**, 521–3.

Richelson, E. (1991). Biological basis of depression and therapeutic relevance. *Journal of Clinical Psychiatry*, **52**, 4–10.

Riddle, M. A., Nelson, J. C., Kleinman, C. S. *et al.* (1991). Sudden death in children receiving Norpramin: a review of three reported cases and commentary. *Journal of the American Academy of Child and Adolescent Psychiatry*, **30**, 104–8.

Riederer, P. & Laux, G. (1992). Therapeutic drug monitoring of psychotropics: report of a consensus conference. *Pharmacopsychiatry*, **25**, 271–2.

Robertson, D. W. & Fuller, R. W. (1991). Progress in antidepressant drugs. *Annual Reviews in Medicinal Chemistry*, **26**, 23–32.

Ross, S. B., Hall, H., Renyi, A. L. & Westerlund, D. (1981). Effects of zimelidine on serotoninergic and noradrenergic neurons after repeated administration in the rat. *Psychopharmacology*, **72**, 219–25.

Ryan, N. D., Puig-Antich, J., Cooper, T. *et al.* (1986). Imipramine in adolescent major depression: plasma level and clinical response. *Acta Psychiatrica Scandinavica*, **73**, 275–88.

Ryan, N. D., Puig-Antich, J., Rabinovich, H. *et al.* (1988). MAOIs in adolescent major depression unresponsive to tricyclic antidepressants. *Journal of the American Academy of Child and Adolescent Psychiatry*, **27**, 755–8.

Saraf, K. R., Klein, D. F., Gittelman-Klein, R. & Groff, S. (1974). Imipramine side effects in children. *Psychopharmacologia*, **37**, 265–74.

Saraf, K. R., Klein, D .F., Gittelman-Klein, R. *et al.* (1978). EKG effects of imipramine treatment in children. *Journal of the American Academy of Child Psychiatry*, **17**, 60–9.

Schroeder, J. S., Mullin, A. V., Elliott, G. R. *et al.* (1989). Cardiovascular effects of desipramine in children. *Journal of the American Academy of Child and Adolescent Psychiatry*, **28**, 376–9.

Schulz, E. & Remschmidt, H. (1988). Pharmakotherapie depressiver Syndrome im Kindes- und Jugendalter. *Zeitschrift für Kinder- und Jugendpsychiatrie*, **16**, 142–54.

Schwartz, J. H. (1985). Molecular steps in synaptic transmission. In *Principles of Neural Science, 2nd edition* (ed. E. R. Kandel, J. H. Schwartz), pp. 167–75, Elsevier Publ. Co., New York, Amsterdam and Oxford.

Shekim, W. O., David, L. G., Bylund, D. R. *et al.* (1982). Platelet MAO in children with attention deficit disorder and hyperactivity. *American Journal of Psychiatry*, **139**, 936–8.

Song, F., Freemantle, N., Sheldon, T. A. *et al.* (1993). Selective serotonin reuptake inhibitors: meta-analysis of efficacy and acceptability. *British Medical Journal*, **306**, 383–7.

Spencer, T., Biederman, J., Wright, V. & Danon, M. (1992). Growth deficits in children treated with desipramine: a controlled study. *Journal of the American Academy of Child and Adolescent Psychiatry*, **31**, 235–43.

Stoff, D. M., Friedman, E., Pollock, L. *et al.* (1989). Elevated platelet MAO is related to impulsivity in disruptive behavior disorders. *Journal of the American Academy of Child and Adolescent Psychiatry*, **28**, 754–60.

Strober, M., Freeman, R. & Rigali, J. (1990). The pharmacotherapy of depressive illness in adolescence. I. An open label trial on imipramine. *Psychopharmacology Bulletin*, **26**, 80–4.

Strober, M., Freeman, R., Rigali, J. *et al.* (1992). The pharmacotherapy of depressive illness in adolescence: II. Effects of lithium augmentation in nonresponders to imipramine. *Journal of the American Academy of Child and Adolescent Psychiatry*, **31**, 16–20.

Trott, E., Friese, H. J., Menzel, M. & Nissen, G. (1992). The use of moclobemide in children with attention deficit hyperactive disorder. *Psychopharmacology* **106**, Suppl., 134–6.

Trott, G. E., Menzel, M., Friese, H. J. & Nissen, G. (1991). Wirksamkeit und VertrÑglichkeit des selektiven MAO-A-Inhibitors Moclobemid bei Kindern mit hyperkinetischem Syndrom. *Zeitschrift für Kinder- und Jugendpsychiatrie*, **19**, 248–53.

Van Harten, J. (1993). Clinical pharmacokinetics of selective serotonin reuptake inhibitors. *Clinical Pharmacokinetics*, **24**, 203–20.

Venkataraman, S., Naylor, M. W. & King, C. A. (1992). Mania associated with fluoxetine treatment in adolescents. *Journal of the American Academy of Child and Adolescent Psychiatry*, **31**, 276–81.

Waldmeier, P. C. (1987). Amine oxidases and their endogenous substrates (with special reference to monoamine oxidase and the brain). *Journal of Neural Transmission* (Suppl.) **23**, 55–72.

Warrington, S. J. (1988). The cardiovascular toxicity of antidepressants. *International Clinical Psychopharmacology*, **3**, (Suppl. 2), 63–70.

Wilens, T. E., Biederman, J., Baldessarini, R. J. *et al.* (1992). Developmental changes in serum concentrations of desipramine and 2-hydroxydesipramine during treatment with desipramine. *Journal of the American Academy of Child and Adolescent Psychiatry*, **31**, 691–8.

Winsberg, B. G., Goldstein, S., Yepes, L. E. & Perel, J. M. (1975). Imipramine and electrocardiographic abnormalities in hyperactive children. *American Journal of Psychiatry*, **132**, 542–5.

Wong, D. T., Horng, J. S., Bymaster, F. P. *et al.* (1974). A selective inhibitor of serotonin uptake: Lilly 110140, 3-(p-trifluoromethylphenoxy)-N-methyl-3-phenyl-propylamine. *Life Sciences*, **15**, 471–9.

Youdim, M. B. H. & Ashkenazi, R. (1982). Regulation of 5-HT catabolism. In *Serotonin in Biological Psychiatry*, (ed. B. T. Ho, J. C. Schoolar, E. Usdin), pp. 35–60. Raven Press, New York.

Young, J. G., Cohen, D. J., Waldo, M. C. *et al.* (1980). Platelet monoamine oxidase activity in children and adolescents with psychiatric disorders. *Schizophrenia Bulletin* **6**, 324–33.

Zametkin, A., Rappoport, J. L., Murphy, D. L. *et al.* (1985). Treatment of hyperactive children with monoamine oxidase inhibitors. *Archives of General Psychiatry*, **42**, 962–6.

Zemlan, F. P. & Garver, D. L. (1990). Depression and antidepressant therapy: receptor dymamics. *Progress in Neuro-Psychopharmacology and Biological Psychiatry*, **14**, 503–23.

References

...

12

The psychotherapeutic management of major depressive and dysthymic disorders in childhood and adolescence: Issues and prospects

Maria Kovacs and Leo J. Bastiaens

INTRODUCTION

In this chapter, we summarise empirical evidence to support the argument that childhood-onset major depression and dysthymia are serious disorders that require aggressive therapeutic management. However, no particular intervention has yet been conclusively documented as efficacious in bringing about symptomatic remission, preventing relapse, and improving the functioning of young patients. The need for effective therapies clearly exists because depressive disorders among school-age children and adolescents have been increasingly identified ever since the Research Diagnostic Criteria (RDC, Spitzer, Endicott & Robins, 1978) and the Diagnostic and Statistical Manual of the American Psychiatric Association (DSM-III and DSM-III-R; APA, 1980, 1987) have gained acceptance. Major depressive disorder and dysthymic or minor depressive disorder, diagnosed according to such operational criteria, have been documented among psychiatrically referred young patients (Strober & Carlson, 1982; Kovacs et al., 1984a,b, 1994a; Geller et al., 1985; Puig-Antich et al., 1985a,b; Ryan et al., 1987; Mitchell et al., 1988), youngsters with a chronic medical illness (Kovacs et al., 1985; Burke et al.,

1989), community and population samples and in primary care paediatric settings (Anderson *et al.*, 1987; Kashani *et al.*, 1987; Bird, *et al.*, 1988; Costello *et al.*, 1988; Lewinsohn *et al.*, 1993), and groups of non-referred and 'at-risk' juveniles (Keller *et al.*, 1988; Warner *et al.*, 1992).

However, the evidence concerning depressive disorders among juveniles has not been uniformly accepted. Much of the criticism has concerned the fact that the diagnostic criteria that were used had been originally designed for adults, and that they were applied in unmodified forms to younger age groups. It has been noted that the DSM-III, DSM-III-R or RDC are not developmentally based, that the diagnoses of depression are not considered in relationship to behaviours that may be normal during a particular stage of maturation or development, and that the criteria do not include age-specific symptoms or features of the disorder (Digdon & Gotlib, 1985; Angold, 1988; Seifer *et al.*, 1989). Based on the development of emotion-recognition, it has been proposed, for example, that different levels of conceptualisation of feelings may be associated with variable depressive symptom clusters among youngsters (Digdon & Gotlib, 1985). This proposal echoes the age-specific classification schemas of childhood-onset depression of the 1960s and 1970s (for a review, see Kovacs & Beck, 1978).

The fact remains, however, that there is no compelling evidence of major age-related changes in the expression of depression during the school-age years. In one study, for example, clinically diagnosed, depressed juveniles at various stages of cognitive and pubertal development did not manifest the hypothesised differences in symptom expression or disorder characteristics (Kovacs & Paulauskas, 1984). According to the findings of three separate investigations, the *core* clinical picture of depressive illness among school-age children and adolescents is very similar to the characteristics of this disorder among adults (Ryan *et al.*, 1987; Mitchell *et al.*, 1988; Kovacs & Gatsonis, 1989), although there is some developmental mediation of symptom expression. The most consistently reported finding in this regard is that sleep disturbance among younger depressed children is more likely to manifest as hyposomnia, whereas the sleep disturbance of depressed adolescents is generally characterized by hypersomnia (Ryan *et al.*, 1987; Mitchell *et al.*, 1988; Kovacs & Gatsonis, 1989).

In advocating for the importance of the aggressive psychotherapeutic management of childhood-onset major depression and dysthymia, we are *not* proposing that developmental considerations are unimportant. Neither are we claiming that the clinical presentation of young depressed children and older adolescents are exactly alike. Developmental considerations are important, particularly in the direct psychiatric examination of the school-age child (Kovacs, 1986) in assessing the social and family consequences of childhood depression and in considering alternative therapeutic strategies. Our stance is that developmental variations in disorder presentation can readily be accommodated by the prototypical nature of existing operational psychiatric diagnostic criteria. Developmental considerations should enrich, but not replace, the use of formal diagnostic strategies to identify depressed children or adolescents. In this regard, it is useful to note that none of the developmentally based alternative classifications of depression in childhood (for a review, see Digdon & Gotlib, 1985) has been validated or became a major impetus for research.

This chapter concerns the problems of children and adolescents who have psychiatrically diagnosable major depressive and dysthymic disorders in particular, and depressive syndromes in general. We review data on the clinical prognosis of youngsters with these conditions and the negative functional concomitants of depressive disorders and depressive syndromes. Then, we present a brief overview of controlled psychotherapy outcome studies of depressed youths. Finally, we discuss major issues that need to be considered in the psychotherapeutic management of depressed youngsters and in attempts to develop effective interventions for them.

CHARACTERISTICS OF MAJOR DEPRESSIVE AND DYSTHYMIC DISORDERS

Clinical picture

Findings from the Pittsburgh Longitudinal Study of youngsters with early-onset depressive disorders have documented that these conditions have a phasic natural history, including high rates of recovery and recurrence. Clinically referred children and adolescents with major depression or dysthymia also are typically characterised by other concurrent (comorbid) psychiatric conditions, including anxiety, conduct, and attention deficit disorders. Nonetheless, on follow-up, such youths continue to be mostly impaired by some form of affective disorder rather than a nonaffective condition.

More specifically, according to data from the Pittsburgh naturalistic follow-up study of clinically referred children, an episode of major depressive disorder (MDD) lasts about 11 months, on average, with a median time to recovery of about 9 months. Recovery is most likely to occur within the first 3 to 12 months after the onset of the episode of major depression, but about 15% of young patients with MDD have a first episode that lasts more than 18 months (Kovacs et al., 1984a, 1994b). Certain clinical subpopulations may even have longer episodes (Geller et al., 1985). Recent findings from studies of nonreferred youths are consistent with and complement the foregoing data, and as would be expected, indicate higher rates of remission and earlier recovery, as compared to clinical samples. Namely, in a study of unreferred youths (Warner et al., 1992), average MDD length was about 10 months (46 weeks), while the median length was 2.7 months (12 weeks). In another sample of unreferred youngsters with major depression, median duration of the episode was reported as 16 weeks (Keller et al., 1988). The fact that childhood-onset major depressive disorders are typically accompanied by multiple disorders also has been reconfirmed in various samples of youths (e.g. Keller et al., 1988; Mitchell et al., 1988).

The type of depression that has been designated in the DSM-III (American Psychiatric Association, 1980) as dysthymic disorder (DD) appears to be a chronic and complicated condition among clinically referred, school-age youths. As documented by data from the Pittsburgh study, the first episode of DD is characterised by early onset (in some children, as early as 5 years of age) and protracted course. The average episode length is close to 4 years, and longitudinal data reveal that recovery is quite gradual. Overall, it takes 8 years from the onset of the dysthymic disorder to reach a 98% recovery rate (Kovacs et al., 1994a). In a small sample of non-referred children ($n = 9$), the course of dysthymia also was reported to be protracted, with a median duration of 5 years (Keller et al., 1988). While the child is still dysthymic, and probably during the first 2 years of dysthymia, he or she is highly likely to have a first episode of major depression (Kovacs et al., 1984b, 1994a). The superimposition of major depression on a chronic dysthymic condition, originally delineated in studies of adults and labelled 'double depression' (Keller & Shapiro, 1982), was first confirmed among youths in the Pittsburgh longitudinal study. Its existence has now been documented in other samples of children and adolescents as well (Kashani et al., 1987; Keller et al., 1988; Mitchell et al., 1988; Lewinsohn et al., 1991).

Early-onset depressive disorders also appear to portend a subsequent chronic history of affective illness. This pattern is very evident among childhood-onset dysthymic patients, of whom about 75% progress to repeated episodes of major depression with a portion developing bipolar illness. Excepting the fact that their depressions tend to start at a younger age, dysthymic children who have had a first episode of MDD are subsequently almost indistinguishable from those youths whose affective disorder history commenced with an episode of MDD. In other words, either DD or MDD in childhood appears to be a marker for subsequent episodes of MDD, bipolarity developing, and other forms of affective illness emerging. These youths move in and out of episodes, spending approximately 30% of their late childhood and adolescent years in some form of affective disorder (Kovacs et al., 1994a).

Youngsters with MDD and/or DD also evidence consistently high rates of suicidal ideation and are increasingly likely to have suicide attempts as they move into adolescence (Kovacs, Goldston & Gatsonis, 1993). This overall unfavourable prognosis for juvenile-onset depression has now been reconfirmed by several follow-up and 'follow-back' studies of clinical samples (Asarnow et al., 1988; Garber et al., 1988; Geller, Fox & Fletcher, 1993; Rao et al., 1993; Strober et al., 1993) and long-term blind re-evaluation of child psychiatric patients (Harrington et al., 1990). Finally, the presentation, course, and outcome of childhood-onset depressive disorders is complicated by the high rates of concurrent, nonaffective disorders, as well as family psychopathology and social strife (see an overview by Kazdin, 1990).

Functional concomitants

There are several ways in which depressive disorders may negatively affect the functioning of youngsters. Negative effects may be secondary to certain depressive symptoms, may derive from the overall impact of the disorder and its duration, and may reflect an interaction of symptomatology and disorder length. Although, in paediatric samples, functional impairment that accompanies depression has been investigated less extensively than its clinical aspects, depressed youths do appear to have problems in scholastic achievement, academic performance, and interpersonal and social functioning. Admittedly, some of the data about functional problems and depression derive from the studies in which self-rated symptom scales or peer-nominations were used to define depression (as opposed to a psychiatric diagnostic interview). Nonetheless, the findings from clinical and nonclinical samples are convergent and can be synthesised.

In general, the evidence suggests that depressed children tend to perform poorly in school, may have to be held back, and have behavioural difficulties in academic settings (for a review, see Kovacs & Goldston, 1991). Although such problems or deficits are not specific to depressed youths (Puig-Antich et al., 1985a,b), the pathways to these negative outcomes may differ according to the child's psychiatric disorder. For example, in the presence of depression, impaired school performance may reflect difficulties with concentration and memory. Indeed, there is some evidence that focused attention may be especially impaired in depression (e.g. Kaslow et al., 1983). Likewise, declining school grades may reflect the reduced interest and lowered hedonic capacity that are hallmarks of depression.

There has been considerable interest in the social and interpersonal consequences of depression, but most of the work has targeted adults (for a review, see Coyne, Burchill & Stiles, 1991). There is some evidence however that, paralleling the findings on depressed adults, children with depressive symptoms and those with diagnosable depressive disorders have problems in social functioning and may elicit negative reactions from school-mates, peers, or parents (for reviews, see Kazdin, 1990; Kaslow & Rehm, 1991; Kovacs & Goldston 1991). In general, the available information suggests that depressed children (as compared to non-depressed peers) are less often selected as playmates, are less liked, more isolated, and have fewer, if any, best friends. In an actual school setting, for example, depressed children were observed as spending more time alone and exhibiting higher rates of negative interactions with schoolmates, compared to non-depressed peers (Altmann & Gotlib, 1988). Other investigators confirmed that depressed schoolchildren tend to be unassertive, isolated, and socially inadequate (Kennedy, Spence & Hensley, 1989), although depression and anxiety may equally contribute to poor peer relationships (Goodyer, Wright & Altham, 1989). Among clinically depressed children and adolescents, notable problems also have been documented in regard to parent–child and peer interactions (Puig-Antich et al., 1985a,b, 1993), and in experimental situations, clinically referred adolescents with depressive disorders are perceived by 'normal' age-mates in unfavourable social terms (Connolly et al., 1992). Most worrisome is evidence that even after recovery from the depression, depressed, clinic-referred youngsters still exhibit residual impairment in the quality of communication and relationship with their mothers (Puig-Antich et al., 1985b).

TREATMENT APPROACHES THAT HAVE BEEN TESTED

Because even one episode of depressive disorder may have serious effects on the functioning of children and adolescents, there is a need for efficacious and age-appropriate interventions. However, treatment development and assessment efforts have not kept pace with the progress in phenomenologic and empiric research. Indeed, as we reviewed the results of controlled psychotherapy trials with depressed juveniles, we found that only three approaches have been subjected to empirical study, namely, behaviour, cognitive-behaviour, and supportive therapies. It is notable that the therapies that have been tested were originally designed for adults. Furthermore, there is no compelling evidence that these interventions have been sufficiently modified to accommodate the developmental characteristics and needs of children and adolescents.

In brief, one of the interventions that has been researched that has its roots in behaviour therapy is Lewinsohn, Biglan & Zeiss' (1976) social skills training. The overall approach emphasises the importance of environmental contingencies and the skills of the person in behavioural outcomes. The basic proposition is that individuals become depressed because they experience a reduced rate of response-contingent positive reinforcement. The low reinforcement rate reflects a combination of poor social skills and external circumstances (e.g. fewer reinforcers). Social skills training, problem-solving strategies, and increasing the frequency of pleasant activities represent the mainstay of Lewinsohn's treatment. Based on the presumed link between stress and depression (Shaw, 1982), relaxation training is another behavioural strategy that has been applied to treat depressed youths. Jacobson's (1929) technique of progressive muscle relaxation is the approach that has been employed. Finally, variations of cognitive-behaviour and cognitive therapies, developed by Rehm (1977) and Beck *et al.* (1979), also have been utilised in the treatment of depressed juveniles. According to the former approach, the core problem in depression is a failure or deficiency in self-control component processes that can be corrected by behavioural strategies (e.g. self-evaluation, self-reinforcement). The treatment developed by Beck *et al.* (1979) reflects a more 'cognitive' perspective and is based on the assumption that depression results from the presence of negative self-referential cognitions and systematic errors in thinking and evaluation. Therefore, the individual's distorted and maladaptive thinking is the core psychological problem in depression (Kovacs & Beck,

1978). Cognitive therapy is used to challenge the erroneous and distorted cognitions, elucidate and correct the underlying negative cognitive schemas, teach the patient a more realistic evaluation of the self, external experiences, and the future, and thereby develop a more adaptive problem-solving repertoire. Finally, supportive therapy, based on psychodynamic or interpersonal theories, also has been used with depressed youths. In general, the focus of supportive therapy has been to enable patients to utilise their assets and coping skills more effectively (Fine *et al.*, 1991). The foregoing cognitive and behavioural therapies have generally been shown to be effective in controlled trials with depressed adults (Steinbrueck *et al.*, 1983; Hollon *et al.*, 1993).

EMPIRICAL TREATMENT-OUTCOME STUDIES

In 1985, Clarizio commented that very little was known about which particular intervention strategies may be effective in the psychological treatment of depression in childhood. Although some information was available regarding behaviour modification and social skills training with depressed youngsters, the evidence was mostly from case reports and small-sample studies. Concomitantly, there were questions as to whether improvement in the target behaviours was accompanied by amelioration of the disorder and whether treatment effects were generalisable. Information about cognitively oriented interventions was likewise confined to case reports (e.g. DiGiuseppe, 1981). Unfortunately, the situation has not changed substantially in recent years.

Clinically diagnosed samples

Since 1980, there have only been two peer-reviewed publications on controlled psychotherapy studies of youths with major depression or dysthymia (Lewinsohn *et al.*, 1990; Fine *et al.*, 1991). In these two studies, a total of 125 clinically depressed, 13- to 18-year-old adolescents received short-term, group-based interventions. At end of treatment, 40 to 50% of the youths reportedly recovered, with equivalent rates of success for social skill training, cognitive techniques, or supportive therapy.

Lewinsohn *et al.* (1990) tested the effectiveness of their 'Coping with Depression' (CWD) course with 14- to 18-year-old symptomatic volunteers. They reported that close to 50% of the treated youths were remitted from their depression at end of treatment, as compared to only 5% of the wait-list controls. The subjects in this study had to meet diagnostic criteria for major depression according to the DSM-III (American Psychiatric Association, 1980), or intermittent or minor depression according to RDC (Spitzer *et al.*, 1978), as determined through structured clinical interviews. Self- and parent-rated symptom scales also were administered. Fifty-nine subjects were randomly assigned to the CWD course, the CWD course with a parent component, or a wait-list control. The protocol involved 14 2-hour sessions during a period of 7 weeks. The two active treatments were identical, except that parents of the subjects in the 'CWD with parent' modality also met once weekly.

In addition to a 50% recovery rate, as determined by structured interviews, the treated groups evidenced significant improvements according to their scores on self- and parent-rated scales. However, according to parental ratings, there were few differences between the CWD and the 'CWD with parent' groups. Participants in both groups continued to improve over the following 2 years, although only 50% of the sample was available for the 2-year follow-up assessment.

Fine *et al.* (1991) compared supportive therapy with social skills training in a sample of 66 13- to 17-year-old adolescent patients, who had DSM-III major depressive or dysthymic disorder, as determined by structured clinical interviews. Supportive therapy involved an emphasis on improving self-concept. The social skill training was operationalised through a manual and focused on recognition of feelings, and assertiveness, feedback, problem-solving, and negotiation skills. Treatment was delivered in a group format during a period of 12 weeks. Fifty per cent of those who received supportive therapy and 40% of the subjects in social skills training experienced significant improvement in mood and hedonic capacity. It should be noted, however, that 41% of the study sample was receiving concomitant psychotherapy or medication. Subjects continued to improve after treatment; approximately 70% evidenced improved mood at the 9-month follow-up. However, 19 subjects did not complete the treatment trial and 7 others dropped out during follow-up.

The above two studies are noteworthy for their methodological rigour. The investigators utilised structured clinical assessments, operational diagnostic criteria, random assignment to groups, operationalised treatments, and follow-up. Nonetheless, the results are disappointing: the response rates at end-of-treatment were comparatively poor, and half or more of the treated cases were still in the midst of a depressive episode. Admittedly, several variables may have obscured or made it difficult to obtain a better response: the nature of the psychiatric diagnoses, comorbidity, the duration of the treatments, the developmental 'readiness' of the patients to benefit from treatment, and the social context of the patients. For example, both studies included subjects with either major depression, dysthymia, or both. These mood disorders entail somewhat different symptoms, are presumed to represent different levels of severity, and have different durations (as discussed earlier in this chapter). Hence, the inclusion of subjects with major depression and dysthymia could have obscured a better response rate possibly associated with one (but not the other) condition.

Additionally, although Lewinsohn et al. (1990) excluded patients with certain conditions (e.g. bipolarity, psychosis, substance abuse, panic disorder), other comorbid disorders such as childhood anxiety disorders, attention deficit disorder, and/or learning disabilities, apparently were not considered. A depressed youngster who has pre-existing attentional or learning problems may be at a disadvantage with an intervention such as the CWD course that incorporates considerable written material and homework assignments. Furthermore, a chronic condition, such as attention deficit/hyperactivity disorder, may continue to play a role in the coping style and interpersonal functioning of the individual, possibly predisposing to relapse or recurrence of the depressive symptoms. Comorbidity may have played a role in the disappointing response rate of the study by Fine et al. (1991) as well.

It is also notable that, considering the average length of a depressive episode in youths, treatment durations were short in both studies. Even though the recovery rates were reported to be 60 to 70% at the 9-month follow-up in one study (Fine et al., 1991), and above 80% at the 24-month follow-up in the other study (Lewinsohn et al., 1990), the rates have to be interpreted in the context of the 'natural' recovery patterns associated with childhood depression. For example, as previously noted, the median recovery (evidenced by 50% of a sample) for an episode of MDD in childhood is about 9 months in clinically referred youths. Therefore, even the approximately 70% recovery rate in the Fine et al. (1991) study may represent no more than a 20% 'gain' over the natural remission rate.

Furthermore, cognitive and social-cognitive developmental issues were apparently not considered in the implementation of the therapies. Given the age span of the patients, there may have been considerable within-sample variability in regards to recognition of emotions and mood, identification of problems and the negative consequences of behaviour, perspective taking, insight, and metacognitive functioning (Digdon & Gotlib 1985; Kovacs, 1986; Leahy, 1988; Shirk, 1988). In so far as treatment gains are mediated by 'developmental readiness' in the foregoing domains, youths at less mature levels may have evidenced comparatively less improvement, and thus negatively affected overall group response rates. Additionally, psychiatrically disturbed youths may already have evidenced delays in reaching cognitive developmental milestones (Szajnberg & Weiner, 1989), that could possibly have interfered with therapeutic learning. Finally, among youths, a potentially favourable treatment response may be adversely affected by contextual factors such as parental psychopathology and adverse family circumstances, including physical or emotional abuse. However, even though Lewinsohn *et al.* (1990) noted the importance of joint sessions of parents and their teenage offspring, the social context of the youths or the mental health of their parents were neither investigated nor targeted for change.

School-based nondiagnosed samples

In addition to the above noted studies, data also are available on the treatment of symptomatically depressed children and adolescents, as reported in five peer-reviewed articles. In these investigations, the therapies were conducted within school settings, students were primarily selected based on cut-off scores on self-rated or parent-rated scales and/or teacher reports, but there were no diagnostic assessments. Treatment response rates appeared to be more favourable than in the studies of clinically diagnosed youths.

Butler *et al.* (1980) published one of the first controlled studies of a school-based treatment of symptomatically depressed fifth and sixth grade students ($n = 56$). The results revealed statistically significant decreases in depressive symptoms and increments in self-esteem for the role-play and cognitive restructuring interventions, compared to control and placebo conditions. The positive changes were mirrored in the reports of teachers. Several years later, Reynolds & Coats (1986) reported on the cognitive-behavioural and relaxation treatment of 30 symptomatically depressed high-school students (mean age of 15.7 years). At end-point, both active treatments were found to be effective: approximately 80% of subjects scored below the clinical cut-off for depression on a self-report scale, while none of the wait-list controls did. Stark, Reynolds & Kaslow (1987) compared self-control therapy and behavioural problem-solving training with 9- to 12-year old middle-school students. The majority of the subjects improved (78% and 60%, respectively). However, there were few significant differences between the two treatments according to subjects' self-reports and parental ratings. Kahn *et al.* (1990) compared cognitive-behavioural, relaxation and self-modelling therapy, and a wait-list condition, with 10- to 14-year-old middle-school students. Subjects in all three treatment groups evidenced similarly significant improvement, as compared to the wait-list controls. However, at one-month follow-up, more of the subjects who were in the self-modelling group (50%) again scored in the dysfunctional ranges on self-report scales, compared to the subjects who were in the cognitive-behavioural and relaxation groups.

Finally, in a school-based study of children who were 7 to 11 years old, and were selected using cut-off scores on a self-rated scale as well as a symptom-based interview, Liddle & Spence (1990) failed to find specific effects for treatment that was delivered during an 8-week period. Children who received group-based social-competence training, attention placebo, or were in a wait-list control group, evidenced similar declines in levels of depression at end of treatment, and by a 2-month post-treatment follow-up assessment.

Although the overall response rates in the above noted school-based studies of symptomatically depressed youths appear to be more favourable than the results with clinically diagnosed samples, the results have to be interpreted with caution. Because the assessments did not include clinical evaluations, data were not available about the primary or comorbid diagnoses of the subjects. Thus, it is not clear whether the findings can be generalised to clinical settings. Furthermore, in at least two investigations (Stark *et al.*, 1987; Kahn *et al.*, 1990), the outcome of assessments by teachers and parents did not coincide with self-reports, raising some questions about the cross-situational generalisability of treatment effects. However, these studies are distinguished by the fact that the interventions were provided in the schools, making it feasible to reach a larger segment of potentially 'needy' youths. Furthermore, in contrast to treatment results with clinical samples, the drop-out rates were generally low, with figures of 0%, 3% and 20%, respectively, in the studies conducted by Kahn *et al.* (1990), Stark *et al.* (1987), and Reynolds & Coats (1986).

CURRENT TRENDS

Clinical trials

Stimulated by the success of treatment development efforts for depressed adults and the paucity of interventions for children and adolescents, several investigators have been developing treatment manuals in conjunction with planned or ongoing clinical trials. Wilkes & Rush (1988) are exploring the use of a cognitive-therapy manual in an open study of depressed adolescent outpatients. Brent *et al.* (1992) are conducting a controlled investigation of the treatment of depressed and suicidal adolescents, using individual cognitive therapy, family therapy, and individual supportive therapy. Lewinsohn's 'Coping With Stress Course' has been modified for adolescents and is being used as a secondary prevention treatment with at-risk populations (Gregory Clarke, personal communication, May, 1993). Interpersonal therapy, originally developed for adults, is currently being modified for use with depressed adolescents (Moreau *et al.*, 1991). Finally, Nguyen *et al.* (1992) have developed a dynamically oriented treatment manual for depressed prepubertal children and their parents, to be employed in conjunction with pharmacotherapy.

The foregoing initiatives attempt to overcome several limitations of previous studies. For example, the newly developed or developing studies are targeted at patients with diagnosable affective illnesses. In several of these studies, attempts are being made to consider factors such as comorbidity and family circumstances, and at least one study includes family therapy as a treatment modality. However, various conceptual and practical issues do not appear to have been addressed. For example, based on our perusal of the treatment manuals, it appears that scant systematic attention has been paid to cognitive and social-cognitive developmental characteristics of young patients, and the impact of such developmental variables on treatment outcome. Also, the inclusion or exclusion of parents in the treatments do not appear to be based on arguments relevant to the onset or maintenance of depression. Finally, with one exception (Nguyen *et al.*, 1992), the new initiatives focus on adolescents and exclude younger, school-age children.

Need for theoretical advances

Although, over the past 15 years, considerable advances have been made in clinical and psychometric assessment, specification of diagnostic criteria, and phenomenologic description of depressed youths, no novel or comprehensive theories of early-onset depressions have been proposed. This may account, in large part, for the general paucity of treatment research with depressed children and adolescents, and the lack of developmental-stage specific intervention strategies.

In the field of adult depression, the most promising and exciting interventions have been based on or were derived from theoretical explanations of the onset and maintenance of depressive symptoms. In contrast, the treatments for depressed youths, briefly noted above, represent 'downward extensions' of therapies for depressed adults: few attempts have been made to examine the 'fit' of the underlying theories of depression to younger age groups. However, the emerging field of developmental psychopathology may eventually give rise to theories of aetiology or causality that are sensitive to age-specific issues (see, for example, Rutter *et al.*, 1986). By integrating perspectives that focus on salient risk and contributory factors (see Office of Technology Assessment, 1987), including parental psychopathology, the impact of the social milieu, sensitive developmental periods, and critical parameters such as attachment (Cicchetti & Schneider-Rosen, 1986), a viable conceptual approach to childhood-onset depressions may emerge. In turn, the identification of presumably important processes or variables could provide the foundation for a theory of early-onset affective illness.

PRACTICAL ISSUES IN THE DELIVERY OF CLINICAL SERVICES

Access to services

Professionals who are committed to helping youths overcome depression are faced with several dilemmas. Firstly, as we discussed above, there is currently no compelling body of evidence supporting the effectiveness of one form of psychotherapy or psychosocial intervention, compared to another, for the amelioration of depression among juveniles. Admittedly, only a limited number of approaches have been subjected to empirical study, and thus, no firm guidelines can be provided regarding the choice of intervention.

However, even if we were to have therapies of 'proven' effectiveness, providing patients access to services remains a critical problem. Indeed, according to recent reports, commissioned by agencies of the government of the USA, the vast majority of children in need of mental health care do not receive it (Office of Technology Assessment, 1987; Institute of Medicine, 1989). Lack of service utilization partly reflects lack of access to service providers.

Therefore, the question arises as to what setting is the most desirable for the delivery of psychotherapy? In this regard, it is noteworthy that the treatment outcome studies of symptomatically depressed youths generally were conducted in school settings (Butler et al., 1980; Reynolds & Coats, 1986; Stark et al., 1987; Kahn et al., 1990). The school is probably the best single location for the early identification and treatment of children and adolescents with depressive disorders. A combination of self-, teacher- and parent-rated scales can provide a first stage screening, followed by more intensive diagnostic evaluations. Cases identified as needing treatment may then be served within the school setting. The feasibility of school-based treatments of depression has been demonstrated as noted above. The large-scale application of such an approach also has been documented in the well-known project of Kolvin et al. (1981).

The advantage of providing treatment in the school setting is that the majority of depressed youths could be reached. Thus, practical problems or other burdens that may prevent parents from bringing a child to a clinic would be overcome. Treatment teams could work closely with teachers and school counsellors to evaluate progress and reinforce new coping skills. Reynolds & Coats (1986) suggested, for example, that the improved academic self-concept of some of the treated students in their study might have reflected the effects of using the school as the treatment milieu. Additionally, some parents may prefer the familiar setting of the school as compared to a clinic or mental health centre in which to obtain help for their children.

Disadvantages of providing treatment in the school-settings may include potential stigmatisation of the student, and difficulties in maintaining privacy and confidentiality. Additionally, because school-based interventions usually take the form of group therapy, they may be not suitable for more severely disturbed youths. Suicidality, psychotic symptoms, or multiple comorbid conditions, that are likely to complicate treatment, would be indicators for referral to a mental health clinic.

Mental health centres or out-patient child psychiatry clinics will probably remain the settings in which much of psychotherapy is delivered. Recently, however, attempts have also been made to provide care in the community at large, using recreational or youth centres that already have established activities (Institute of Medicine, 1989). The use of such community centres could be ideal for some cultural and ethnic groups that may be uncomfortable with, or distrustful of 'mainstream' institutional environments. Finally, partial hospitalisation programmes and in-patient units continue to be necessary to provide care for youths with incapacitating depressive disorders. At the present time, there are no adequate treatment outcome studies with populations in such settings (Pruitt & Kiser, 1991; Woolston, 1991).

The treatment modality

With some modifications, most psychotherapeutic interventions can be delivered in one of several ways: individual therapy, group therapy, family therapy, or any combination of the foregoing. Each modality has advantages and disadvantages. Individual therapy, for example, provides the patient with more attention and a more favourable 'therapy over time' ratio. Possibly, it also enhances the therapeutic alliance that is an important ingredient of any intervention (Barbanel, 1982). Concomitantly, more 'private' feelings, thoughts and behaviours can be explored. Individual therapy also makes it possible to respond within the session to crises and emergencies, such as those that can arise with a potentially suicidal patient. The major disadvantage of individual therapy is that it is expensive, labour-intensive, and cannot accommodate all those who are potentially in need of help.

In contrast, group therapy for childhood depressive disorders is more cost-effective. Additionally, it provides access to care to a larger number of youths at any given point in time. Its structure also provides patients with peer support and the opportunity to practice social and coping skills. However, some of the disadvantages of group therapy include the lack of individual privacy, difficulty maintaining the same group over time, and constraints on the therapist's ability to attend to the needs of more severely depressed youths.

Family therapy likewise shares several of the advantages and disadvantages that characterise group and individual therapy. But it may be particularly advantageous if members of the family unit are directly implicated in the onset or maintenance of the youth's depression. Stark *et al.* (1987) noted, for example, that many of the children in their study identified family problems as a source of their difficulties. However, because traditional family therapies are process- and interaction-oriented, it is not clear in what fashion a depressed youngster's specific needs could be accommodated.

The duration of treatment

As long ago as 1959, Levitt, Beiser & Robertson have posed the question as to what time period or number of hours should constitute 'a course of psychotherapy'. Because children are in the process of growth and maturation, the duration of therapy takes on a degree of importance for which there is no precedence in the literature on adults. Therefore, decisions about what constitutes a course of treatment should be made empirically. For example, as noted, the existing information suggests that an episode of dysthymic disorder in childhood lasts about 4 years, on average (Kovacs *et al.*, 1994*b*). Attenuation, reversal, or remediation of such a chronic condition is not likely to be accomplished over a short time-period. It would therefore seem sensible that disorder duration be one variable guiding decisions about treatment length.

Additionally, the ability to evidence a positive and lasting treatment response may be mediated by level of social and interpersonal maturity of the young patient. Therefore, the extent of the depressed child's developmental stage, or delay, as opposed to chronological age alone, may be another variable that could guide treatment duration, with more immature or 'delayed' youngsters requiring longer courses of treatment. Finally, the goals of most therapeutic systems embrace learning new ways of behaving, perceiving relationships, and interpreting interpersonal and other events of relevance. In so far as learning requires rehearsal, repeated execution of the target behaviours across multiple settings, and 'internationalisation' of the new rules, developmental-stage specific learning trajectories may provide additional guidance for selecting optimal treatment durations.

TOPICS THAT REQUIRE FURTHER ATTENTION

The role of parents in treatment

The ambiguous role of parents in studies of the psychotherapy of depressed youngsters is a notable aspect of the literature; just as it is a problem in child psychotherapy research in general (Kovacs & Lohr, 1995). The omission of parents from most treatment trials may partly reflect the fact that many studies were carried out in school settings. However, the sparse attention paid to parents persists in several currently available drafts of psychotherapy treatment manuals, and is remarkable in light of practical and clinical issues.

First, the political and social reality is that children and adolescents have limited legal rights. In the USA, federal laws recognise the family 'as a zone of privacy' and the fundamental right of parents to be protected from governmental interference in family decisions (Melton & Wilcox, 1989). Additionally, as a service, psychotherapy (at least in the USA) usually involves financial considerations, whereas youths do not have independent financial resources. Therefore, in most instances, the parents or caretaking adults are the 'gatekeepers' with respect to initial referral and financial coverage. At a practical level, parental cooperation is therefore critical to the treatment of their offspring.

Second, parental mental health is likely to be a significant moderator of children's response to and compliance with treatment. There exists considerable literature suggesting that parents who have an affective or other mental disorder (as compared to those who do not) are more likely to have children who have dysfunctional behaviours or psychiatric illness, including depression (e.g. Harder et al., 1980; Beardslee et al., 1983; Cantwell & Baker, 1984; Turner, Beidel & Costello, 1987). Conversely depressed children and adolescents who are clinically referred have parents with elevated rates of psychopathology (e.g. Strober & Carlson, 1982; Puig-Antich et al., 1989). Therefore, treatment of the parents' own disorders should be seriously considered in tandem with the psychotherapy of a youngster. It is difficult to see how one could expect a positive and *lasting* treatment response from a child whose parent is disturbed and is thereby probably unable to meet the youngster's needs.

Third, assuming reasonable parental mental health, the omission of parents from treatment trials diminishes the educational and psychological roles they play in their children's lives. Treatment studies of conduct disordered youths have documented that parents can be important agents of behaviour change in the home (e.g. Dadds, Schwartz & Sanders, 1987; Kazdin et al., 1987). Furthermore, Harter (1990) has demonstrated that positive parental attitude is a powerful contributor to self-worth in childhood and adolescence. At the very least, therefore, including the parents in some aspect of their offspring's therapy may help parents to become more effective in the subsequent care of young patients.

Finally, in actual clinical practice, children and adolescents are rarely treated completely on their own. According to a recent overview, most therapists who work with children do involve the parents at some level as well (Fauber & Long, 1991), although the nature and scope of parental involvement have not been well documented. Empirical treatment studies of depressed youths may therefore contribute to clinical practice by providing explicit practical and/or theoretical rationales for parental participation and clear guidelines regarding the nature of their involvement in their children's treatment. Thereby, the results of treatment outcome studies also may become more meaningful and relevant to clinical practitioners.

Parent–child interactions and depression

We propose that a major factor that contributes to the surprisingly long episodes of depression and associated functional impairment among clinically referred youths is the disruptive effect of the depression on the parent–child relationship and on the behaviour of the parent. As noted above, empirical observations suggest that diagnosed or symptomatic depressed children are less socially adept than their peers and their interactions are generally negative in tone (Blechman et al., 1986; Altmann & Gotlib, 1988).

Clinically, one of the notable features of depressed children and adolescents is the nonreciprocity of their interpersonal interactions, coupled with an unwillingness or inability to verbalise their affective experience. The affective dysregulation frequently presents as irritability, impatience, crankiness, and anger (Kovacs et al., 1994a). Concomitantly, it is reasonable to assume that depressed youngsters stop providing positive reinforcement to their parents or other caretakers. In return, the parents can be expected to withhold emotional support, guidance, and expressions of affection, or to become inconsistent with their offspring in these regards. Because juveniles are almost entirely dependent on their parents with respect to most areas of their functioning, behaviour that consistently alienates or does not reinforce the parent is likely to have extremely negative repercussions. A downward spiral may be established that, in turn, reinforces the depression of the child. This scenario may be particularly likely if the depressed child lives in a single-parent household, and if the parent him/herself is depressed.

Most importantly, the negative effects of the child on the parent, and the eventual recursive nature of these consequences may undermine the attachment relationship between them. From a developmental viewpoint, the attachment bond or relationship between parent and child remains an important crucible for maturation and the growth of the child's self-esteem. Following the reasoning of Bowlby (1973, 1980), Cicchetti and associates have pointed out that 'attachment' is an ongoing process (e.g. Cicchetti & Schneider-Rosen, 1986; Cummings & Cicchetti, 1990). Children and adolescents need to receive affectionate caregiving in order to master successfully the developmental tasks they encounter, and to negotiate an age-appropriate balance between attachment and autonomy at each developmental phase. Thus, preservation of the attachment relationship, that is a crucial developmental task, is probably disrupted by the depression of the offspring.

Coyne has outlined an interactional perspective on depression and has elaborated its implications (Coyne et al., 1991). He has emphasised that depressed individuals are likely to precipitate negative mood in others, and provoke reactions that further reinforce their sense of rejection, unhappiness, or low self-esteem, leading to increasingly conflictual interactions. Such negative interactions also have been detected between depressed children and their parents, particularly the alienation of the mothers (Puig-Antich et al., 1985a,b; Cole & Rehm, 1986). Thus, the reestablishment or preservation of parent–child attachment may need to be a salient goal of the psychotherapy of depressed youths.

The link between developmental issues and treatment strategies

The level of cognitive, emotional, and social maturity of depressed children and adolescents represent realistic constraints on the delivery of psychotherapy (e.g. DiGiuseppe, 1981; Barbanel, 1982; Kazdin, 1990). Three developmental issues have been noted most often in the literature, as discussed in detail elsewhere (Kovacs, 1986; Kovacs & Paulauskas,

1986). First, there is consensus that the nonvoluntary nature of child and adolescent 'patienthood' typically results in an initially uncooperative or fearful attitude that must be resolved for positive changes to occur. Second, the limited capacity of juveniles to introspect and monitor internal distress and psychological motives put constraints on the topics that can be explored, and the therapeutic strategies that can be utilised. Third, school-age children and some adolescents have limited skills with regard to 'abstract' thinking, interpersonal perspective-taking, or verbal disputation, that must also be taken into account in the selection of a therapy. However, developmental considerations have only been minimally integrated into the therapies that have been tested. And there still is a dearth of assessment methods and tools focusing on the relevant skills and abilities that could be used in treatment studies to categorise young subjects.

Cognitive development is one area that requires more detailed attention. Because Piaget's theory still represents the most comprehensive view of the unfolding of cognitive capacities, authors in the field usually note the importance of having to distinguish the young child, whose thinking is 'concrete' and pre-operational, from the child aged 12 or above, presumably characterised by the ability to think abstractly (e.g. DiGiuseppe & Bernard, 1983; Kazdin, 1991). However, such a dichotomy is an oversimplification because the presence of depression may already have resulted in cognitive impairment or delay, making it difficult to infer developmental stage from chronological age alone. Furthermore, even in the absence of psychopathology, chronological age is not a surrogate for cognitive stage, and many individuals may not even attain the stage of formal operational thinking (Neimark, 1975). Additionally, the 'Piagetian' stage of formal operations encompasses diverse 'operations' and 'substages', and development can be uneven across presumably equivalent domains. The belief that adolescents can readily engage in logical, abstract reasoning also may be incorrect (e.g. Elkind, 1967). Thus, certain cognitive distortions, or conclusions contrary to evidence, that would be targeted for change in the context of interpersonal, cognitive, or rational-emotive therapy, for example, may possibly be developmentally normal operations during the late teen years. Although cognitive theories of the nature of depression have not been modified to include such developmental considerations, empirical research may serve to clarify their applicability and suitability to children (Hammen & Zupan 1984; Kaslow, Rehm & Siegel, 1984; Seligman et al., 1984; Asarnow, Carlson & Guthrie, 1987).

301

Another developmental issue that requires further study is the ability of children and adolescents to form a therapeutic alliance. A positive relationship between patient and therapist is usually considered to be an essential ingredient for successful treatment outcome. In turn, establishing a therapeutic relationship partly depends on the ability of the patient to recognise the therapist as a helping agent, an expectation that his/her problems can be solved, having confidence and trust in the therapist, and willingness to self-disclose (for an overview, see Kovacs, 1986).

Although the interpersonal aspects of psychotherapy with youngsters are not usually articulated in such terms, it is widely accepted that the therapist's relationship to the child is 'key' to treatment outcome (Barbanel, 1982). Irrespective of one's theoretical orientation, being able 'to engage the patient's trust and confidence' (McDermott & Char, 1984) has been considered a most important 'first stage' in the psychotherapy of juveniles. However, because of their level of cognitive and social development, children may have limited ability to engage effectively in psychotherapy (Kovacs & Paulauskas, 1986). For example, according to the developmental literature, establishing a trusting relationship with younger children may require that the therapist engage in overt action on their behalf or provide them with gifts, the latter of which has been discussed with some reluctance (Barbanel, 1982).

Attempts to integrate up-to-date empirical developmental research and the conduct of psychotherapy are illustrated by a recent book, entitled *Cognitive development and child psychotherapy* (Shirk, 1988). The implications of developmental stages in self-understanding, social perspective taking, and the identification of emotions, among others, are discussed with regard to 'broad' categories of interventions. Such approaches also may serve to better understand developmental constraints on the ability of youths to form and maintain a therapeutic alliance and the extent to which depression may further impede this process.

Populations with special needs

An overview of psychotherapy for depressed school-age children and adolescents has to call attention to populations with special needs or characteristics. This general category includes children whose lives are complicated by extreme poverty and homelessness, parental substance abuse, and human immunodeficiency virus infection, and the increasing cohort of children with chronic medical disorders. Depressed, homeless children, for instance, are unlikely to have access to individual psychotherapy, and family support systems for them may be non-existent. Indeed, many of the issues raised in the present chapter may be irrelevant in the face of the multiple deprivations such children have to endure, and the fact that their unstable environments probably negate any long-term interventions. For these youths, psychotherapeutic strategies would have to be part of a comprehensive social-service 'module' that can be offered in the form of crisis-intervention.

The needs of juveniles who have a chronic medical disorder also require attention. Increased understanding of the pathogenesis of various childhood-onset diseases, including insulin-dependent diabetes mellitus, asthma, or cystic fibrosis, and concomitant advances in their medical management have led to reduced mortality and better prognosis. However, youngsters with medical problems *and* depression (or other emotional problems) have generally been ignored in child psychotherapy research and treatment development. Existing treatment approaches will need to be modified in order to take into account functional issues and psychological concerns that are specific to the chronically ill, and to facilitate these youngsters' medical management in tandem with their psychotherapy.

CONCLUSIONS

In this chapter, we summarise empirical evidence that depressive disorders in childhood are serious and disabling conditions that require aggressive therapeutic management. In the juvenile years, episodes of major depression and dysthymia are more protracted than hitherto thought, they are associated with high rates of comorbid psychiatric disorders and impairment in various areas of functioning, and they appear to portend future bouts of affective illness. Although the need for effective interventions clearly exists, data are scant in regard to what form of psychotherapy may be most appropriate to bring about symptomatic remission, prevent relapse, and improve the functioning of young patients. We also discussed a number of issues that have not received sufficient consideration in treatment-outcome studies of depressed youths, and still remain to be addressed in current treatment development efforts.

Mental health professionals who treat depressed youths are faced with several challenges. These challenges include not only the lack of information about efficacious treatments, but also the fact that the pool of professionals is not sufficiently large to meet the mental health needs of our juvenile population. Under these circumstances, what is to be done? From a practical viewpoint, the evidence about the treatment of depressed youths together with information on psychotherapies that have been documented as effective with depressed adults can provide some guidelines. Thus, for example, it would appear that structured, goal-directed, or problem-solving oriented interventions that focus on symptom reduction, enhancement of self-esteem, and social/interpersonal skill development are appropriate for depressed juveniles. The best implementation of available strategies may, however, require a closer collaboration between clinicians and academically oriented developmental psychologists. Additionally, if the literature on the treatment of depressed adults is any indication, it would seem advisable to provide youths with some form of 'maintenance' psychotherapy as well, in order to reinforce the skills they have learned, and to prevent relapse. Possibly, the concomitant use of antidepressant pharmacotherapy also could be considered, although that form of intervention is beyond the scope of our chapter.

In the treatment of depressed youths, we would also argue for the systematic involvement of the parents or primary caretakers. This involvement should occur on at least two levels. First, parents should be assessed to determine if they themselves suffer from some form of emotional or mental disorder: those who are symptomatic should be treated. Second, parents should be engaged, whenever possible, as agents of change in the treatment of their own children. Such involvement may not only help to reestablish or strengthen attachment bonds, but may teach parents some skills to better manage their offspring in the future.

To meet the needs of the population of depressed children and adolescents, treatment goals may have to vary depending on the setting in which services can be delivered. As we discussed, although school-settings or community-based centers may allow easier access to more youths, certain youngsters may not be adequately served in such places. Possibly, multistage screening coupled with alternative forms of intervention could be implemented in nonclinical settings. However, even as more effective therapies and forms of service delivery are developed and possibly new theories of early-onset depression emerge, the best solution will require a better understanding of risk and predisposing factors, in order to make primary prevention possible.

ACKNOWLEDGEMENTS

Preparation of this chapter was supported in part by Grant MH33990 from the National Institute of Mental Health, Rockville, MD, USA. We thank Barbara Bridge for secretarial assistance.

REFERENCES

Altmann, E. O. & Gotlib, I. H. (1988). The social behavior of depressed children: An observational study. *Journal of Abnormal Child Psychology*, **16**, 29–44.

American Psychiatric Association. (1980). *Diagnostic and statistical manual of mental disorders* (3rd edn). Author, Washington, DC.

American Psychiatric Association. (1987). *Diagnostic and statistical manual of mental disorders* (3rd edn revised). Author, Washington, DC.

Anderson, J. C., Williams, S., McGee, R. & Silva, P. A. (1987). DSM–III disorders in preadolescent children. *Archives of General Psychiatry*, **44**, 69–76.

Angold, A. (1988). Childhood and adolescent depression. II. Research in clinical populations. *British Journal of Psychiatry*, **153**, 476–92.

Asarnow, J. R., Carlson, G. A. & Guthrie, D. (1987). Coping strategies, self-perceptions, hopelessness, and perceived family environments in depressed and suicidal children. *Journal of Consulting and Clinical Psychology*, **55**, 361–6.

Asarnow, J. R., Goldstein, M. J., Carlson, G. A. *et al.* (1988). Childhood-onset depressive disorders. A follow-up study of rates of rehospitalization and out-of-home placement among child psychiatric inpatients. *Journal of Affective Disorders*, **15**, 245–53.

Barbanel, L. (1982). Short-term dynamic therapies with children. In *The handbook of school psychology* (ed. C. R. Reynolds & T. B. Gutkin), pp. 554–569. John Wiley and Sons, New York.

Beardslee, W. R., Bemporad, J., Keller, M. B. & Klerman, G. L. (1983). Children of parents with major affective disorder: A review. *American Journal of Psychiatry*, **140**, 825–32.

Beck, A. T., Rush, A. J., Shaw, B. F. & Emery, G. (1979). *Cognitive therapy of depression*. Guilford Press, New York.

Bird, H. R., Canino, G., Rubio-Stipec, M. *et al.* (1988). Estimates of the prevalence of childhood maladjustment in a community survey in Puerto Rico. *Archives of General Psychiatry*, **45**, 1120–26.

Blechman, E. A., McEnroe, M. J., Carella, E. T. & Audette, D. P. (1986). Childhood competence and depression. *Journal of Abnormal Psychology*, **95**, 223–7.

Bowlby, J. (1973). *Separation: anxiety, and anger*. Basic Books, New York.

Bowlby, J. (1980). *Attachment and loss. Volume III: Loss*. Basic Books, New York.

Brent, D. A., Kolko, D. J., Boylan, B. *et al.* (1992). Cognitive therapy in depressed suicidal adolescents. Abstract presented at the 39th annual meeting of the American Academy of Child and Adolescent Psychiatry. *Scientific Proceedings*, **8**.

Burke, P., Meyer, V., Kocoshis, S. *et al.* (1989). Depression and anxiety in pediatric inflammatory bowel disease and cystic fibrosis. *Journal of the American Academy of Child and Adolescent Psychiatry*, **28**, 948–51.

Butler, L., Miezitis, S., Friedman, R. & Cole, E. (1980). The effect of two school-based intervention programs on depressive symptoms in pre-adolescents. *American Educational Research Journal*, **17**, 111–19.

Cantwell, D. P. & Baker, L. (1984). Parental mental illness and psychiatric disorders in 'at risk' children. *Journal of Clinical Psychiatry*, **45**, 503–7.

Cicchetti, D. & Schneider-Rosen, K. (1986). An organizational approach to childhood depression. In *Depression in young people: Developmental and clinical perspectives* (ed. M. Rutter, C. E. Izard, & P. B. Read), pp. 71–134. Guilford Press, New York.

Clarizio, H. F. (1985). Cognitive-behavioral treatment of childhood depression. *Psychology in the Schools*, **22**, 308–22.

Cole, D. A. & Rehm, L. P. (1986). Family interaction patterns and childhood depression. *Journal of Abnormal Child Psychology*, **14**, 297–314.

Connolly, J., Geller, S., Marton, P. & Kutcher, S. (1992). Peer responses to social interaction with depressed adolescents. *Journal of Clinical Child Psychology*, **21**, 365–70.

Costello, E. J., Costello, A. J., Edelbrock, C. *et al.* (1988). Psychiatric disorders in pediatric primary care. *Archives of General Psychiatry*, **45**, 1107–16.

Coyne, J. C., Burchill, S. A. L., & Stiles, W. B. (1991). An interactional perspective on depression. In *Handbook of social and clinical psychology: The health perspective* (ed. C. R. Snyder & D. R. Forsyth), pp. 327–349. Pergamon Press, New York.

Cummings, E. M. & Cicchetti, D. (1990). Toward a transactional model of relations between attachment and depression. In *Attachment in the preschool years. Theory, research, and intervention* (ed. M. T. Greenberg, D. Cicchetti & E. M. Cummings), pp. 339–372. The University of Chicago Press, Chicago.

Dadds, M. R., Schwartz, S. & Sanders, M. R. (1987). Marital discord and treatment outcome in behavioral treatment of child conduct disorders. *Journal of Consulting and Clinical Psychology*, **55**, 396–403.

Digdon, N. & Gotlib, I. H. (1985). Developmental considerations in the study of childhood depression. *Developmental Review*, **5**, 162–99.

DiGiuseppe, R. A. (1981). Cognitive therapy with children. In *New directions in cognitive therapy* (ed. G. Emery, S. D. Hollon, & R. C. Bedrosian), pp. 50–67. Guilford Press, New York.

DiGiuseppe, R. & Bernard, M. E. (1983). Principles of assessment and methods of treatment with children: Special considerations. In *Rational-emotive approaches to the problems of childhood* (ed. A. Ellis, & M. E. Bernard), pp. 45–88. Plenum Press, New York.

Elkind, D. (1967). Egocentrism in adolescence. *Child Development*, **38**, 1025–33.

Fauber, R. L. & Long, N. (1991). Children in context: The role of the family in child psychotherapy. *Journal of Consulting and Clinical Psychology*, **59**, 813–20.

Fine, S., Forth, A., Gilbert, M. & Haley, G. (1991). Group therapy for adolescent depressive disorder: A comparison of social skills and therapeutic support. *Journal of the American Academy of Child and Adolescent Psychiatry*, **30**, 79–85.

Garber, J., Kriss, M. R., Koch, M. & Lindholm, L. (1988). Recurrent depression in adolescents: A follow-up study. *Journal of the American Academy of Child and Adolescent Psychiatry*, **27**, 49–54.

Geller, B., Chestnut, E. C., Miller, M. D. *et al.* (1985). Preliminary data on DSM-III associated features of major depressive disorder in children and adolescents. *American Journal of Psychiatry*, **142**, 643–4.

Geller, B., Fox, L. W. & Fletcher, M. (1993). Effect of tricyclic antidepressants on switching to mania and on the onset of bipolarity in depressed 6- to 12-year-olds. *Journal of the American Academy of Child and Adolescent Psychiatry*, **32**, 43–50.

Goodyer, I. M., Wright, C. & Altham, P. M. E. (1989). Recent friendships in anxious and depressed school age children. *Psychological Medicine*, **19**, 165–74.

Hammen, C. & Zupan, B. A. (1984). Self-schemas, depression, and the processing of personal information in children. *Journal of Experimental Child Psychology*, **37**, 598–608.

Harder, D. W., Kokes, R. F., Fisher, L. & Strauss, J. S. (1980). Child competence and psychiatric risk. IV. Relationships of parent diagnostic classifications and parent psychopathology severity to child functioning. *Journal of Nervous and Mental Disease*, **168**, 343–7.

Harrington, R., Fudge, H., Rutter, M. *et al.* (1990). Adult outcomes of childhood and adolescent depression. I: Psychiatric status. *Archives of General Psychiatry*, **47**, 465–73.

Harter, S. (1990). Causes, correlates and the functional role of global self-worth: A life-span perspective. In *Competence considered* (ed. R. J. Sternberg & J. Kolligian), pp. 67–97. Yale University Press, New Haven, CT.

Hollon, S. D., Shelton, R. C. & Davis, D. D. (1993). Cognitive therapy for depression: Conceptual issues and clinical efficacy. *Journal of Consulting and Clinical Psychology*, **61**, 270–5.

Institute of Medicine. (1989). *Research on children and adolescents with mental, behavioral & developmental disorders: Mobilizing a national initiative.* National Academy Press, Washington, DC.

Jacobson, E. (1929). *Progressive relaxation.* University of Chicago Press, Chicago.

Kahn, J. S., Kehle, T. J., Jenson, W. R. & Clark, E. (1990). Comparison of cognitive-behavioral, relaxation, and self-modeling interventions for depression among middle-school students. *School Psychology Review*, **19**, 196–211.

Kashani, J. H., Carlson, G. A., Beck, N. C. *et al.* (1987). Depression, depressive symptoms, and depressed mood among a community sample of adolescents. *American Journal of Psychiatry*, **144**, 931–4.

Kaslow, N. J. & Rehm, L. P. (1991). Childhood depression. In *The practice of child therapy* (ed. T. R. Kratochwill & R. J. Morris), pp. 43–75. Pergamon Press, New York.

Kaslow, N. J., Rehm, L. P., & Siegel, A. W. (1984). Social-cognitive and cognitive correlates of depression in children. *Journal of Abnormal Child Psychology*, **12**, 605–20.

Kaslow, N. J., Tanenbaum, R. L., Abramson, L. Y. *et al.* (1983). Problem-solving deficits and depressive symptoms among children. *Journal of Abnormal Child Psychology*, **11**, 497–501.

Kazdin, A. E. (1990). Childhood depression. *Journal of Child Psychology and Psychiatry*, **31**, 121–60.

Kazdin, A. E. (1991). Effectiveness of psychotherapy with children and adolescents. *Journal of Consulting and Clinical Psychology*, **59**, 785–98.

Kazdin, A. E., Esveldt-Dawson, K., French, N. H. & Unis, A. S. (1987). Effects of parent management training and problem-solving skills training combined in the treatment of antisocial child behavior. *Journal of the American Academy of Child and Adolescent Psychiatry*, **26**, 416–24.

Keller, M. B., Beardslee, W., Lavori, P. W. *et al.* (1988). Course of major depression in non-referred adolescents: A retrospective study. *Journal of Affective Disorders*, **15**, 235–43.

Keller, M. B. & Shapiro, R. W. (1982). 'Double depression': Superimposition of acute depressive episodes on chronic depressive disorders. *American Journal of Psychiatry*, **139**, 438–42.

Kennedy, E., Spence, S. H. & Hensley, R. (1989). An examination of the relationship between childhood depression and social competence amongst primary school children. *Journal of Child Psychology and Psychiatry*, **30**, 561–73.

Kolvin, I., Garside, R. F., Nicol, A. R. *et al.* (1981). *Help starts here. The maladjusted child in the ordinary school.* Tavistock Publications, New York.

Kovacs M. (1986). A developmental perspective on methods and measures in the assessment of depressive disorders: The clinical interview. In *Depression in young people* (ed. M. Rutter, C. E. Izard & P. B. Read), pp. 435–465. Guilford Press, New York.

Kovacs, M., Akiskal, H. S., Gatsonis, C. & Parrone, P. L. (1994*a*). Childhood-onset dysthymic disorder: Clinical features and prospective naturalistic outcome. *Archives of General Psychiatry*, **51**, 365–74.

Kovacs, M. & Beck, A. T. (1978). Maladaptive cognitive structures in depression. *American Journal of Psychiatry*, **135**, 525–33.

Kovacs, M., Feinberg, T. L., Crouse-Novak, M. A. *et al* (1984*a*). Depressive disorders in childhood. I. A longitudinal prospective study of characteristics and recovery. *Archives of General Psychiatry*, **41**, 229–37.

Kovacs, M., Feinberg, T. L., Crouse-Novak, M. *et al*. (1984*b*). Depressive disorders in childhood. II. A longitudinal study of the risk for a subsequent major depression. *Archives of General Psychiatry*, **41**, 643–9.

Kovacs, M., Feinberg, T. L., Paulauskas, S. *et al*. (1985). Initial coping responses and psychosocial characteristics of children with insulin-dependent diabetes mellitus. *Journal of Pediatrics*, **106**, 827–34.

Kovacs, M. & Gatsonis, C. (1989). Stability and change in childhood-onset depressive disorders: Longitudinal course as a diagnostic validator. In *The validity of psychiatric diagnosis* (ed. L. N. Robins & J. E. Barrett), (pp. 57–75). Raven Press, New York.

Kovacs, M., Gatsonis, C., Voti, L. & Parrone, P. L. (1994*b*). Major depressive and dysthymic disorders in childhood: Clinical and sociodemographic factors related to recovery from the first episode. Unpublished manuscript, University of Pittsburgh.

Kovacs, M. & Goldston, D. (1991). Cognitive and social cognitive development of depressed children and adolescents. *Journal of the American Academy of Child and Adolescent Psychiatry*, **30**, 388–92.

Kovacs, M., Goldston, D. & Gatsonis, C. (1993). Suicidal behaviors and childhood-onset depressive disorders: A longitudinal investigation. *Journal of the American Academy of Child and Adolescent Psychiatry*, **32**, 8–20.

Kovacs, M. & Lohr, W. D. (1995). Research on psychotherapy with children and adolescents: An overview of evolving trends and current issues. *Journal of Abnormal Child Psychology,* **23**, 11–30.

Kovacs, M. & Paulauskas, S. L. (1984). Developmental stage and the expression of depressive disorders in children: An empirical analysis. In *Childhood Depression* (ed. D. Cicchetti & K. Schneider-Rosen). (New Directions for Child Development, no. 26) pp. 59–80. Josey-Bass, San Francisco.

Kovacs, M. & Paulauskas, S. (1986). The traditional psychotherapies. In *Psychopathological disorders of childhood* (ed. H. C. Quay & J. S. Werry), pp. 496–522. John Wiley & Sons, New York.

Leahy, R. (1988). Cognitive therapy of childhood depression. In *Cognitive development and child psychotherapy* (ed. S. R. Shirk), pp. 187–202. Plenum Press, New York.

Levitt, E. E., Beiser, H. R. & Robertson, R. E. (1959). A follow-up evaluation of cases treated at a community child guidance clinic. *American Journal of Orthopsychiatry*, **29**, 337–49.

Lewinsohn, P. M., Biglan, A. & Zeiss, A. M. (1976). Behavioral treatment of depression. In *The behavioral management of anxiety, depression and pain* (ed. P. O. Davidson), pp. 91–146. Brunner/Mazel, New York.

Lewinsohn, P. M., Clarke, G. N., Hops, H. & Andrews, J. (1990). Cognitive-behavioral treatment for depressed adolescents. *Behavior Therapy*, **21**, 385–401.

Lewinsohn, P. M., Rohde, P., Seeley, J. R, & Fischer, S. (1993). Age-cohort changes in the lifetime occurrence of depression and other mental disorders. *Journal of Abnormal Psychology*, **102**, 110–20.

Lewinsohn, P. M., Rohde, P., Seeley, J. R. & Hops, H. (1991). Comorbidity of unipolar depression: I. Major depression with dysthymia. *Journal of Abnormal Psychology*, **100**, 205–13.

Liddle, B. & Spence, S. H. (1990). Cognitive-behaviour therapy with depressed primary school children: A cautionary note. *Behavioural Psychotherapy*, **18**, 85–102.

McDermott, J. F. & Char W. F. (1984). Stage-related models of psychotherapy with children. *Journal of the American Academy of Child Psychiatry*, **23**, 537–43.

Melton, G. B. & Wilcox, B. L. (1989). Changes in family law and family life. *American Psychologist*, **44**, 1213–16.

Mitchell, J., McCauley, E., Burke, P. M. & Moss, S. J. (1988). Phenomenology of depression in children and adolescents. *Journal of the American Academy of Child and Adolescent Psychiatry*, **27**, 12–20.

Moreau, D., Mufson, L., Weissmam, M. M. & Klerman, G. L. (1991). Interpersonal psychotherapy for adolescent depression: Description of modification and preliminary application. *Journal of the American Academy of Child and Adolescent Psychiatry*, **30**, 642–51.

Neimark, E. D. (1975). Intellectual development during adolescence. In *Review of child development research, vol. 4* (ed. F. D. Horowitz, E. M. Hetherington, S. Scarr-Salapatek, & G. M. Siegel), pp. 541–594. University of Chicago Press, Chicago.

Nguyen, N., Scimeca, K., Mills, D. *et al.* (1992). Children's treatment manual: Time-limited supportive-expressive/psychoeducational group therapy for depressed children. Unpublished manuscript, The University of Oklahoma Health Sciences Center, Oklahoma City.

Office of Technology Assessment. (1987). *Children's mental health. Problems and services*. Duke University Press, Durham, NC.

Pruitt, D. B. & Kiser, L. J. (1991). Day treatment: Past, present, and future. In *Child and adolescent psychiatry. A comprehensive textbook* (ed. M. Lewis), pp. 878–889. Williams & Wilkins, Baltimore.

Puig-Antich, J., Goetz, D., Davies, M. *et al.* (1989). A controlled family history study of prepubertal major depressive disorder. *Archives of General Psychiatry*, **46**, 406–18.

Puig-Antich, J., Kaufman, J., Ryan, N. D. *et al.* (1993). The psychosocial functioning and family environment of depressed adolescents. *Journal of the American Academy of Child and Adolescent Psychiatry*, **32**, 244–53.

Puig-Antich, J., Lukens, E., Davies, M. *et al.* (1985a). Psychosocial functioning in prepubertal major depressive disorders. I. Interpersonal relationships during the depressive episode. *Archives of General Psychiatry*, **42**, 500–7.

Puig-Antich, J., Lukens, E., Davies, M. *et al.* (1985b). Psychosocial functioning in prepubertal major depressive disorders. II. Interpersonal relationships after sustained recovery from the affective episode. *Archives of General Psychiatry*, **42**, 511–17.

Rao, U., Weissman, M. M., Martin, J. A. & Hammond, R. W. (1993). Childhood depression and risk of suicide: A preliminary report of a longitudinal study. *Journal of the American Academy of Child and Adolescent Psychiatry*, **32**, 21–7.

Rehm, L. P. (1977). A self-control model of depression. *Behavior Therapy*, **8**, 787–804.

Reynolds, W. M. & Coats, K. I. (1986). A comparison of cognitive-behavioral therapy and relaxation training for the treatment of depression in adolescents. *Journal of Consulting and Clinical Psychology*, **54**, 653–60.

Rutter, M., Izard, C. E. & Read, P. B. (eds.). (1986). *Depression in young people. Developmental and clinical perspectives*. Guilford Press, New York.

Ryan, N. D., Puig-Antich, J., Ambrosini, P. *et al.* (1987). The clinical picture of major depression in children and adolescents. *Archives of General Psychiatry*, **44**, 854–61.

Seifer, R., Nurcombe, B., Scioli, A. & Grapentine, W. L. (1989). Is major depressive disorder in childhood a distinct diagnostic entity? *Journal of the American Academy of Child and Adolescent Psychiatry*, **28**, 935–41.

Seligman, M. E. P., Peterson, C., Kaslow, N. J. *et al.* (1984). Attributional style and depressive symptoms among children. *Journal of Abnormal Psychology*, **93**, 235–8.

Shaw, B. F. (1982). Stress and depression: A cognitive perspective. In *Psychological stress and psychopathology* (ed. R. W. J. Neufeld), pp. 125–146. McGraw-Hill, New York.

Shirk, S. (1988). Children's understanding of therapeutic interpretations. In *Cognitive development and child psychotherapy* (ed. S. R. Shirk), pp. 53–87. Plenum Press, New York.

Spitzer, R. L., Endicott, J. & Robins, E. (1978). Research diagnostic criteria: Rationale and reliability. *Archives of General Psychiatry*, **35**, 773–82.

Stark, K. D., Reynolds, W. M. & Kaslow, N. J. (1987). A comparison of the relative efficacy of self-control therapy and a behavioral problem-solving therapy for depression in children. *Journal of Abnormal Child Psychology*, **15**, 91–113.

Steinbrueck, S. M., Maxwell, S. E. & Howard, G. S. (1983). A meta-analysis of psychotherapy and drug therapy in the treatment of unipolar depression with adults. *Journal of Consulting and Clinical Psychology*, **51**, 856–63.

Strober, M. & Carlson, G. (1982). Bipolar illness in adolescents with major depression: Clinical, genetic, and psychopharmacologic predictors in a three- to four-year prospective follow-up investigation. *Archives of General Psychiatry*, **39**, 549–55.

Strober, M., Lampert, C., Schmidt, S. & Morrell, W. (1993). The course of major depressive disorder in adolescents: I: Recovery and risk of manic switching in a follow-up of psychotic and nonpsychotic subtypes. *Journal of the American Academy of Child and Adolescent Psychiatry*, **32**, 34–42.

Szajnberg, N. M. & Weiner, A. (1989). Children's conceptualization of their own psychiatric illness and hospitalization. *Child Psychiatry and Human Development*, **20**, 87–97.

Turner, S. M., Beidel, D. C. & Costello, A. (1987). Psychopathology in the offspring of anxiety disorders patients. *Journal of Consulting and Clinical Psychology*, **55**, 229–35.

Warner, V., Weissman, M. M., Fendrich, M. *et al.* (1992). The course of major depression in the offspring of depressed parents. Incidence, recurrence, and recovery. *Archives of General Psychiatry*, **49**, 795–801.

Wilkes, T. C. R. & Rush, A. J. (1988). Adaptations of cognitive therapy for depressed adolescents. *Journal of the American Academy of Child and Adolescent Psychiatry*, **27**, 381–6.

Woolston, J. L. (1991). Psychiatric inpatient services for children. In *Child and adolescent psychiatry: A comprehensive textbook* (ed. M. Lewis), pp. 890–894. Williams & Wilkins, Baltimore.

13

Longitudinal perspectives and affective disorder in children and adolescents

Richard Harrington and Panos Vostanis

INTRODUCTION

In all areas of medicine the natural history of a disorder is an important feature, both because it guides treatment and because it gives an estimate of prognosis. In psychiatry, where diagnoses must necessarily be based mostly on the clinical picture, the course of a disorder is also a major validating criterion. Indeed, the classification of the functional psychoses is dominated by Kraepelin's division into schizophrenia and manic-depression, which was mainly based on differences in prognosis. Kraepelin considered that a poor outcome with severe impairments was a defining characteristic of schizophrenia and separated it from manic-depression. However, although Kraepelin's dichotomy is sometimes taken to mean that affective disorders have a good outcome, this is only when they compared with schizophrenia. Recent research has shown that adult depressive disorders are in fact highly recurrent (Coryell & Winokur, 1992). As a result there has been increasing interest in long-term approaches to treatment (Guze & Freedman, 1991; Klerman & Weissman, 1992; Lancet, 1992), which are now being developed (Kupfer, 1992).

Longitudinal research on affective disorders arising in childhood and adolescence is at a much earlier stage, if only because of the relatively recent identification of depressive disorders in this age group using standardised methods of assessment. Nevertheless, over the past 10 years or so data have been accumulating steadily on the course and outcome of juvenile affective conditions. The main purpose of this chapter is to review these studies. The chapter begins with an outline of the methodological issues encountered in this area. Next, the research findings are reviewed. Finally, some prospects for future progress are outlined.

ISSUES

Samples

The first point to be made is that much of the research on the course of affective disorder in young people has been based on subjects who had been referred for treatment of active illness. Since many researchers were based at tertiary referral centres, the sample of patients available to them may have been biased towards cases with relatively recurrent and disabling illness. Indeed, research on the course of depressive disorder in non-referred samples (Keller et al., 1988; McGee & Williams, 1988; Hammen et al., 1990a; Warner et al., 1992; Cohen, Cohen & Brook, 1993a; Fleming, Boyle & Offord, 1993; Lewinsohn et al., 1993) has generally found less strong temporal continuities than found among clinical cases (Kovacs et al., 1984a,b; Zeitlin, 1986; Harrington et al., 1990).

Samples have also varied in the extent to which they may have been biased by non-participation and this problem has often been compounded by lack of information on non-respondents. In addition, very few studies mentioned sample size justification. This omission can be partly understood by the fact that in only one study (Kovacs et al., 1984a,b) was the original sample selected for the specific purpose of determining the outcome of depressive disorders. Multivariate within-group analyses that were performed in order to examine prognostic factors were often therefore based on inadequate sample sizes and few studies provided confidence limits to help in the interpretation of the results.

It is also notable that the studies were often heterogeneous in the age of the sample studied. In the study of Kovacs and her colleagues (Kovacs et al., 1984a), for example, the age at onset of depression ranged from 6 to 14 years, whereas in the study of King and Pittman (1970) the age range was 12 to 19 years.

Definitions and measurement

Definitions were also heterogenous. In particular, there have been marked inconsistencies in the use of the term 'recovery'. Thus, in some studies recovery included states in which there was still much psychopathology (Shain *et al.*, 1991), while in others recovery was defined as the absence of all but a few subclinical symptoms (Kovacs *et al.*, 1984*a*). One study defined recovery as 'no mental state abnormalities' whatsoever (Goodyer *et al.*, 1991).

The definition of 'relapse' has been more uniform, being defined in most studies as a return of symptoms satisfying the full syndrome criteria. However, a problem has arisen because relapse has usually been regarded as an all-or-nothing phenomenon. Few investigators have attempted to study what has happened *after the first relapse*. Indeed, it has now become commonplace to use methods of statistical analysis, namely survival methods, that *remove* cases from the analysis when the first relapse has occurred. The problem is that these methods make it difficult to distinguish between cases who had just one further episode and those who had multiple ones. This distinction is important not only because of the clinical implications (cases with multiple further episodes will of course require much more treatment) but because the risk mechanisms for long-term, recurrent depressive disorders may be different from those for less recurrent forms (Rodgers, 1990).

The problems of defining recovery and relapse are formidable enough, but a further problem in the interpretation of follow-ups of depressed children arises from the definition of 'caseness'. It is sometimes assumed that the diagnosis of major depression, which in most of the studies considered here was made using DSM-III criteria (American Psychiatric Association, 1980), will result in a homogeneous group of disorders. Manifestly it does not. The heterogeneity of the diagnosis is perhaps most obvious when the difference between bipolar and non-bipolar major depressions is considered. Thus, although in adults the phenomenology of the two types of depression is very similar (Brockington *et al.*, 1982), they differ markedly in the extent to which genetic influences are involved (McGuffin & Katz, 1986). It would not be surprising, therefore, to find that the prognosis also differed. More importantly, since the DSM-III diagnosis of major depression had no requirement about the level of social impairment (it was based solely on the number and duration of symptoms) it is likely that cases included in follow-ups were very heterogeneous with regard to severity of illness. We shall see later that social impairment is itself a strong predictor of subsequent outcome.

It must also be remembered that the concept of disorder categories that 'recover' may itself be misconceived. Instead, as many psychologists have argued, it could be that depressive disorder is best thought of as the extreme end of an affective continuum. According to this viewpoint, there is no qualitative discontinuity between the states of 'disorder' and 'recovery', but rather quantitative variations along a dimension. Surprisingly, there has been no research comparing the validity of dimensional and categorical approaches to defining recovery and/or relapse of juvenile affective conditions. Such research is much needed as it is by no means self-evident which time point should be used to label the onset or offset of the disorder. Indeed, relapse of major depression in children has been found in many cases to be superimposed on a prolonged period of chronic dysthymia (Kovacs et al., 1984b). Should the point of relapse be regarded as the first time the low grade symptoms appeared, the first appearance of major depressive symptoms, the first point that the diagnostic criteria for major depression were met, or the time when there was first social impairment? Of course, the precise timing of the relapse may not matter if it is being treated dimensionally. However, accurate timing becomes crucial when longitudinal designs are being used to study *temporal* associations between risk factors and categorical states, such as the timing of episodes of maternal and child depression (Hammen, Burge & Adrian, 1991).

Much of the research reviewed in this chapter has used standardised instruments to assess depression. The use of such instruments has led to great advances in the field, but there are many unresolved difficulties. For instance, there is often only moderate agreement between the child and the parent on the presence of disorder, and child and parent evaluations of recovery are also frequently discrepant (Goodyer et al., 1991). It is not at all clear how these differences should be handled when the results are analysed and reported.

General issues in longitudinal research

Investigators of the outcome of depression in young people have had to contend not only with these complex problems of definition, but also with the other difficulties that are encountered generally by longitudinal researchers. In particular, long interval follow-ups have had to deal with the fact that methods and theoretical concerns regarding depression in children have changed a great deal over the past 20 years. So, for example, in our adult follow-up of depressed children (Harrington et al., 1990) we had to rely initially on measures and concepts of depression that were devised many years ago (Pearce, 1974, 1978). In addition, types of treatments and rates of possible precipitating and maintaining factors (e.g. unemployment, divorce) for depression have altered greatly since the first follow-ups of depressed children were published. These kinds of effects, commonly known as **period effects**, mean that it cannot automatically be assumed that the course of depression will be the same now as it was 25 years ago.

A related issue concerns changes in affective phenomena that occur with age, or **ageing effects**. There has, for instance, been much debate in the literature on whether prepubertal major depression shows the same continuity with depression in adult life as depressions with an onset during or after puberty. The question seems simple enough, but there are in fact major difficulties in ensuring that the measures at different ages are comparable and in using comparable periods of follow-up. Thus, in order to equate the two disorders it would obviously be desirable that they were followed up for equal time periods. However, since most follow-ups take place at a single time point this will often mean that the outcomes were assessed at different ages.

Straightforward longitudinal studies cannot disentangle ageing and period effects. Depressed children aged 8 in 1990 may differ from the same people age 15 in 1997 because of changes over the time period as well as in age.

Statistical analysis

The choice of statistical methods that have been used in the studies also requires brief comment. One issue is whether or not depression was regarded as a categorical or dimensional variable. In most studies depression was analysed as a time-limited categorical variable, using techniques such as survival analysis. Such procedures provide a natural way of dealing with what are called 'censored' observations, the occurrence of individuals who have not yet exhibited the event of interest but for whom it might yet occur. However, in other studies depression was also analysed as a continuous variable, even when categorical measures of depressive disorder were available (Hammen, Adrian & Hiroto, 1988; McGee & Williams, 1988). These different methods of analysis can sometimes lead to different results (Brown, Harris & Lemyre, 1991).

A further statistical consideration is that the impression given of the strength of continuity over time depends greatly on the method of analysis employed (Rutter, 1977) and on how the results are interpreted. It is often assumed that the finding of a low correlation means that there is little continuity. However, it must be remembered that correlations are really only an index of the proportion of variance explained and that the size of the correlation will therefore depend greatly on the base rate of the disorder in question. It is perfectly possible for an independent variable to have a substantial effect but to have only a modest correlation with the criterion. Consider, for example, our follow-up of depressed children into adulthood (Harrington *et al.*, 1990). Depression in childhood showed a relatively low correlation with major depression in adult life ($\emptyset = 0.29$). Yet, the relative risk of developing major depression in adulthood was nearly six fold higher for the childhood depressed group compared with the control group!

Confounding variables

Longitudinal research provides a powerful way of approaching the problem of whether or not a variable is simply a risk indicator or whether it represents a risk mechanism. However, every student is aware that just because variable A precedes variable B does not necessarily mean that A causes B. Thus, we shall see later that many studies showed that depression in young people was associated with an increased risk of subsequent depression, but it may not be the case that this risk stemmed specifically from the earlier depression. In fact, it is common for affective disorders among young people to be associated with other psychiatric conditions, such as conduct disorder and anxiety (Caron & Rutter, 1991; Harrington *et al.*, 1991; Brady & Kendall, 1992). These associated factors, rather than the depression, may constitute the main psychiatric risk for subsequent difficulties. It was very unusual for follow-ups of depressed children to have taken into account comorbidity, and in many studies it was not even documented.

Considerations of associated *disorders* by no means exhausts the possibilities of confounding variables. Depression in young people is also associated with much impairment of social functioning, including problems in interpersonal relationships (Puig-Antich *et al.*, 1985a). We need, therefore, to consider the possibility that predictors such as depression may be epiphenomena or markers of the severity of disorder, rather than posing a specific psychiatric risk. In other words, it could be that childhood depression predicts adolescent depression because it is a marker of severe childhood psychosocial problems, not because there is direct continuity. The continuity may in fact stem from deficiencies in interpersonal relationships. Again, very few studies have attempted to tackle this issue.

CONTINUITY AND RECURRENCE

Risk of subsequent episodes of depression

For all these reasons, it is necessary to be cautious in interpreting the follow-ups published so far. Nevertheless, one conclusion seems reasonably secure: *young people diagnosed as depressed are at increased risk of subsequent episodes of depression.* Thus, many early uncontrolled studies reported that children who had one episode of depression were at risk of another (Poznanski, Kraheneuhl & Zrull, 1976; Cantwell, 1983; Eastgate & Gilmour, 1984). More recently, several controlled studies have reported that by comparison with non-depressed subjects, young people diagnosed as depressed were at increased risk of further episodes of depression. Thus, two studies of pre-adolescent children meeting DSM-III criteria for depression showed that depression in childhood often recurred (Kovacs et al., 1984b; McGee & Williams, 1988). For example, Kovacs and colleagues (1984b), undertook a systematic follow-up of child patients with a major depressive disorder, a dysthymic disorder, an adjustment disorder with depressed mood, and some other psychiatric disorder. The development of subsequent episodes of depression was virtually confined to children with major depressive disorders and dysthymic disorders. Thus, within the first year at risk, 26% of children who had recovered from major depression had had another episode; by 2 years this figure had risen to 40%; and by 5 years the cohort ran a 72% risk of another episode! Similarly, Asarnow and co-workers (1988) found that children who had been hospitalised with major depression were at increased risk of re-hospitalisation because of suicidal behaviour or increasing depression. Within a little less than 2 years 45% were re-hospitalised, a rate that was not significantly different from that found for children with schizophrenia spectrum disorders.

Two studies have examined recurrence rates of major depression in the children of depressed parents (Hammen et al., 1990a; Warner et al., 1992). As might be expected, the rate of recurrence was a little lower than in studies of referred samples (23 and 16%, over 2 and 3 years respectively). However, in both studies the risk of subsequent depressive disorder in depressed cases exceeded that found in non-depressed cases.

Surveys of community samples have generally confirmed that depressive disorders among young people tend to be recurrent (McGee & Williams, 1988; Fleming *et al.* 1993; Lewinsohn *et al.*, 1993). For instance, Lewinsohn *et al.* (1993) found that the 1-year relapse rate for unipolar depression (18.4%) was much higher than the relapse rate found in most other disorders. Only one study has failed to find significant continuity for depressive disorder (Cohen *et al.*, 1993*a*), but confidence in this study's diagnostic methods is limited by the fact that it reported an equal sex ratio for depressive disorder in early adulthood (Cohen *et al.*, 1993*b*). This finding runs counter to the results of many other investigations.

Investigators of the short-term stability of questionnaire ratings of depressive *symptoms* in community samples of young people have also found significant correlations over time (Garrison *et al.*, 1990; Larsson *et al.*, 1991; Edelsohn *et al.*, 1992; Stanger, McConaughy & Achenbach, 1992). Larsson *et al.* (1991), for instance, found that the correlation over a 4 to 6-week period on the Beck Depression Inventory was 0.66. Garrison *et al.* (1990) reported that the stability of adolescents' self-reports of depression was 0.53 at 1 year and, as described earlier, 0.36 at 2 years after the initial assessment.

Adult outcomes

None of these studies has yet extended beyond mid-adolescence, but a similarly high rate of subsequent psychiatric morbidity has been reported in follow-up studies of depressed adolescents that have extended into late adolescence or early adult life (Strober & Carlson, 1982; Kandel & Davies, 1986; Garber *et al.*, 1988). These studies have suggested both that self-ratings of depression in adolescent community samples predict similar problems in early adulthood (Kandel & Davies, 1986) and that adolescent patients with depressive disorders are at increased risk of subsequent major affective disturbance (Strober & Carlson, 1982; Garber *et al.*, 1988). Although the findings of these studies were limited by issues such as the uncertainty regarding the connection between depression questionnaire scores and clinical depressive disorder (Kandel & Davies, 1986) and high rates of sample attrition

(Garber *et al.*, 1988), they clearly suggest that adolescents with depression are at increased risk of depression in early adult life.

Moving still further into adult life, Harrington *et al.* (1990) followed up 63 depressed children and adolescents, on average 18 years after their initial contact. The depressed group had a substantially greater risk of depression after the age of 17 years than a control group who had been matched on a large number of variables, including non-depressive symptoms and measures of social impairment. This increased risk was maintained well into adulthood and was associated with significantly increased rates of attending psychiatric services and of using medication as compared to the controls. Depressed children were no more likely than the control children to suffer non-depressive disorders in adulthood, suggesting that the risk for adult depression was specific and unrelated to comorbidity with other psychiatric problems.

Subsequent social impairment

There are a number of reasons for thinking that early-onset depressive disorder might not only predict further episodes of depression, but also could be associated with effects on social and cognitive functioning. Thus, depression in young people is frequently accompanied by social withdrawal and irritability, and so depressed youngsters may find it more difficult to establish and maintain social relationships. In addition, symptoms such as loss of concentration and psychomotor retardation may interfere with the process of learning. This in turn might lead to low self-esteem and so on to further academic failure. Kovacs & Goldston (1991) pointed out that young people suffering from major depression are impaired for a significant proportion of the life span and they are handicapped at a time when learning takes place rapidly. Perhaps, then, they will eventually show cognitive as well as social delays.

Several studies have examined the social outcomes of depressed young people. Puig-Antich and his colleagues (Puig-Antich *et al.*, 1985*a,b*) found that impairment of peer relationships persisted several months after recovery from depression. In the longer term, Kandel & Davies (1986) reported that self-ratings of dysphoria in adolescence were associated with heavy cigarette smoking, greater involvement in delinquent activities, and impairment of intimate relationships as young adults. Garber *et al.* (1988) found that depressed adolescent in-patients reported more marital and relationship problems when they were followed up 8 years after discharge than non-depressed psychiatric control subjects.

These findings have important theoretical as well as clinical implications since they suggest that the social isolation and lack of a supporting relationship that have been found in cross-sectional studies of adult depression (Brown & Harris, 1978) may reflect social selection as much as social causation (Kandel & Davies, 1986). However, none of these studies excluded the effects that childhood conduct problems, which are commonly associated with adolescent depression, could have on these outcomes. Harrington *et al.* (1991) found that juvenile depression seemed to have little direct impact on social functioning in adulthood, whereas comorbid conduct disorder was a strong predictor of subsequent social maladjustment. The implication is that it is important to differentiate the course of depressive disorder from the course of other, comorbid disorders.

Subsequent suicidality

The most serious complication of depression is of course suicide. Depressed young people very commonly have suicidal thoughts and some of them make suicidal attempts (Andrews & Lewinsohn, 1992). Ryan *et al.* (1987), for instance, found that about 60% of children and adolescents with major depression had suicidal ideation. Mitchell *et al.* (1988) reported that 67% of depressed young people had suicidal thoughts, and nearly 40% had made a suicide attempt. Conversely, it seems that suicidal children are at increased risk of depression. For example, Pfeffer *et al.* (1991) found that young people who had attempted suicide were ten fold more likely to have a mood disorder during the 6- to 8-year follow-up period than young people who had not made an attempt.

Myers *et al.* (1991) examined the risk factors for suicidality in the depressed sample described by Mitchell *et al.* (1988). Three variables predicted later suicidality: severity of initial suicidality, anger, and age. Kienhorst *et al.* (1991) also found that previous suicidality was a predictor of subsequent attempts, as were features of the initial depression, a broken home, and feelings of hopelessness. In a review of this topic, Pfeffer (1992) found that the risk indicators for suicidal attempts among depressed young people included previous suicidality, suicidal ideation, hopelessness, comorbid problems such as substance abuse and anger, easy access to the method, and lack of social support. The importance of comorbidity with conduct disturbance and/or substance abuse is underlined by the findings of Kovacs, Goldston & Gatsonis (1993). They reported that the presence of these problems more than doubled the risk of suicide attempts among depressed child patients.

Relatively little is known about the risk of completed suicide in depressed young people. In our follow-up of 80 depressed probands (Harrington *et al.*, 1990) all three deaths in adulthood were due to 'unnatural causes', of which two were definite suicides. Although no statistical weight can be attached to these small numbers, they are clearly far in excess of those expected in the general population of young adults. Similarly, in a preliminary communication from a longitudinal study of the depressed children and adolescents initially studied by Puig-Antich and his group, Rao *et al.* (1993) reported that seven (4.4%) had committed suicide. There were no suicides in the psychiatric control group.

Another way of looking at the relationship between depression and suicide is through 'psychological autopsy' studies of young people who have killed themselves. Such studies involve the interviewing of relatives and the collection of data from a variety of other sources in order to make a diagnostic assessment on the suicide victim. Several recent psychological autopsy studies of suicide in young people found high rates of affective disorders (Brent *et al.*, 1988; Shaffer, 1988; Marttunen *et al.*, 1991). It is, however, important to note that other mental disorders may also be relevant in suicide. For instance, Marttunen *et al.* (1991) found that nearly one-fifth of suicides aged between 13 and 19 years had a conduct disorder or anti-social personality, and that a quarter abused alcohol or drugs. Brent *et al.* (1990) found that among those depressed patients who had attempted suicide, the degree of intent was associated with conduct disorder and comorbid substance abuse. Perhaps, then, it is the combination of depression and certain personality characteristics, such as aggression or the propensity to take risks, that is especially likely to lead to suicide in young people. There seems to be an important relationship between comorbid disorders and depressive disorders with respect to suicidal risk.

Predictors of continuity of depression

The **characteristics of the index depressive episode** appear to be important to the extent that children with DSM-III 'double depression' (major depression and dysthymic disorder) have a worse short-term outcome than children with major depression alone (Kovacs *et al.*, 1984*b*;

321

Asarnow *et al.*, 1988; Warner *et al.*, 1992). Continuity to adulthood seems best predicted by a severe 'adult-like' depressive presentation and, interestingly, by the absence of conduct disorder (Harrington *et al.*, 1990, 1991). The latter finding was all the more striking because children with conduct disorder had high rates of many kinds of adversity in adulthood, such as marital problems and trouble with the police. However, neither anxiety disorder nor conduct disorder appear to influence the short-term risk of relapse of a depressive syndrome (Kovacs *et al.*, 1988, 1989). Two studies have found that older depressed children had a worse prognosis than younger depressed children (Kovacs *et al.*, 1989; Harrington *et al.*, 1990).

The importance of **family variables** as predictors of the outcome of early-onset depressive disorders has been shown by data from several different types of investigations. Thus, many high risk studies of the children of depressed parents have found an increased risk of affective disorders among the offspring (for example, Beardslee *et al.*, 1983; Grigoroiu-Serbanescu *et al.*, 1991; Radke-Yarrow *et al.*, 1992; Weissman *et al.*, 1992). Similarly, two studies have reported that a family history of mental illness was itself a predictor of recurrence within samples of adolescents with affective conditions (King & Pittman, 1970; Strober & Carlson, 1982).

The mechanisms underlying this predictive power are not known. The finding of specific familial links between depression in children and depression in their parents (Harrington *et al.*, 1993) supports the idea of genetically mediated mechanisms. Indeed, there is no doubt that there is a substantial genetic component to the severe bipolar disorders of adults (McGuffin & Katz, 1986) and it seems that earlier age of onset is associated with an increased familial loading for depression (Strober, 1992a).

However, the relevance of environmental links has also been demonstrated in numerous cross-sectional studies (Rutter, 1990). Thus, for example, it seems that children of unipolar depressed mothers actually have a *higher* risk of depression than children from bipolar depressed mothers (Hammen *et al.*, 1990a; Radke-Yarrow *et al.*, 1992), a finding that runs counter to the genetic prediction that risk should be higher in bipolar families. Moreover, longitudinal investigations have underscored the importance of environmental factors in mediating continuities. Thus, Hammen *et al.* (1991) found a close *temporal* relationship between depression in parents and their offspring. Asarnow *et al.* (1993) found that child in-patients with depressive disorders who returned to homes where the parents had high levels of expressed emotion (EE) had a much higher risk of relapse than depressed patients who returned to low EE homes.

Several studies have suggested that other ongoing *adversities*, such as problems in peer relationships (Goodyer *et al.*, 1991) and/or adverse life events (Garrison *et al.*, 1990; Burge & Hammen, 1991) predict continuity. It is possible that there is an interaction between family variables and these adversities such that one increases the risk of the other. Thus, Goodyer *et al.* (1993) reported that the families of depressed girls seemed to become life event prone as a result of parental psychopathology. Perhaps, then, young people become depressed when depressed parents are no longer able to protect them from adversity.

Mechanisms involved in continuity and recurrence

What processes could underpin these strong continuities over time? The first thing to say here is that the strength and specificity of the continuities clearly support the idea that there may be *direct* persistence of the initial disorder. For example, perhaps individuals are changed in one way or another by the first episode so that they become more vulnerable to subsequent ones. This notion, often referred to as '*scarring*', has attracted a good deal of attention from investigators of the neurobiological (Post, 1992) and psychological (Rohde, Lewinsohn & Seeley, 1990) processes that may be involved in the relapsing and remitting course of depression in adults. The idea of scarring has yet to be systematically evaluated in depressions occurring in children and adolescents. It is important because it suggests that much greater attention should be paid to the recognition and treatment of the *first episode* of depression. Since late adolescence is a common period for the onset of adult depressive disorders (Burke *et al.*, 1990) the implication is that child and adolescent psychiatry could have an important part to play in the prevention of depression in adulthood. Indeed, there are plenty of developmental examples of the ways in which early disorders that are not managed appropriately can lead to permanent changes in both the biology of individuals and in their psychosocial functioning (Wolkind & Rutter, 1985).

Scarring should be distinguished from the related concept of **vulnerability**, in which the predisposition to depression *precedes* the first episode. There are a large number of *psychological* theories about the factors that may make some individuals vulnerable to depression, but perhaps the most influential among investigators of childhood depression have been the so-called 'cognitive theories' of depression. These are dealt with in other parts of this book and so they need not be considered in detail here. For the purposes of this chapter, however, it is worth noting that negative cognitions such as self criticism can be remarkably stable (Koestner, Zuroff & Powers, 1991) and several longitudinal studies have shown that they may precede depressive *symptoms* in young people (Seligman & Peterson, 1986; Reinherz *et al.*, 1989; Nolen-Hoeksema, Girgus & Seligman, 1992). However, different results have been obtained when depressive *disorders* have been studied. Thus, in an investigation that included the offspring of women with affective disorders, Hammen *et al.* (1988) found that depression at follow-up was best predicted by initial symptoms and life events but not by negative attributions. Similarly, Asarnow and Bates (1988) found that in-patient children whose depressive disorder had remitted did not show negative attributional patterns. These findings suggest that negative attributional style may be a state-dependent symptom of depressive disorder rather than a trait-like predisposition.

The search for evidence of **biological traits** has up to now been focused almost exclusively on the kinds of markers that have been studied in depressed adults, such as the Dexamethasone Suppression Test (Casat & Powell, 1988), the Thyroid Releasing Hormone Test (Kutcher *et al.*, 1991), and sleep encephalography (Emslie *et al.*, 1990; Kutcher *et al.*, 1992). There have, however, been difficulties in replicating positive findings obtained with these measures (see Ferguson & Bawden, 1988; Goetz *et al.*, 1991). Moreover, as developmentalists we must remember that continuities over time frequently do not stem from the unchanging persistence of 'trait-like' dispositions. It could be that the observed continuities for depression stem as much from continuity in *process*, as occurs for example in the concept of **social competence**. The idea here is that competence in one developmental period will exert a positive influence towards achieving competence in the next and, conversely, early incompetence will predispose to later maladaptation. So, continuity of depression may occur because at each developmental level the individual lacks the social and emotional competencies that are important to achieving adaptation (Sroufe, 1979; Cicchetti & Schneider-Rosen, 1986).

Environmentally mediated mechanisms could also be relevant. Perhaps, for instance, continuity arises because there is **constancy of adverse family environments**. There is no doubt that some kinds of family adversity, such as marital discord, can be highly persistent (Richman,

Stevenson & Graham, 1982; Rutter & Quinton, 1984) and there is growing evidence of the relevance of these factors to continuities of depressive disorders in young people (Hammen, 1991; Asarnow et al., 1993; Warner et al., 1992). Alternatively, there may be stability because individuals *select adverse environments.* Brown, Harris & Bifulco (1986) found that in some women early lack of care was linked to early pregnancy and thence to depression. Early adverse experiences seemed to make it more likely that young people would act in ways that resulted in their selecting adverse environments, and so increase their risk of depression. In our research (Harrington et al., 1991), however, children with depression and conduct disorder, who had high rates of social adversity in adulthood (such as marital problems and lack of friendships) had relatively low levels of major depression in adult life.

In summary, the findings thus far do not give rise to any overarching conclusion on the processes involved in the continuities of juvenile depressive disorders. If the available evidence is put together, it seems probable that early onset depression is associated with subsequent depression through several different mechanisms, though knowledge on their relative importance is lacking. Clearly, the strength and specificity of the links point to a relatively uninterrupted form of continuity, as would occur in the direct persistence of the initial disorder. There appears to be a substantial self-perpetuating quality to juvenile depressive disorders, with severe 'typical' depressions having the strongest continuity. Nevertheless, even these kinds of disorders do seem to remain susceptible to environmental influences, particularly those that occur within families. Probably there are circular processes in which the effects of social experiences change the child's views of him/herself and the world, which in turn leads to depression, which then alters the child's experiences of the environment.

DISCONTINUITY AND RECOVERY

Developmental discontinuities

The findings thus far suggest that juvenile depressive disorders show substantial continuities over time. Nevertheless, the available data also suggest that many depressed young people will *not* go on to have another episode, and so it is important to consider briefly the reasons for *discontinuity*. There is a surprising lack of knowledge on this issue, but some limited evidence is available.

The first point to make is that there may be *developmental* differences in the continuity of depressive disorders. Interest in the possibility of such differences has been increased by the finding of marked age differences in the prevalence of affective phenomena such as depression, suicide and attempted suicide (Harrington, 1992, 1994). Thus, for example, it seems that depressive disorders show an increase in frequency during early adolescence (Fleming, Offord & Boyle, 1989; Velez, Johnson & Cohen, 1989; McGee *et al.*, 1992). The reasons for these age trends are still unclear (Rutter, 1991), but there is some evidence that they are accompanied by developmental differences in *continuity*. Thus, in our child to adult follow-up of depressed young people, continuity to major depression in adulthood was significantly stronger in pubescent/postpubertal depressed probands than in prepubertal depressed subjects. All five cases of bipolar disorder in adulthood occurred in the postpubertal group. Similarly, Kovacs *et al.* (1989) reported that among cases who had recovered from their index episode of major depression, older children would go into a new episode faster than younger ones.

What do these differences mean? Clearly, the association with age and/or puberty suggests that maturational factors could play an important part. For example, perhaps the relative cognitive immaturity of younger children protects them from the development of cognitive 'scars' arising from an episode of depression. Or, it may be that the massive changes in sex hormone production that occur around the time of puberty are involved. However, it would be unwise to dismiss the effects of environment altogether. After all, puberty is associated not only with maturational changes but also with marked changes in social/family environment (Buchanan, Eccles & Becker, 1992). Indeed, we shall see in the next section that environmental factors could play an important part in explaining discontinuities and there may be age differences in some of the social adversities that precipitate and/or maintain depression.

Recovery from an episode of depression

It is important to distinguish between long-term continuities/discontinuities in the course of depressive disorders and the prognosis for the index attack. Indeed, the available data suggest that the majority of children with major depression will recover within 2 years. For example, Kovacs *et al.* (1984a) reported that the cumulative probability of recovery from major depression by one year after onset was 74% and by 2 years was 92%. The median time to recovery was about 28 weeks. This study included many subjects who had previous emotional-behavioural problems and some form of treatment, and might therefore have been biased towards the most severe cases. However, very similar results were reported by Keller *et al.* (1988) in a retrospective study of recovery from first episode of major depression in young people who had mostly not received treatment (Keller *et al.*, 1991), and by Warner *et al.* (1992) in a study of the children of depressed parents. The probability of recovery for adolescent in-patients with major depression also appears to be about 90% by 2 years (Strober *et al.*, 1993), though those with long-standing depressions seem to recover less quickly than those whose presentation was acute (Shain *et al.*, 1991).

Although these results clearly provide some grounds for optimism regarding the short-term outcome of early-onset depressions, it is worth noting that the speed of recovery found in the study of Strober *et al.* appeared to be slower than that reported in comparable studies of depressed adults (see Strober *et al.*, 1992). Moreover, both Kovacs *et al.* (1984*a*) and Warner *et al.* (1992) reported that an earlier age at onset predicted a longer time to recovery. In addition, it seems that a significant proportion of cases will become 'chronic' to the extent that recovery takes many months or even years. Thus, Shain *et al.* (1991) found that about 10% of severe cases of adolescent-onset depression became 'chronic' to the extent that they had not recovered by 1 year. Ryan *et al.* (1987) estimated that nearly one half of depressed children and adolescents in their clinical sample had been 'ill' for over 2 years. Clearly, all these findings challenge the common belief that children have only transient depressions.

How do young people recover from an episode of depression? The paucity of systematic studies among the young makes it impossible to draw firm conclusions about this issue. Indeed, even the adult literature is sparse and has for the most part been concerned with recovery in the context of treatment trials rather than with the process itself. It has provided, however, a number of pointers about the mechanisms that could be involved in young people. It may be, for instance, that environmental circumstances change. For example, perhaps there is a *reduction in adversity*. Alternatively, it could be that some kind of *positive event* needs to occur before depression will abate (see, for example, Needles & Abramson, 1990; Brown, Lemyre & Bifulco, 1992).

There are also a number of *biological explanations* for the periodicity of affective disorders. It could be, for instance, that the physiological systems involved in recurrent affective conditions oscillate 'endogenously'. The recovery phase occurs because homeostatic mechanisms come into force in order to correct underlying biochemical imbalances. Or, it might be that there is some kind of external photic or temperature-related seasonal cue that leads to cycling. Recovery occurs when the external biological cue has ceased.

Treatment may also influence recovery from depression. There is now impressive evidence from numerous controlled trials that tricyclic antidepressants are superior to placebo in alleviating the symptoms of depressive disorders in adults (Paykel, 1989). However, it remains to be seen whether such treatments will be effective in juvenile major depression. The published trials have failed so far to show any significant benefits of medication over placebo (Harrington, 1992*b*).

COURSE OF EARLY ONSET BIPOLAR DISORDERS

Bipolar disorder in adults is usually recurrent, though there is marked individual variability in episode duration and cycle length (Goodwin & Jamison, 1984). The interval between attacks shows a tendency to shorten as the disorder progresses (Goodwin & Jamison, 1984) and in about 10% of cases rapid cycling (four or more affective episodes per year) occurs (Bauer & Whybrow, 1991).

Unfortunately, little is known about the course of bipolar disorder in adolescents (Strober, 1992*b*). The available data suggest that the prognosis is probably no better than that of cases arising later in life (Carlson, Davenport & Jamison, 1977). However, Werry, McClellan & Chard (1991) reported that the outcome of bipolar disorder seemed to be better than early onset schizophrenia. In this study the strongest predictor of future functioning was premorbid adjustment (Werry & McClellan, 1992).

A proportion of adolescent patients who present with depression will go on to develop mania. Strober *et al.* (1992) found that five out of 58 adolescents with major depression developed manic or hypomanic episodes during the 24-month follow-up period. In line with the findings from other follow-up studies (Akiskal *et al.*, 1983) all of these cases had psychotic features during their depressive episode.

PROSPECTS

Future directions for longitudinal research into depression among young people have been touched on at various points in this chapter. Too many questions remain for it to be helpful to review them all comprehensively. In conclusion, therefore, we shall try to highlight just a few of the key unresolved issues and outline some of the research avenues that seem to be a priority.

Since *long-interval* follow-up research on juvenile depressive disorders is still at an early stage, perhaps the most immediately pressing need is for more studies designed to replicate the main findings of the research reviewed here. Thus, it should be possible within the next few years to mount long-term prospective follow-ups of children diagnosed as depressed using standardised interviews and present-day diagnostic criteria. Indeed, several ongoing research programmes have systematic data on depressed children who were first seen in the late 1970s and early 1980s. New generations of child to adult longitudinal studies could be based on these children.

Such studies will be relatively expensive but they need to be undertaken. Their starting point should be a reconsideration of some of the important issues that have been raised by the existing studies, such as the strength of the links between adolescent and adult depressions and the impact of comorbidity on prognosis. It will be important to control for symptomatology other than depression, as it is becoming clear that the effects of early depression need to be distinguished from the effects of comorbid difficulties. It will also be necessary to use larger samples, especially when subgroups are the focus of interest. Two subgroups stand out as particularly in need of further investigation: (1) children with depression and conduct disorder, and (2) prepubertal depressed children. Children with depression and conduct disorder need to be studied further because of the uncertainties regarding the meaning of the overlap between these two conditions. Prepubertal depressed children are of interest not only in their own right but also because of the provocative finding from our research that they seem to differ from depressed adolescents in regard to adult prognosis (Harrington *et al.*, 1990).

There is, however, also a need for further *short interval* follow-ups with a duration of no more than a year or two. Such studies are relatively inexpensive and could provide important clues about mediating mechanisms. Indeed, for many purposes short-interval longitudinal studies are preferable to long-interval ones. They are especially useful when it is necessary to date risk factors and episodes of depression accurately. *Multiple cohort longitudinal* designs would seem to be a particularly promising way of investigating juvenile depressive disorders. As was described earlier, there is now good evidence that depression increases in prevalence during early adolescence, but the reasons for these age trends remain poorly understood. So, short interval longitudinal studies covering some of the key transitions (such as puberty or the transition to secondary school) could tell us much about the aetiology of depression at all ages. For example, they could be used to study within-individual developmental sequences. Of course, there are a large number of possible mechanisms that could explain these age trends and so it will be necessary to study many potential aetiological factors, including hormones, social networks, depressive cognitions/self-esteem and adversities of one kind or another. It is not possible to discuss all of these here. The important point is that the age changes in depression that occur during adolescence constitute an important natural experiment with which to test ideas about the processes that lead to the disorder.

The recurrent nature of early-onset depressive disorders also underlines the need to move beyond the study of the acute precipitants of one episode in order to study adversities as they occur *over time*. In particular, as Rutter and Sandberg (1992) pointed out, we need to know where the acute adversities that are highly prevalent in the lives of depressed children (Harrington *et al.*, 1993) come from. In a few children, depression occurs in response to acts of fate such as disasters. However, a glance through lists of adverse events that have been studied in depressed young people (e.g., de Wilde *et al.*, 1992) shows that very few of them can be regarded as completely independent of the child or his family.

The importance of *family factors* in determining the course of early-onset depressive disorders has been touched on by several investigators (Hammen, Burge & Stansbury, 1990*b*; Hammen *et al.*, 1991; Warner *et al.*, 1992; Asarnow *et al.*, 1993) and clearly needs further investigation. There is evidence pointing towards the importance of environmentally mediated mechanisms (see above), but much more also needs to be known about the role of genetic factors. Unfortunately, there have been no systematic twin studies of early-onset depressive disorders. Such investigations are much needed, though they are going to be difficult to accomplish because of the rarity of twins who have severe depressive conditions with an onset in childhood or adolescence. In the first place, therefore, it might be necessary to conduct these studies retrospectively in centres where systematic twin registers and cases records have been kept over many years. Such retrospective designs present formidable methodological difficulties but have the great advantage that they necessarily involve a longitudinal component. Thus concordance within monozygotic and within dizygotic twin pairs could be analysed according to psychiatric status in both childhood and adult life, as well as by persistence across those two age periods. It should also be possible to assess genetic shaping of the environment by examining concordance for environmental factors in adulthood.

Another issue relates to the kinds of *samples* that are going to be needed for these studies. Clinical samples are still required for longitudinal research into juvenile affective conditions if only because of the need to study young people with uncommon but potentially highly informative disorders such as bipolar conditions. Thus, for instance, a systematic follow-up of a large sample of adolescents with bipolar disorders is long overdue. In addition, we need to know much more about the early signs of relapse of unipolar depressive conditions in young people.

There are, however, several outstanding issues that are best tackled using an epidemiological approach. For instance, the longitudinal course of depression and comorbid disorders needs further investigation in community samples, because samples referred to clinics may be biased towards severe, comorbid cases. Community samples will also be required to conduct the kinds of multiple cohort studies that were described above.

It will continue to be important to study high risk samples, such as the children of depressed parents (Dodge, 1990; Rutter, 1990). However, it must be remembered that since most depressed children do not have an affectively ill parent (Strober *et al.*, 1988; Kutcher & Marton, 1991; Harrington *et al.*, 1993) such studies may overestimate the role of parental depressive disorder in childhood depressive conditions. Much could therefore be gained from the study of other high risk groups, such as children exposed to chronic adversity.

Finally, we should return to the issue of measurement. There is no doubt that the use of adult-like diagnostic criteria together with standardised interviews has led to important advances in our ability to measure affective conditions in young people. At the same time, however, we must acknowledge that current diagnostic concepts regarding juvenile depressive conditions are no more than working hypotheses that will need to be revised in line with ongoing research on validity. It fol-

331

lows that any commitment in a longitudinal study to the classification that prevails at the time of the study's inception may turn out to be premature. Initial data sets need therefore to be organised according to symptoms and behaviours, rather than diagnoses, so that the investigator can return to them some years later in order to reconstruct diagnostic distinctions. In practice, this will mean using diagnostic interviews that collect data at a symptom rather than a syndrome level (Harrington & Shariff, 1992). In addition, it will be necessary to collect and organise data so that a broad range of baseline symptoms and outcomes are assessed. It will be impossible to study the impact of comorbidity on outcome if too narrow a range of measures is used.

It will also be essential to pay greater attention to the measurement of 'recovery' and 'recurrence'. As noted in the introduction to this chapter, it is not at all clear where the line should be drawn between these two states. Indeed, different studies are likely to need different definitions. For example, investigators who are interested in identifying relapses at a very early stage so that treatment can be prescribed, might wish to use a criterion that was based solely on the recurrence of mild symptoms for a brief period. On the other hand, researchers wishing to identify relapses retrospectively in order to chart the course of the disorder might want to have a more robust criterion for relapse (such as substantial social impairment lasting for at least a week), because mild symptoms are notoriously unreliable when rated retrospectively (Harrington et al., 1988).

The implication is that measures of psychopathology should be able to cover several different concepts of relapse or recovery. Different definitions could then be tested empirically. For example, Frank et al. (1991) have argued that the duration criterion that is necessary to define recovery can be established by finding out where the 'point of rarity' lies beyond which very few patients experience a return of the full syndrome. Such a point would then be regarded as defining the duration criterion for 'recovery'. Clearly, however, to accomplish this goal psychiatric instruments are going to have to cover the onset and offset of individual symptoms in a great deal more detail than they do now.

It may also be necessary to combine information from a variety of different sources, so as to minimise the bias arising from any single source. It could be, for example, that the predictive power of child ratings for a subsequent episode of depression differs from that of parent ratings. Indeed, there is evidence that source of information can have an effect on the apparent strength of continuities over time (Stanger et al., 1992).

CONCLUSIONS

In our discussion of the methodological issues involved in longitudinal research on juvenile depressive disorders we have pointed to the large number of difficulties that investigators working in this area have had to contend with. It is scarcely likely, therefore, that the studies would give rise to identical conclusions. Nevertheless, it is striking that there has been widespread agreement on the finding that juvenile affective disorders tend to be recurrent. This finding is important because it has been taught for many years that while behavioural difficulties such as conduct disorders show strong continuity over time, 'emotional' problems among the young tend to be short-lived. The studies described here suggest that this view is mistaken, at least so far as clinical cases of depressive disorders are concerned. They are associated with considerable impairment of psychosocial functioning and in severe cases vulnerability extends into adult life.

What, then, are the clinical implications that arise from these findings? The clearest conclusions apply to the long-term management of juvenile depressive disorders. It is sometimes assumed that the rapid recovery of depressed children means that treatment endeavours need only focus on the short-term. The evidence reviewed here firmly contradicts this sanguine view. It is apparent that both assessment and treatment need to be viewed as extending over a prolonged period of time. Young people with depressive disorders are likely to have another episode and so it is important that we develop effective maintenance and/or prophylactic treatments. Thus, for example, it may be necessary in severe cases of adolescent-onset depressive disorder to consider long-term medication and/or psychological treatment. In milder cases who are relatively well between episodes it is important that we teach the child and his parents early recognition of the signs of a relapse, and encourage them to return to us when the first symptoms appear.

Since severe forms of early-onset depressive disorder seem to have a significant self-perpetuating quality there is clearly a need to help individuals to develop coping strategies that will enable them to deal with the illness in the long-term. However, there is also evidence that relapses are linked to changes in environmental circumstances, especially family disturbances such as parenting difficulties and mental illness. Accordingly, clinicians treating young people with depressive disorders need to assess the extent to which these factors are relevant. It may be possible to intervene therapeutically to improve patterns of family relationships. Parents who are depressed or suffering from some other form of mental disorder also need to be helped. In other words, there needs to be a concern with the family as a whole and not just with the patient as an individual.

The evidence on the course of early-onset depressive disorders also has implications for preventive policies. For example, it may be that intensive work with at-risk groups such as the children of depressed parents will reduce the risk of depression in the children. Unfortunately, so far data are lacking on the extent to which primary preventive interventions are in fact protective, so it may be better to concentrate on the early recognition and intensive treatment of the first episode of depression. There is some evidence that in adults the earlier the intervention the shorter the episode (Kupfer, Frank & Perel, 1989) and it could be that the same will be found to occur in juvenile depressions.

Finally, the multiple problems of the depressed young person make it especially important that multimodal approaches to treatment are used. Reduction of depression is a legitimate focus of treatment but should not distract from the treatment of comorbid difficulties. Some of these difficulties, such as problems in peer relationships, may play a part in prolonging depression (Goodyer *et al.*, 1991). Others, such as conduct disorder, appear to exert an independent influence on the prognosis (Harrington *et al.*, 1991). Depressed young people therefore require a range of therapeutic interventions. It remains to be seen whether these will alter the long-term outcome.

REFERENCES

Akiskal, H. S., Walker, P., Puzantian, V. R. *et al.* (1983). Bipolar outcome in the course of depressive illness: phenomenologic, familial, and pharmacologic predictors. *Journal of Affective Disorders*, **5**, 115–28.

American Psychiatric Association. (1980). *Diagnostic and statistical manual of mental disorders – DSM-III* (3rd edn). American Psychiatric Association, Washington DC.

Andrews, J. A. & Lewinsohn, P. M. (1992). Suicidal attempts among older adolescents: prevalence and co-occurrence with psychiatric disorders. *Journal of the American Academy of Child Psychiatry*, **13**, 655–62.

Asarnow, J. R. & Bates, S. (1988). Depression in child psychiatric inpatients: cognitive and attributional patterns. *Journal of Abnormal Child Psychology*, **16**, 601–15.

Asarnow, J. R., Goldstein, M. J., Carlson, G. A. *et al.* (1988). Childhood-onset depressive disorders. A follow-up study of rates of rehospitalization and out-of-home placement among child psychiatric inpatients. *Journal of Affective Disorders*, **15**, 245–53.

Asarnow, J. R., Goldstein, M. J., Tompson, M. & Guthrie, D. (1993). One-year outcomes of depressive disorders in child psychiatric inpatients: evaluation of the prognostic power of a brief measure of expressed emotion. *Journal of Child Psychology and Psychiatry*, **34**, 129–37.

Bauer, M. S. & Whybrow, P. C. (1991). Rapid cycling bipolar disorder: clinical features, treatment, and etiology. In *Advances in neuropsychiatry and psychopharmacology*, Vol. 2: *Refractory depression* (ed. J. D. Amsterdam), pp. 191–208. Raven Press, New York.

Beardslee, W. R., Bemporad, J., Keller, M. B. & Klerman, G. L. (1983). Children of parents with major affective disorder: a review. *American Journal of Psychiatry*, **140**, 825–32.

Brady, E. U. & Kendall, P. C. (1992). Comorbidity of anxiety and depression in children and adolescents. *Psychological Bulletin*, **111**, 244–55.

Brent, D. A., Kolko, D. J., Allan, M. J. & Brown, R. V. (1990). Suicidality in affectively disordered adolescent inpatients. *Journal of the American Academy of Child Psychiatry*, **29**, 586–93.

Brent, D. A., Perper, J. A., Goldstein, C. E. *et al.* (1988). Risk factors for adolescent suicide. A comparison of adolescent suicide victims with suicidal inpatients. *Archives of General Psychiatry*, **45**, 581–8.

Brockington, I. F., Altman, E., Hillier, V. *et al.* (1982). The clinical picture of bipolar affective disorder in its depressed phase. A report from London and Chicago. *British Journal of Psychiatry*, **141**, 558–62.

Brown, G. W. & Harris, T. (1978). *Social origins of depression*. Tavistock Publications, London.

Brown, G. W., Harris, T. O. & Bifulco, A. (1986). Long-term effects of early loss of parent. In *Depression in young people: Developmental and clinical perspectives* (ed. M. Rutter, C. E. Izard, & P. B. Read), pp. 251–96. Guilford Press, New York.

Brown, G., Harris, T. & Lemyre, A. (1991). Problems of choosing between categories and dimensions in longitudinal research. In *Stability and change: Methods and models for data treatment* (ed. D. Magnusson, L. Bergman, & G. Rudinger), pp. 67–94. Cambridge University Press, Cambridge.

Brown, G. W., Lemyre, L. & Bifulco, A. (1992). Social factors and recovery from anxiety and depressive disorders. A test of specificity. *British Journal of Psychiatry*, **161**, 44–54.

Buchanan, C. M., Eccles, J. S. & Becker, J. B. (1992). Are adolescents the victims of raging hormones: evidence for activational effects of hormones on moods and behaviour at adolescence. *Psychological Bulletin*, **111**, 62–107.

Burge, D. & Hammen, C. (1991). Maternal communication: predictors of outcome at follow-up in a sample of children at high and low risk for depression. *Journal of Abnormal Psychology*, **100**, 174–80.

Burke, K. C., Burke, J. D., Regier, D. A. & Rae, D. S. (1990). Age at onset of selected mental disorders in five community populations. *Archives of General Psychiatry*, **47**, 511–8.

Cantwell, D. P. (1983). Childhood depression: issues regarding natural history. In *Affective disorders in childhood and adolescence. An update* (ed. D. P. Cantwell & G. A. Carlson), pp. 266–78. MTP Press, Lancaster.

Carlson, G. A., Davenport, Y. B. & Jamison, K. (1977). A comparison of outcome in adolescent and late onset bipolar manic depressive illness. *American Journal of Psychiatry*, **134**, 919–22.

Caron, C. & Rutter, M. (1991). Comorbidity in child psychopathology: concepts, issues and research strategies. *Journal of Child Psychology and Psychiatry*, **32**, 1063–80.

Casat, C. D. & Powell, K. (1988). The dexamethasone suppression test in children and adolescents with major depressive disorder: a review. *Journal of Clinical Psychiatry*, **49**, 390–3.

Cicchetti, D. & Schneider-Rosen, K. (1986). An organisational approach to childhood depression. In *Depression in young people: Developmental and clinical perspectives* (ed. M. Rutter, C. Izard, & P. B. Read), pp. 71–134. Guilford Press, New York.

Cohen, P., Cohen, J., & Brook, J. (1993a). An epidemiological study of disorders in late childhood and adolescence – II. Persistence of disorders. *Journal of Child Psychology and Psychiatry*, **34**, 869–77.

Cohen, P., Cohen, J., Kasen, S. *et al.* (1993b). An epidemiological study of disorders in late childhood and adolescence – I. Age- and gender-specific prevalence. *Journal of Child Psychology and Psychiatry*, **34**, 851–67.

Coryell, W., & Winokur, G. (1992). Course and outcome. In E. S. Paykel (Ed.), *Handbook of affective disorders* (2nd edn), pp. 89–108. Churchill Livingstone, Edinburgh.

Dodge, K. A. (1990). Developmental psychopathology in children of depressed mothers. *Developmental Psychology*, **26**, 3–6.

Eastgate, J. & Gilmour, L. (1984). Long-term outcome of depressed children: a follow-up study. *Developmental Medicine and Child Neurology*, **26**, 68–72.

Edelsohn, G., Ialongo, N., Werthamer-Larsson, L. *et al.* (1992). Self-reported depressive symptoms in first-grade children: developmentally transient phenomena? *Journal of the American Academy of Child Psychiatry*, **31**, 282–90.

Emslie, G. J., Rush, A. J., Weinberg, W. A. *et al.*(1990). Children with major depression show reduced rapid eye movement latencies. *Archives of General Psychiatry*, **47**, 119–24.

Ferguson, H. B. & Bawden, H. N. (1988). Psychobiological measures. In *Assessment and diagnosis in child psychopathology* (ed. M. Rutter, A. H. Tuma, & I. S. Lann), pp. 232-63. Guilford Press, New York.

Fleming, J. E., Boyle, M. H., & Offord, D. R. (1993). The outcome of adolescent depression in the Ontario Child Health Study follow-up. *Journal of the American Academy of Child Psychiatry*, **32**, 28–33.

Fleming, J. E., Offord, D. R. & Boyle, M. H. (1989). Prevalence of childhood and adolescent depression in the community: Ontario child health study. *British Journal of Psychiatry*, **155**, 647–54.

Frank, E., Prien, R. F., Jarrett, R. B. *et al.* (1991). Conceptualisation and rationale for consensus definitions of terms in major depressive disorder. Remission, recovery, relapse, and recurrence. *Archives of General Psychiatry*, **48**, 851–5.

Garber, J., Kriss, M. R., Koch, M. & Lindholm, L. (1988). Recurrent depression in adolescents: a follow-up study. *Journal of the American Academy of Child Psychiatry*, **27**, 49–54.

Garrison, C. Z., Jackson, K. L., Marsteller, F. *et al.* (1990). A longitudinal study of depressive symptomatology in young adolescents. *Journal of the American Academy of Child Psychiatry*, **29**, 581–5.

Goetz, R. R., Puig-Antich, J., Dahl, R. E. *et al.* (1991). EEG sleep of young adults with major depression: a controlled study. *Journal of Affective Disorders*, **22**, 91–100.

Goodwin, F. K. & Jamison, K. R. (1984). The natural course of manic-depressive illness. In *The neurobiology of mood disorders* (ed. R. M. Post, & J. C. Ballenger), pp. 20-37. Williams & Wilkins, Baltimore.

Goodyer, I. M., Germany, E., Gowrusankur, J. & Altham, P. (1991). Social influences on the course of anxious and depressive disorders in school-age children. *British Journal of Psychiatry*, **158**, 676–84.

Goodyer, I. M., Cooper, P. J., Vize, C. & Ashby, L. (1993). Depression in 11 to 16 year old girls: the role of past parental psychopathology and exposure to recent life events. *Journal of Child Psychology and Psychiatry*, **34**, 1103–15.

Grigoroiu-Serbanescu, M., Christodorescu, D., Magureanu, S. *et al.* (1991). Adolescent offspring of endogenous unipolar depressive parents and of normal parents. *Journal of Affective Disorders*, **21**, 185–98.

Guze, B. H. & Freedman, B. X. (1991). Psychiatry (Commentary). *Journal of the American Medical Association*, **265**, 3164–5.

Hammen, C. (1991). *Depression runs in families. The social context of risk and resilience in children of depressed mothers*. Springer-Verlag, New York.

Hammen, C., Adrian, C. & Hiroto, D. (1988). A longitudinal test of the attributional vulnerability model in children at risk for depression. *British Journal of Clinical Psychology*, **27**, 37–46.

Hammen, C., Burge, D., Burney, E. & Adrian, C. (1990*a*). Longitudinal study of diagnoses in children of women with unipolar and bipolar affective disorder. *Archives of General Psychiatry*, **47**, 1112–7.

Hammen, C., Burge, D. & Stansbury, K. (1990*b*). Relationship of mother and child variables to child outcomes in a high risk sample: a causal modelling analysis. *Developmental Psychology*, **26**, 24–30.

Hammen, C., Burge, D. & Adrian, C. (1991). Timing of mother and child depression in a longitudinal study of children at risk. *Journal of Consulting and Clinical Psychology*, **59**, 341–5.

Harrington, R. C. (1994). Affective disorders. In *Child and adolescent psychiatry: Modern approaches*, 3rd edn (ed. M. Rutter, L. Hersov, & E. Taylor), pp. 330–50. Blackwell Scientific, Oxford.

Harrington, R. C. (1992). Annotation: the natural history and treatment of child and adolescent affective disorders. *Journal of Child Psychology and Psychiatry*, **33**, 1287–302.

Harrington, R. C. & Shariff, A. (1992). Choosing an instrument to assess depression in young people. *Newsletter of the Association for Child Psychology and Psychiatry*, **14**, 279–82.

Harrington, R. C., Hill, J., Rutter, M. *et al.* (1988). The assessment of lifetime psychopathology: a comparison of two interviewing styles. *Psychological Medicine*, **18**, 487–93.

Harrington, R. C., Fudge, H., Rutter, M. *et al.* (1990). Adult outcomes of childhood and adolescent depression: I. Psychiatric status. *Archives of General Psychiatry*, **47**, 465–73.

Harrington, R. C., Fudge, H., Rutter, M. *et al.* (1991). Adult outcomes of childhood and adolescent depression: II. Risk for antisocial disorders. *Journal of the American Academy of Child Psychiatry*, **30**, 434–9.

Harrington, R. C., Fudge, H., Rutter, M. *et al.* (1993). Child and adult depression: a test of continuities with family-study data. *British Journal of Psychiatry*, **162**, 627–33.

Kandel, D. B. & Davies, M. (1986). Adult sequelae of adolescent depressive symptoms. *Archives of General Psychiatry*, **43**, 255–62.

Keller, M. B., Beardslee, W., Lavori, P. W. *et al.* (1988). Course of major depression in non-referred adolescents: a retrospective study. *Journal of Affective Disorders*, **15**, 235–43.

Keller, M. B., Lavori, P. W., Beardslee, W. R. *et al.* (1991). Depression in children and adolescents; new data on 'undertreatment' and a literature review on the efficacy of available treatments. *Journal of Affective Disorders*, **21**, 163–71.

Kienhorst, C. W. M., Wilde, E. J. D., Diekstra, R. F. W. & Wolters, W. H. G. (1991). Construction of an index for predicting suicide attempts in depressed adolescents. *British Journal of Psychiatry*, **159**, 676–82.

King, L. J. & Pittman, G. L. (1970). A six-year follow-up study of 65 adolescent patients. Natural history of affective disorders in adolescence. *Archives of General Psychiatry*, **22**, 230–6.

Klerman, G. L., & Weissman, M. M. (1992). The course, morbidity, and costs of depression. *Archives of General Psychiatry*, **49**, 831–4.

Koestner, R., Zuroff, D. C. & Powers T. A. (1991). Family origins of adolescent self-criticism and its continuity into adulthood. *Journal of Abnormal Psychology*, **100**, 191–7.

Kovacs, M., Feinberg, T. L., Crouse-Novak, M. A. *et al.* (1984a). Depressive disorders in childhood. I. A longitudinal prospective study of characteristics and recovery. *Archives of General Psychiatry*, **41**, 229–37.

Kovacs, M., Feinberg, T. L., Crouse-Novak, M. *et al.* (1984b). Depressive disorders in childhood. II. A longitudinal study of the risk for a subsequent major depression. *Archives of General Psychiatry*, **41**, 643–9.

Kovacs, M., Gatsonis, C., Paulauskas, S. & Richards, C. (1989). Depressive disorders in childhood. IV. A longitudinal study of comorbidity with and risk for anxiety disorders. *Archives of General Psychiatry*, **46**, 776–82.

Kovacs, M. & Goldston, D. (1991). Cognitive and social cognitive development of depressed children and adolescents. *Journal of the American Academy of Child Psychiatry*, **30**, 388–92.

Kovacs M., Goldston D., Gatsonis C (1993) Suicidal behaviours and childhood onset depressive disorders: a longitudinal investigation. *The Journal of the American Academy of Child and Adolescent Psychiatry*, **32**, 8–20.

Kovacs, M., Paulauskas, S., Gatsonis, C. & Richards, C. (1988). Depressive disorders in childhood. III. A longitudinal study of comorbidity with and risk for conduct disorders. *Journal of Affective Disorders*, **15**, 205–17.

Kupfer, D. (1992). Maintenance treatment in recurrent depression: current and future directions. *British Journal of Psychiatry*, **161**, 309–16.

Kupfer, D., Frank, E. & Perel J. M. (1989). The advantage of early treatment intervention in recurrent depression *Archives of General Psychiatry*, **46**, 771–5.

Kutcher, S., Malkin, D., Silverberg, J. *et al.* (1991). Nocturnal cortisol, thyroid stimulating hormone, and growth hormone secretory profiles in depressed adolescents. *Journal of the American Academy of Child Psychiatry*, **30**, 407–14.

Kutcher, S. & Marton, P. (1991). Affective disorders in first-degree relatives of adolescent onset bipolars, unipolars, and normal controls. *Journal of the American Academy of Child Psychiatry*, **30**, 75–8.

Kutcher, S., Williamson, P., Marton, P. & Szalai, J. (1992). REM latency in endogenously depressed adolescents. *British Journal of Psychiatry*, **161**, 399–402.

Lancet. (1992). Depression and suicide: are they preventable? *Lancet*, **340**, 700–1.

Larsson, B., Melin, L., Breitholtz, E. & Andersson, G. (1991). Short-term stability of depressive symptoms and suicide attempts in Swedish adolescents. *Acta Psychiatrica Scandinavica*, **83**, 385–90.

Lewinsohn, P. M., Hops, H., Roberts, R. E. *et al.* (1993). Adolescent psychopathology: I. Prevalence and incidence of depression and other DSM-III-R disorders in high school students. *Journal of Abnormal Psychology*, **102**, 133–44.

Marttunen, M. J., Aro, H. M., Henriksson, M. M. & Lonnqvist, J. K. (1991). Mental disorders in adolescent suicide. DSM-III-R axes I and II diagnoses in suicides among 13- to 19-year-olds in Finland. *Archives of General Psychiatry*, **48**, 834–39.

McGee, R., Feehan, M., Williams, S. & Anderson, J. (1992). DSM-III disorders from age 11 to age 15 years. *Journal of the American Academy of Child Psychiatry*, **31**, 50–9.

McGee, R. & Williams, S. (1988). A longitudinal study of depression in nine-year-old children. *Journal of the American Academy of Child Psychiatry*, **27**, 342–48.

McGuffin, P. & Katz, R. (1986). Nature, nurture and affective disorder. In *The Biology of Depression* (ed. J. F. W. Deakin), pp. 26-52. Royal College of Psychiatrists, London.

Mitchell, J., McCauley, E., Burke, P. M. & Moss, S. J. (1988). Phenomenology of depression in children and adolescents. *Journal of the American Academy of Child Psychiatry*, **27**, 12–20.

Myers, K., McCauley, E., Calderon, R. & Treder, R. (1991). The 3-year longitudinal course of suicidality and predictive factors for subsequent suicidality in youths with major depressive disorder. *Journal of the American Academy of Child Psychiatry*, **30**, 804–10.

Needles, D. J. & Abramson, L. Y. (1990). Positive life events, attributional style, and hopefulness: testing a model of recovery from depression. *Journal of Abnormal Psychology*, **99**, 156–65.

Nolen-Hoeksema, S., Girgus, J. S. & Seligman, M. E. P. (1992). Predictors and consequences of childhood depressive symptoms: a 5-year longitudinal study. *Journal of Abnormal Psychology*, **101**, 405–22.

Paykel, E. S. (1989). Treatment of depression: the relevance of research for clinical practice. *British Journal of Psychiatry*, **155**, 754–63.

Pearce, J. B. (1974). Childhood Depression. M.Phil thesis, London.

Pearce, J. B. (1978). The recognition of depressive disorder in children. *Journal of the Royal Society of Medicine*, **71**, 494–500.

Pfeffer, C. R. (1992). Relationship between depression and suicidal behaviour. In *Clinical guide to depression in children and adolescents* (ed. M. Shafii & S. L. Shafii), pp. 115–26. American Psychiatric Press, Washington.

Pfeffer, C., Klerman, G. L., Hunt, S. W. *et al.* (1991). Suicidal children grown up: demographic and clinical risk factors for adolescent suicidal attempts. *Journal of the American Academy of Child Psychiatry*, **30**, 609–16.

Post, R. M. (1992). Transduction of psychosocial stress into the neurobiology of recurrent affective disorder. *American Journal of Psychiatry*, **149**, 999–1010.

Poznanski, E. O., Kraheneuhl, V. & Zrull, J. P. (1976). Childhood depression – a longitudinal perspective. *Journal of the American Academy of Child Psychiatry*, **15**, 491–501.

Puig-Antich, J., Lukens, E., Davies, M. *et al.* (1985a). Psychosocial functioning in prepubertal major depressive disorders. I. Interpersonal relationships during the depressive episode. *Archives of General Psychiatry*, **42**, 500–7.

Puig-Antich, J., Lukens, E., Davies, M. *et al.* (1985b). Psychosocial functioning in prepubertal major depressive disorders. II. Interpersonal relationships after sustained recovery from affective episode. *Archives of General Psychiatry*, **42**, 511–17.

Radke-Yarrow, M., Nottelmann, E., Martinez, P. *et al.* (1992). Young children of affectively ill parents: a longitudinal study of psychosocial development. *Journal of the American Academy of Child Psychiatry*, **31**, 68–77.

Rao, U., Weissman, M., Martin, J. A. & Hammond, R. W. (1993). Childhood depression and risk of suicide: preliminary report of a longitudinal study. *Journal of the American Academy of Child Psychiatry*, **32**, 21–7.

Reinherz, H. Z., Stewart-Berghauer, G., Pakiz, B. *et al.* (1989). The relationship or early risk and current mediators to depressive symptomatology in adolescence. *Journal of the American Academy of Child Psychiatry*, **28**, 942–7.

Richman, N., Stevenson, J. & Graham, P. (1982). *Pre-school to school: a behavioural study*. Academic Press, London.

Rodgers, B. (1990). Influences of early-life and recent factors on affective disorder in women: an exploration of vulnerability models. In *Straight and Devious Pathways from Childhood to Adulthood* (ed. L. N. Robins, & M. Rutter), pp. 314–27. Cambridge University Press, Cambridge.

Rohde, P., Lewinsohn, P. M. & Seeley, J. R. (1990). Are people changed by the experience of having an episode of depression? A further test of the scar hypothesis. *Journal of Abnormal Psychology*, **99**, 264–71.

Rutter, M. (1977). Prospective studies to investigate behavioural change. In *The origins and course of psychopathology* (ed. J. S. Strauss, H. M. Babigian, & M. Roff), pp. 223–47. Plenum, New York.

Rutter, M. (1990). Commentary: some focus and process considerations regarding effects of parental depression on children. *Developmental Psychology*, **26**, 60–67.

Rutter, M. (1991). Age changes in depressive disorders: some developmental considerations. In *The development of emotion regulation and dysregulation* (ed. J. Garber, & K. A. Dodge), pp. 273–300. Cambridge University Press, Cambridge.

Rutter, M. & Quinton, D. (1984). Parental psychiatric disorder: effects on children. *Psychological Medicine*, **14**, 853–80.

Rutter, M. & Sandberg, S. (1992). Psychosocial stressors: concepts, causes and effects. *European Child and Adolescent Psychiatry*, **1**, 3–13.

Ryan, N. D., Puig-Antich, J., Ambrosini, P. *et al.* (1987). The clinical picture of major depression in children and adolescents. *Archives of General Psychiatry*, **44**, 854–61.

Seligman, M. E. P. & Peterson, C. (1986). A learned helplessness perspective on childhood depression: theory and research. In *Depression in young people: developmental and clinical perspectives* (ed. M. Rutter, C. E. Izard, & P. B. Read), pp. 223–50. Guilford Press, New York.

Shaffer, D. (1988). The epidemiology of teen suicide: an examination of risk factors. *Journal of Clinical Psychiatry*, **49**, (Suppl. 9), 36–41.

Shain, B. N., King, C. A., Naylor, M. & Alessi, N. (1991). Chronic depression and hospital course in adolescents. *Journal of the American Academy of Child Psychiatry*, **30**, 428–33.

Sroufe, L. A. (1979). The coherence of individual development. *American Psychologist*, 34, 834–41.

Stanger, C., McConaughy, S. H. & Achenbach, T. M. (1992). Three-year course of behavioural/emotional problems in a national sample of 4- to 16-year-olds: II. Predictors of syndromes. *Journal of the American Academy of Child Psychiatry*, **31**, 941–50.

Strober, M. (1992*a*). Relevance of early age-of-onset in genetic studies of bipolar affective disorder. *Journal of the American Academy of Child Psychiatry*, **31**, 606–10.

Strober, M. (1992*b*). Bipolar disorders: natural history, genetic studies, and follow-up. In *Clinical guide to depression in children and adolescents* (ed. M. Shafii & S. L. Shafii), pp. 251–68. American Psychiatric Press, Washington, DC.

Strober, M. & Carlson, G. (1982). Bipolar illness in adolescents with major depression: clinical, genetic and psychopharmocologic predictors in a three- to four-year prospective follow-up investigation. *Archives of General Psychiatry*, **39**, 549–55.

Strober, M., Morrell, W., Burroughs, J. *et al.* (1988). A family study of bipolar I disorder in adolescence. Early onset of symptoms linked to increased familial loading and lithium resistance. *Journal of Affective Disorders*, **15**, 255–68.

Strober, M., Lampert, C., Schmidt, S. & Morrell, W. (1992). The course of major depressive disorder in adolescents: I. Recovery and risk of manic switching in a 24-month prospective, naturalistic follow-up of psychotic and nonpsychotic subtypes. *Journal of the American Academy of Child Psychiatry*, **32**, 34–42.

Velez, C. N., Johnson, J. & Cohen, P. (1989). A longitudinal analysis of selected risk factors for childhood psychopathology. *Journal of the American Academy of Child Psychiatry*, **28**, 861–4.

Warner, V., Weissman, M. M., Fendrich, M. *et al.* (1992). The course of major depression in the offspring of depressed parents. Incidence, recurrence, and recovery. *Archives of General Psychiatry*, **49**, 795–801.

Weissman, M. M., Fendrich, M., Warner, V. & Wickramaratne, P. (1992). Incidence of psychiatric disorder in offspring at high and low risk for depression. *Journal of the American Academy of Child Psychiatry*, **31**, 640–8.

Werry, J. S. & McClellan, J. M. (1992). Predicting outcome in child and adolescent (early onset) schizophrenia and bipolar disorder. *Journal of the American Academy of Child Psychiatry*, **31**, 147–50.

Werry, J. S., McClellan, J. M. & Chard, L. (1991). Childhood and adolescent schizophrenic, bipolar, and schizoaffective disorders: a clinical and outcome study. *Journal of the American Academy of Child Psychiatry*, **30**, 457–65.

Wilde, E. J. de, Kienhorst, I. C. W. M., Diekstra, R. F. W. & Wolters, W. H. G. (1992). The relationship between adolescent suicidal behaviour and life events in childhood and adolescence. *American Journal of Psychiatry*, **149**, 45–51.

Wolkind, S. & Rutter, M. (1985). Separation, loss and family relationships. In *Child and adolescent psychiatry: Modern approaches* (ed. M. Rutter, & L. Hersov), pp. 34–57. Blackwell, Oxford.

Zeitlin, H. (1986). *The natural history of psychiatric disorder in children.* Oxford University Press, Oxford.

Index

Page numbers for figures and tables are in italics

social support, life events and risk of
depression, 179–80
solipsistic knowledge and emotion, 33
somatostatin and growth hormone in
adolescent depression, 197, 198,
200
Soranus on melancholy and manic states, 9
spleen, 5
historical terminology, 4
Standard Psychiatric Assessment modified
for children, 119
Stress
coping, and early attachments, 62
effect on hypothalamic–pituitary–
adrenal axis, 204
see also life events
stressors
and development of emotional
regulation and response, 71–3
family, physiological and environmental,
98
substance abuse and suicide, 321
and parental depression, 142
suicide, suicidal
attempted (parasuicide), 225
behaviour
in adolescents, 225–51
anxiety, 241
behavioural factors, 241–2
cognitive distortions and coping,
235–6
cognitive factors, 235
concepts and methods, 230
correlates, 230–43
and depression, 225–6, 233, 240
longitudinal perspectives, 320–1
developmental changes, 242–3
developmental stage, 234–43
differences between mother and
father, 233
emotional states, 239
environmental factors, 232–3
gender differences, 243
hopelessness, 240
ideation and future attempts, 237
imitation, 238–9
impulsiveness, 236–8
intent, 231
lack of planning, 236–8
learning, 239
method, 231
physical changes, 242–3
psychological and psychopathological
factors, 233
reasons, 231
reflective behaviour, 237
terminology, 225

continuum of suicidality, from ideation
to completion?, 229–30
definitions, 225
drawing attention, 231
epidemiology, 226–30
age range, 226–7
attempts, statistics, 227–8
correlates of trends, 227
increase among adolescents, 227
prognosis for world suicide rates,
227
rare in children under 12, 226
statistics, 226
suicidal thoughts, 228–9
idea
and dysthymic disorder, 285
and major depressive disorder, 285
ideation, 225
prevention, 243–4
relation to depression, 17–19, 225, 233,
240
supportive therapy
for major depression and dysthymia,
results, 288–92
in major depressive disorders, 287–8

temperament
and attachment, 59–60
characteristics of depressed children,
56–7
in the developmental process, 55–7
continuity and stability of traits over
time, 55–6
genetic determination, 55
and the 'difficult' child, 55
terminological and conceptual confusion,
historical, 4, 5–6
thoughts, suicidal, 228–9
thymergastic reactions, full-fledged, 15
thyroid hormone and adolescent
depression, 200–4
basal secretion, 201–2
developmental considerations, 201
levels of T4 in depressed relatives, 202
regulation, 200
TRH Stimulation Test, 202–4
TSH stimulation and release, 200–1,
202–4
thyroid-stimulating hormone levels in
depression, 90
toloxatone, MAO-A selective inhibitor,
267
tranylcypromine, irreversible MAO
inhibitor, side-effects, 269
tricyclic antidepressant drugs
dosage regimens, 256–7
side-effects, 257–8

Index